Get *Well* & *Stay Well*

Optimal Health through Transformational Medicine®

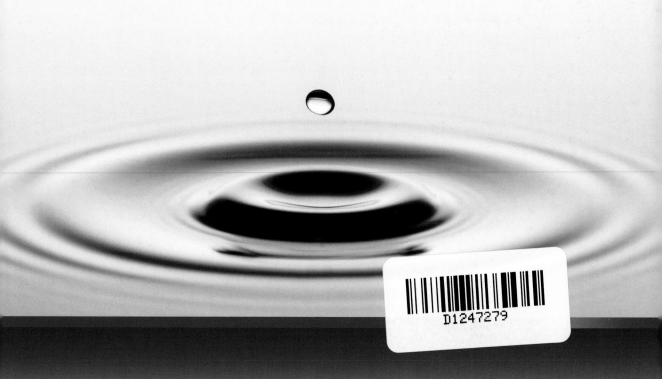

Get *Well* & Stay *Well*

Optimal Health through Transformational Medicine®

STEVE AMOILS, M.D.

SANDI AMOILS, M.D.

Integrative Medicine Foundation
www.IntegrativeMedFoundation.org

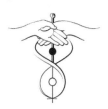

Transformational Medicine is a registered trademark of Steve and Sandi Amoils, M.D.s.

ACE Healing Treatment is a registered service mark of the Alliance Institute for Integrative Medicine.

Library of Congress Control Number: 2011939925

ISBN: 978-0-9852719-1-6

Designed by Grannan Design Ltd., www.grannandesign.com
Artwork by Kristin Luther, www.luthermultimedia.com and Abbey Urbas, www.abbeyurbas.com
Cover photo © Alamy / Johner Images
Authors photo by David Ziser, www.ziser.com

Manufactured in the United States of America

Printed by BookMasters, Ashland, Ohio

First edition

Even more praise for *Get Well & Stay Well*

Get Well & Stay Well is necessary for everyone, but *essential* for athletes. When Steve and Sandi Amoils aren't there, *Get Well & Stay Well* is. It's a bible on well-being—riveting, easy to understand, and life-affirming.

—Johnny G, founder, Spinning® and Kranking®; author, *Romancing the Bicycle*

Get Well & Stay Well will change the way you think about health. In fact, it just may save your life. Getting to the underlying cause of disease and preventing disease in the first place is key to transforming medicine. The Amoils have the key!

—Mimi Guarneri, M.D., founder and Medical Director, Scripps Center for Integrative Medicine, La Jolla, California; President, American Board of Integrative and Holistic Medicine; author, *The Heart Speaks*

Drawing on their wealth of knowledge and clinical experience, Drs. Steve and Sandi Amoils provide deep insights and practical ways for readers to take charge and transform their health and well-being.

—Brian Berman, M.D.; Professor, Family and Community Medicine, Founder and Director, Center for Integrative Medicine, University of Maryland School of Medicine; Founder, Institute for Functional Medicine; President, Institute for Integrative Health; co-author, *Own Your Health: Choosing the Best from Alternative & Conventional Medicine*

This is simply a *wonderful* book! The authors, Dr. Steve and Dr. Sandi Amoils, synthesize the best possibilities from many, many disciplines of medicine—ancient and traditional as well as conventional—into a methodology that will help you, the reader, find your unique pathway to a personalized door that you can open and enter on your own journey to healing. Through their story of discovery and dedication to their calling as doctors, the authors illuminate and point the way for your own journey of transformation.

—David S. Jones, M.D.; President and Director of Medical Education, Institute for Functional Medicine

Personalized transformation of your health and your life is a goal for which we should all strive. Dr. Steve and Dr. Sandi Amoils provide a masterful and scientific path to this goal in this incredible book. It is a look into the medicine of the future that achieves the symphony of optimal health in mind, body, and spirit.

—Mark Houston M.D., MS, ABAARM, FACP, FAHA, FASH; Associate Clinical Professor of Medicine, Vanderbilt University School of Medicine; Director, Hypertension Institute of Nashville; author, *What Your Doctor May Not Tell You About Hypertension* and *What Your Doctor May Not Tell You About Heart Disease.*

In this exceptionally written book, Dr. Steve and Dr. Sandi Amoils synthesize a wealth of information—combining the rigor of conventional medicine, the wisdom of ancient healing, and the science of lifestyle modification—creating a practical guide that will truly transform the way you feel and function.

—Daniel A. Monti, M.D.; Executive and Medical Director of the Jefferson and Myrna Brind Center for Integrative Medicine; Associate Professor of Psychiatry and Emergency Medicine at Jefferson Medical College; coauthor, *The Great Life Makeover* and *Integrative Psychiatry*

Contributing Authors

Steve Bleser, D.C.

Senior Chiropractor, Alliance Institute for Integrative Medicine. Past President, Ohio State Chiropractic Association. Past President and Board Member Emeritus, Ohio State Board of Chiropractic Examiners. Fellow, International College of Chiropractic. Examiner, National Board of Chiropractic Examiners.

Claudia Harsh, M.D.

Integrative Gynecologist in Dallas, Texas (www.graceandbalance.com; www.livingwelldallas.com). Bravewell Fellow, University of Arizona Integrative Medicine Program. Former Director of Integrative Gynecology at the Alliance Institute for Integrative Medicine.

Jim Leonard, M.D.

Orthopedic Surgeon at Wellington Orthopedics, Cincinnati, Ohio. Former Director of Musculoskeletal Medicine at the Alliance Institute for Integrative Medicine. Clinical Instructor for the Helms Medical Acupuncture program.

John Sacco, M.D.

Integrative Oncology consultant at the Alliance Institute for Integrative Medicine. Fellow, University of Arizona Integrative Medicine Program. Radiation Oncologist with Oncology Hematology Care in Cincinnati, Ohio.

Keith Wilson, M.D.

Associate Professor. Director, Division of Head and Neck Surgery, Department of Otolaryngology–Head and Neck Surgery, University of Cincinnati. Bravewell Fellow, University of Arizona Integrative Medicine Program.

Liz Woolford, M.D.

Family and Integrative Medicine Physician. Director of Physician Education and the Integrative Medicine Physicians of Excellence program through the Alliance Institute for Integrative Medicine and the Integrative Medicine Foundation.

Proceeds from this book will go to the Integrative Medicine Foundation, a nonprofit 501(c)(3) corporation, to fund low-cost or free integrative care for underserved patients and to fund integrative medicine training for physicians and health care providers. For more information, see **www.integrativemedfoundation.org.**

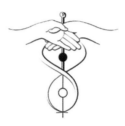

This book is printed on green paper.

Dedication

TO OUR PATIENTS
Whose illnesses we have struggled with, whose successes have inspired us, and whose acknowledgment has nourished us.

TO OUR FRIENDS AND FAMILY
Who have sustained us, nurtured us, and supported us.

TO FREDRIC AND JULIE HOLZBERGER
Who help make dreams come true.

and finally,

TO YOU, THE READER
May this book inspire you to improve your health and well-being.
May your new-found vitality inspire you to make positive changes in your world.

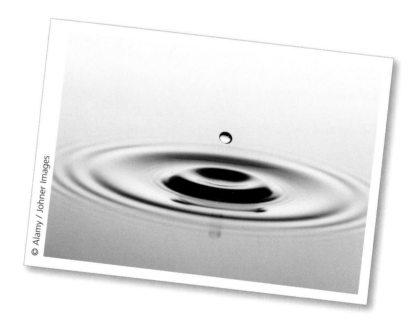

© Alamy / Johner Images

Contents

How do you **really feel** about your health?

- Are you tired, moody, or overwhelmed by life?

- Are you bloated or overweight?

- Are you aching, with no real way to address the pain?

- Do you miss the sense of well-being you once had?

- Are you sick . . . or just not feeling your best?

- Are you looking for a cure when you really need to learn how to heal?

- Do you feel powerless to change your health?

Our approach will help you **take charge of** your health.

It includes exercise, mind-body techniques, and ways to combine conventional medicine with integrative therapies to reduce pain, overcome stress, and normalize your weight, blood pressure, cholesterol, and blood sugar.

This same approach will help you treat your current problems, heal your old ones, and prevent future ones. What's more, it will promote vitality and may even prolong your life.

We call it Transformational Medicine®.

Transformational Medicine teaches you how to transform your life and your health. And it can be tailored just for you.

We invite you to **discover how to** get well, live well, and stay well.

Transformational Medicine® and the Evolution of Medical Care

How a Journey into the Heart of Healing Led to a New Vision of Health

The word heal derives from the root "to make whole." This book offers insight on healing and tools you can use to move toward wholeness. We'll explore how you can use your symptoms or your current illness to create change in your life—on your journey toward health and well-being.

A Patient's Story

Imagine a teenage competitive swimmer who suddenly finds himself breaking state records at training sessions, week after week. It is the middle of the off-season, and he has high hopes that he will set national records when summer comes. Excited at the prospect, he decides to devote additional hours each day to pushing his training to the limit. In order to keep up his grades, he foregoes a few hours of sleep each night. And on weekends, he still goes out with his friends. (Heaven forbid that a teenager would sacrifice his social life.)

One day he gets out of bed feeling tired and dizzy. He quickly realizes that he is not just tired—he is bone-weary—totally exhausted. Walking up stairs, his pulse rate shoots up so high that he feels as if his heart is jumping out of his throat. Initially, he expects that he will feel better soon, but the malaise continues for weeks, then months. He feels listless and beaten, almost to the point of tears. He begins to have fainting episodes if he stands too long, especially in the heat. His training suffers significantly. His morale plummets.

His father, a doctor, confers with his grandfather and his uncle, both highly respected physicians. They decide the boy should see a specialist. The specialist examines him, runs a battery of lab tests, and then sends him for an EKG to check his heart and for a chest x-ray. All are normal. Finally, the specialist says to him gently, "Son, I think this is all in your head."

Devastated, the boy turns to other sources for help. A world-famous bodybuilder begins to give him advice on taking care of his body. A yoga teacher instructs him on stretching and meditation. Finally, he goes to see an acupuncturist, who simply feels his pulse and then asks him, "How did you get so exhausted?" Unlike the medical experts, his new mentors appear to have a deep respect and understanding for what he is feeling.

He begins to take their advice. For months, he practices yoga and meditation daily and receives regular acupuncture treatments. Little by little, his energy begins to return.

Four years later, having completely recovered, he decides to pursue a career as a physician. Despite the grueling schedule of medical school, he is able to maintain his health and energy. As he later explained, "I sometimes get sleepy, maybe a little tired, but I don't ever remember feeling exhausted."

While in medical school he falls in love with a classmate, his future wife. She too becomes interested in alternative approaches to healing. They realize that their passion in medicine lies in discovering what makes patients truly heal.

The patient in this story is me—Steve Amoils. My experience of burnout in high school taught me that none of us expect to get sick. We want to ignore illness, or just have it fixed by a doctor should it arise. But what if your illness can't be ignored or easily fixed?

Despite my initial disillusion with conventional medicine, I decided that this was the career I wanted to pursue. It was in medical school that I began to understand clearly the value of conventional medicine. The rigor and discipline of scientific thought bring standardization to the healing profession that is extremely useful in dealing with medical conditions.

> The path to healing often begins with a personal crisis, a disaster, or an illness. Although it is initially stressful, this time of introspection often leads to a journey of self-discovery.

More Questions than Answers

At medical school in Johannesburg, South Africa, I met Sandi, my future wife. We realized that we shared a similar philosophy of openness to different treatment modalities, no matter what they were. As study partners, we would swap stories of our experiences treating patients. For example, some of our patients with back pain reported that they had seen a chiropractor as a last resort before surgery, only to have all their pain resolve permanently. We were equally aware, however, of patients who had seen a medicine man and been given a strange concoction of herbs, only to develop kidney failure. There were also patients who had seen an alternative practitioner and were told not to worry about their heartburn, only to suffer a heart attack weeks later.

For us, the evidence pointed to the idea that a rational balance between conventional medicine and the safest, most effective alternative therapies could result in an economical, patient-oriented form of medicine. Deep down, this just made sense to both of us. Without realizing it, we were embarking on what would become a life's journey of learning to assess and integrate alternative therapies with conventional medicine. Later, Dr. Andrew Weil would describe this as Integrative Medicine. When we started in the late 1970s, all we knew was that we wanted to learn more.

> We wanted to know what made people get well. Why did they feel better? Was it the therapy or their belief in it? Why had some therapies persisted in cultures for generations?

Sandi and I began seeking out anyone in the healing arts who was achieving superior results. We interviewed everyone with open but skeptical minds. We studied with the most highly skilled of these healers. For instance, once a week we spent a half-day with a well-known

---

What Is Integrative Medicine?

Integrative medicine respects and treats the whole person—body, mind, and spirit. The integrative approach is grounded in modern scientific medicine, but makes use of all effective therapies, both conventional and alternative. Integrative medicine emphasizes therapeutic partnerships for treating health problems and for promoting better health and the prevention of illness.

doctor trained in both osteopathy and naturopathy. He was highly respected for curing patients with complex conditions. We listened in amazement as patient after patient told us how he had resolved their problems. His methods were inexpensive, simple, safe, and effective. We realized that we needed to open our eyes to a new vision, to expand our paradigm beyond what we knew, in order to broaden the resources for healing in our medical practice.

We were also lucky to be able to spend time with a famous African medicine man named Credo Mutwa, who helped us see disease from a different point of view. As physicians, we treat epileptic seizures with medication to stop and prevent them. Credo had a different perspective. He told us, "In our culture, having a seizure is called *tswala*, the calling to become a medicine man." He went on to explain how they felt the seizure opened up an area in the brain necessary to become a shaman. What a different way of viewing a disease! We certainly don't espouse this, but marveled at how a different paradigm could give a whole new dimension to a health problem.

During our medical education, we decided that we wanted to travel around the world to meet healers from different cultures and healing traditions who were able to successfully heal conditions considered untreatable. We decided that if we could not explain how someone had gotten better, we would follow up on it. Almost as soon as we decided this, people came to us with stories of famous healers and miraculous cures around the world. For our purposes, we defined a "miraculous cure" as one that defied conventional medical outcomes. With this as our new agenda, we left South Africa in 1984 for a trip overseas that would last two years.

The Journey Begins

Our travels took us through Australia, the Philippines, Hong Kong, Taiwan, Japan, Hawaii, the United States, the United Kingdom, and Europe. Open to healers of all sorts and shapes, we met aboriginal healers, psychic surgeons, acupuncturists, tai chi and chi gong masters, faith healers, energy healers, homeopaths, and herbalists. Along the way, we encountered enlightened people and charlatans, masters and magicians. For us, certain questions remained: why were some of these people getting clinical results and what could we learn from them? How could we tell the difference between a quack and a true master?

Consider our visit with an acupuncture master in Australia, who took Sandi's hand and began taking her pulse (one of the traditional Chinese forms of medical diagnosis). He looked over at me, smiled, and said gently, "Your wife is ovulating today." I stood back, astounded, as he then turned to her and said, "Your sunny disposition belies a great sadness."

He was correct. Sandi's father had died suddenly a few years earlier, right in the middle of our final medical school examinations. Forced to continue with her exams in order to complete medical school, she had never really adequately grieved his death. Later that day, the master took us to his office for an acupuncture treatment. "You will feel good," he told me before my treatment, "but Sandi's sadness will need to come out." Sandi later described the feeling of a "tap being turned on" when he stuck a needle in her ear. The waves of tears and sadness continued to pour out for days after the treatment, only to be replaced by a sense of love and connectedness to her late father. We knew then that we wanted to learn how to do this. A short treatment had changed our lives forever!

We visited the Philippines, intent on getting closer to the truth about the healers known as psychic surgeons. Many were located in an area close to Baguio City. Dismissed by many Western scientists as nothing more than charlatans and magicians, these psychic surgeons saw thousands of patients each day. Were they helping, or were they simply a hoax? We wanted to see this phenomenon for ourselves.

We found ourselves journeying out of Baguio into the valley below on a bus filled with chickens, dogs, and a myriad of local Philippine people. Our goal was to visit a psychic surgeon known only as Rosa, who took no money and offered her "treatment" as a spiritual service. Sandi asked her if she would treat an unattractive, raised purple scar on her foot, which had not changed over the prior three years. Rosa answered that she could not take the scar away, but she could take away the infection underneath. Quickly, painlessly, and with a sleight-of-hand maneuver, she seemed to pull some flesh out of the scar. Interestingly, the scar—swollen and purple—shrank and turned pink overnight. It remains that way to this day.

We stayed for weeks, watching hundreds of patients receive this form of healing. One patient in particular still sticks in our minds. He was a famous American actor who had gone to the Philippines to try this healing for lung cancer, which had spread to his brain, paralyzing one side of his body. He initially made some startling improvements. One day after a

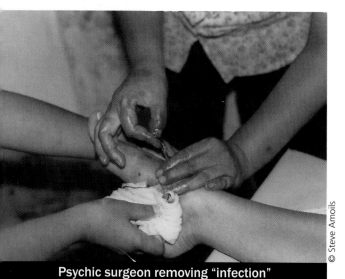

Psychic surgeon removing "infection" from a scar in Sandi's foot.

Steve and Sandi with their calligraphy.

treatment, he had a seizure. One hour later, he got up and began walking around. He was convinced he was cured. Unfortunately, he died two weeks later.

Traditional Studies in Japan

In Japan, we were fortunate to be chosen to participate in a seminar on traditional Japanese arts. We lived in a small traditional village near Kyoto, where we immersed ourselves in centuries-old Japanese culture. We wore traditional Japanese garb and studied various arts such as the tea ceremony, calligraphy, flower arrangement, Noh drama, and a martial art similar to aikido. Ultimately, through our contacts there, we met and studied with a true master of acupuncture, Mii Sensei.

Sensei means doctor, master, or teacher in Japanese. Each day in his Osaka office, together with his seven students, Mii Sensei saw up to a hundred patients. Decades before there was research evidence to confirm acupuncture's effectiveness, we watched as Mii Sensei reversed asthma symptoms, removed pain, treated strokes, and seemingly fixed a whole host of other problems, quite effortlessly. He was able to achieve these improvements in his patients simply by performing an acupuncture diagnosis and then inserting fine acupuncture needles at highly specific points on the body.

As a teacher, he had an innate sense of how his students were feeling. On days we were discouraged and down, he was nurturing and supportive. However, if he felt we were becoming overconfident, he would quickly bring us back to earth.

Mii Sensei would teach us about the origins of Oriental medicine, as well as its focus on prevention and well-being. He often reminded us, "In ancient China, in every village it was the responsibility of the physician to keep the community well. The doctor was only paid if people were well. Once they got sick, he stopped getting paid. It was therefore the job of the physician to teach people to stay well and to stop disease before it arose."

Mii Sensei also taught us something that has become a guiding principle for us with every patient we see: "At each visit you must treat

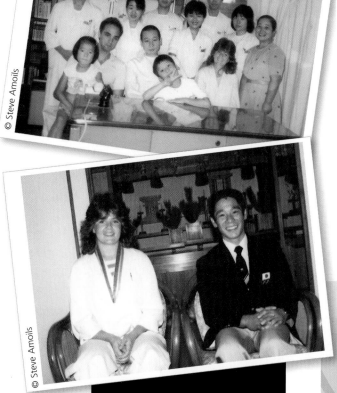

© Steve Amoils

Top: Mii Sensei and his students, children and wife complete the picture. Mii Sensei is seated in the middle front row, flanked by Sandi and Steve.

Middle: Koji Gushiken, winner of the men's gymnastic Gold Medal at the 1984 Olympics, attributed his good health to Mii Sensei's acupuncture treatments.

Left: Mindfulness: Sandi preparing for a ceremony by washing her hands.

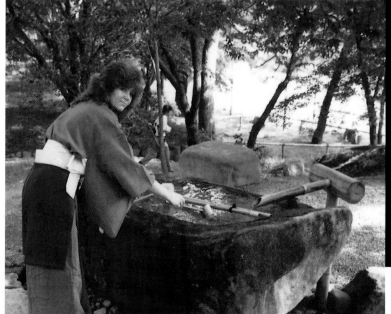

© Steve Amoils

the patient's current symptoms and illness, heal their previous illnesses and simultaneously prevent future illness. You must do all three, in order to practice good medicine."

Celebrities from all over the world came to consult with Mii Sensei. Rock stars, wealthy businessmen, members of the Japanese parliament, athletes, and commoners were all treated with the same dignity, compassion, and integrity. When Koji Gushiken, the "old man" of men's gymnastics at twenty-six years of age, returned to Japan with his Olympic gold medal, he brought it to Mii Sensei, attributing his health to the acupuncture master.

Our First Integrative Practice

We returned to South Africa in 1986, and I began working in a large family practice in Johannesburg. During this time, I began to see the benefit of combining complementary therapies with conventional approaches. One day, a muscular metalworker came in, bent over and moaning and groaning in pain from a sprained back. He was anxious to get back to work and implored me to do more than just give him painkillers or send him for physical therapy. I explained manipulative therapies and acupuncture to him. Not quite sure what to think, he nodded in agreement, desperate to get some relief. Thirty minutes later, after I had treated him, he walked back into the waiting room, completely pain free. He began to dance for the front office staff and the people in the waiting room, cavorting exuberantly.

My integrative practice began right there. This particular case resulted in an onslaught of patients who began to come to me for many different pain conditions. Seeing how effectively these therapies worked to resolve our patients' health crises—and how

quickly they worked—helped me realize that what we had learned around the world could be applied in a conventional medical clinical setting.

A few months later, a senior partner asked what I was doing that was so successful. In just one day I had treated three celebrity athletes—a runner who was a world record holder in the 800 meter hurdles, a soccer goalkeeper with Manchester United, and a tennis player who had won the Wimbledon doubles title many times. I explained that people seemed to want a treatment that was effective, yet quicker, cheaper, and less invasive than the traditional methods they had come to expect. Acupuncture, manipulative therapies, massage, and energy healing were proving to be an efficacious combination. Because what I was doing was working, he gave me his full encouragement.

Since those early days, Sandi and I have had the honor of treating hundreds of athletes, many of them world-class, including members of the U.S. women's gymnastics team. We had come full circle from watching our acupuncture

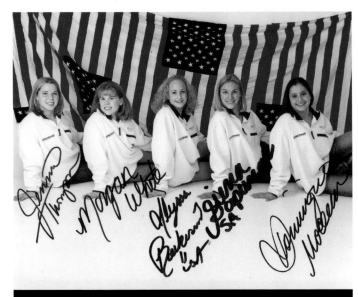

Photo given to us by members of the U.S. Women's Gymnastics Team.

sensei in Japan treat an Olympic gymnast to treating Olympic athletes ourselves.

The Journey's Culmination

Sandi and I immigrated to the United States in 1987. After completing our family medicine residencies at the University of Cincinnati, we worked with several family practice groups that ultimately merged into one. As board-certified primary care doctors, we began incorporating effective complementary therapies into our family practice. In 1999, at the request of the five-hospital group for which we worked, we opened the Alliance Institute for Integrative Medicine. In 2004, our center was chosen as one of the leading clinical centers of integrative medicine in the United States by the Bravewell Collaborative (www.Bravewell.org). As such, we are able to work in partnership with national leaders in the field of integrative medicine, doing research and learning where integrative medicine is working—and where it is not. We have developed substantial clinical experience in this area. Our center has averaged over twenty thousand visits a year for the last ten years.

Sandi's Story

While writing this book, Sandi and I went out for a ride on our bicycles one balmy evening. We hadn't ridden a mile when we slowed down at a four-way stop. I went through and turned around to make sure Sandi had followed me. To my absolute shock, I saw her lying face down in a pool of blood. A piece of wood had jammed her front wheel, causing her to plummet face-first into the road. This devastating accident knocked out six of her front teeth. In addition, she had ankle and finger fractures, a concussion, neck and spine injuries, and multiple soft tissue injuries.

Her courageous recovery from this dreadful accident was augmented and accelerated by the use of a truly integrative approach.

On the mainstream side, she has been blessed to have a superb prosthodontist and oral surgeon who started working on her within an hour of the accident. They were able to salvage much of the remaining oral tissue. Her orthopedic surgeon ably dealt with her concussion and her fractures.

Her journey of recovery was also enhanced by the most incredible team of healers, who provided synergistic complementary therapies.

I watched with amazement the first day when her face, swollen like a soccer ball, literally shrank back almost to normal after five hours of a treatment using frequency specific microcurrent (FSM) together with energy healing. She received massages, acupuncture, energy healing, and chiropractic treatments, rotated on a daily basis. Each day she showed small but definite improvement.

Sandi remained remarkably positive throughout the process, choosing to focus on the fact that she was alive and healing, frequently acknowledging that her injuries could have been much worse. Even when looking at her beautiful face, she was able to joke about her lack of front teeth. She faced gum grafts, dental implants, and lip revision surgeries with the same courage and upbeat outlook. Her fractures healed remarkably quickly. Her soft tissue injuries, which in some people can be devastating and produce long-lasting pain, slowly melted away.

Sandi has been a role model for the lifestyle we espouse. She was fit and healthy and has always eaten a healthful diet. Because her pre-accident condition was so good, her tissue resilience allowed her to bounce back quickly.

The transformational process she has experienced has been truly amazing. The accident, while life-altering for her, also turned out to be life-affirming—an opportunity to transform her life. She has a new glow, an inner strength that shines through. My nickname for her is Sandi 2.0. She has reassessed many of the values in her life, reprioritizing what is truly important. Her life has a new spiritual dimension. Her physical and emotional healing process has reaffirmed for me that she is a true example of what we aspire to do in our medical model. Despite what she has been through, her life is in many ways richer and better!

Synergistic Goals and Complementary Talents: The Evolution of a Philosophy

Sandi and I have been fortunate to have been influenced and taught by the astute minds of philosophers, physicians, and healers who have been able to think out of the box. In our current age, the ability to produce data is often confused with science. The law of gravity was present long before Newton "discovered" it. Similarly, our bodies seem to behave in ways that have been observed for centuries, even though scientific techniques may not yet have "validated" them. Diagnostic and therapeutic techniques will continue to evolve, and we will continue to incorporate that progress into our practice. The rest of this book, however, is based upon what we and our contributing authors have learned from centuries of medical traditions, wise teachers, decades of clinical experience, and thousands of patients. These unchanging concepts give you insight into your body's hardware and software—and help you view your health and life in a new way.

Transforming Your Life

We have seen the ability to bounce back from stress in many of our most successful mentors, friends, and patients. When they do, they have come out stronger, wiser, and more successful. They have taken a problem that might devastate most people and used it to make them-

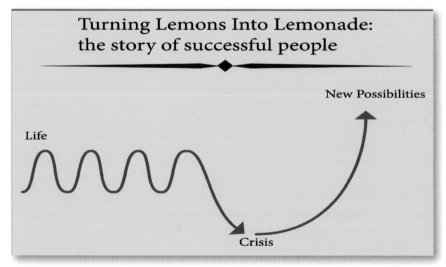

Turning Lemons Into Lemonade: the story of successful people

Life

New Possibilities

Crisis

Figure P1

Crisis and Transformation

selves—and the world—a better place. To use a well-known phrase, they have turned lemons into lemonade.

In Transformational Medicine, our goal is to optimize physical function, psychological transformation, and spiritual growth to attain true healing.

Healing is a dynamic process. Often the starting point is the diagnosis of a disease or the persistence of symptoms even after treatment. Transformational Medicine usually means working with a health care team. At the center is a physician with whom you can openly discuss both your symptoms and your fears—a doctor you can trust to do an appropriate medical workup and who will refer you to appropriate medical specialists if necessary. However, Transformational Medicine also means looking at other options beyond conventional medicine. Depending on your needs, other health care providers may become part of your team. In our practice, we work with chiropractors, acupuncturists, energy healers, massage therapists, and others who provide healing care.

We have come to realize that we all can move toward well-being by transforming our symptoms of dis-ease or dis-comfort into a new state of better health—and this is an approach we can each apply to our life on a daily basis.

In other words, we would like you to reinterpret your illness as a reminder that you may need to change. This approach will enable you to use each of life's major problems as a turning point or inflection point to self-correct. We all have the option of changing our trajectory toward either well-being or disease. With this book, we would like to give you the tools to expand your options to create healing and achieve positive change in your life.

Transformational Medicine and the Evolution of Medical Care: A Solution to the Escalating Burden of Chronic Illness

To explain how and why we want you to change your life, we need you to understand how medicine arrived at its current status. Today, patients, especially those with chronic conditions, get a lot of medical treatment—office visits, tests of all sorts, many prescriptions for drugs, physical therapy, weight-loss counseling and more—yet their health is no better. How can we have so much medicine while also having more and more people with chronic conditions that only get worse despite aggressive treatment?

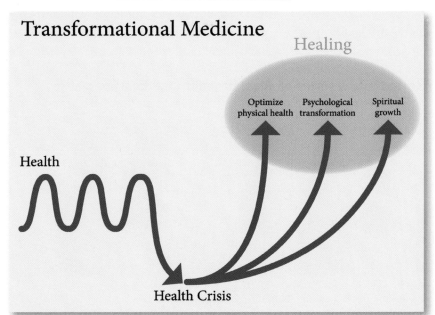

Transformational Medicine

Healing

Optimize physical health

Psychological transformation

Spiritual growth

Health

Health Crisis

Figure P2

The Healing Goals of Transformational Medicine.

The Development of Modern Medicine and the Legacy of Flexner

One hundred years ago, there was a need for standardization in medicine. At the time, there were a multitude of approaches to medicine. Many were worthless and others were harmful. It was the time of snake-oil salesmen. There was no FDA, there were no standards, and there were no protections against medicines that were contaminated or ineffective. It was simply an open market. Medical schools varied widely in how well they taught their students—in some schools, students who didn't even have a high school education could get a diploma after just two years.

To rectify the problem, the Carnegie Foundation commissioned Abraham Flexner, a professional educator, to study medical schools and the drug industry and make recommendations for improvements. The recommendations in *The Flexner Report* of 1910 set high standards and established a level of consistency within medicine and the emerging pharmaceutical industry. The report set the stage for safer medical protocols and standards of practice as we know them today.

Unfortunately, this internal housecleaning within American medicine also resulted in a degree of overstandardization. Many disciplines focusing on prevention and health promotion were eliminated. As these other forms of medicine began to fade away, the concept of "healing" became associated with drugs and surgery.

The Age of the Silver Bullet

The era of antibiotics began soon after World War II, when penicillin became widely available. The focus of medicine then became finding the correct microbe that was causing the disease and killing it with the correct antibiotic. This quest for a singular cause extended to other areas of medicine as well. Scientists began to break down a problem into its smallest components and look for a way to remedy these. It became a system of "anti"-dotes—hence our emphasis today on antibiotics, anti-inflammatories, and anticancer agents. Patients want that silver bullet and expect a quick fix when it comes to their health.

Medical Silos

The same thought pattern entered medicine. Different specialties arose as independent fields, treating independent parts of the body. The presumption is that with higher specialization comes improved care. Is this true? Yes, if your problem calls for someone who is highly specialized in one area. But what if a specialist acts in a "silo," without seeing all aspects of

Physicians are sorted into a series of silos, based on medical specialty.

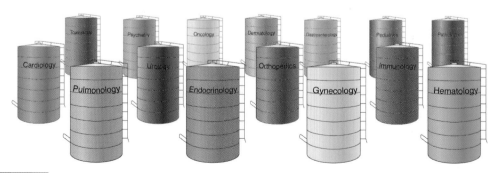

| Figure P3 | Medical Specialization Leads to a Silo Mentality. |

Faith's Story

Faith, a 46-year-old woman, came to see us soon after the onset of constant, throbbing headaches at the back of her head, worse on the left. She had been to see her doctor three times with no success. The headache was not relieved by any over-the-counter medication, nor by any of the medications her doctor had prescribed. In desperation, she came to our center to try acupuncture for the pain.

On closer questioning, Faith described a very subtle intermittent blurring of her peripheral vision. She had no previous history of severe headaches or any family history of migraine. She had no other symptoms that would point to another source of the headache: no trauma, fever, weight loss, or rash and no depression or increased stress. Both her recent intense headaches and her subtle neurological symptoms were red flags to us, pointing to something more serious.

We sent her for an urgent MRI (magnetic resonance imaging) and MRA (magnetic resonance angiogram). Fortunately, this test identified a clotted internal carotid artery, and she was rushed into surgery. She did very well and recovered completely after the surgery. As it turned out, Faith didn't need our integrative medicine approach. She was helped by our taking a traditional, thorough medical history and then being treated with the latest high-tech imaging and surgery techniques.

---

your health or discussing your care with your other physicians? That is where problems arise. An orthopedic surgeon may prescribe anti-inflammatories without knowing a patient has kidney problems. The results can be disastrous. In some areas of the United States, the average patient takes six to seven prescription drugs. In addition, patients often use herbal remedies or supplements without telling their doctor, risking potentially dangerous drug interactions. And while there are good studies on the effects of single drugs, there are no good studies on what happens when patients take multiple drugs at the same time.

Where Medicine Succeeds

You don't need to look far to be impressed by the miracles of modern medicine. What is working is working very well. The benefits of Western medicine range from newer, better medications and less invasive surgeries to high-tech trauma centers and state-of-the-art intensive care units.

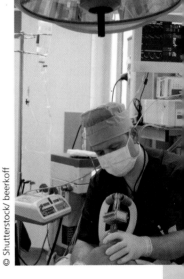

© Shutterstock/ beerkoff

If you pause to think about these advances, though, you realize that most of them deal with acute care, highly technical care, less invasive and safer surgery, and the effect of blockbuster drugs on conditions like high cholesterol, heart disease, depression, heartburn, hypertension, inflammation, and psychosis. Western medicine especially excels in acute conditions such as infection, trauma, or heart attacks. The medications developed to treat these conditions are fast-acting and can be life-saving, and modern trauma care is without parallel in the history of medicine. In acute situations, there is no better place to be than in the hands of a physician who has made a correct diagnosis and is prescribing the correct treatment.

Chronic Illness and Conventional Medicine

As Faith's story shows, the Western medical approach works well in areas that deal with acute conditions. By accurately defining a problem, medical practitioners can provide the best treatment to save lives.

The problem is that this approach isn't working as well for chronic health issues such as obesity, type 2 diabetes, high blood pressure, chronic pain conditions such as arthritis and back pain, gastrointestinal disorders, autoimmune diseases, and other problems, especially if someone has more than one condition.

Chronic health problems are seldom easy to treat. As a result, they are crippling our medical system. More than half of all adults in the United States have some form of chronic illness. In addition, 65 percent of Americans are overweight or obese and at serious risk of type 2 diabetes. The need for a system of health care that addresses chronic conditions has become more important than ever.

Care for chronic disorders can be extremely frustrating for both physicians and patients, with our medical system being built around a specific-drugs-for-a-specific-disorder model. This is aggravated by the time pressure placed on primary care physicians. Given the economic and time constraints, mainstream medicine forces primary care physicians to become technicians, relying on algorithms. Patients may feel that they are not being heard, and doctors may inadvertently dismiss important complaints. Treatment tends to focus on symptoms that are the expression of underlying problems, rather than on the problems themselves. For example, high cholesterol is not a disease, but an expression of an underlying malfunction that may or may not lead to heart disease.

Despite all of the technology, the puzzle of chronic illness has not been easy to decipher.

In 1989, Kurt Kroenke, a medical researcher, tracked the progress of one thousand patients in an Army outpatient medical clinic over a three-year period. He looked at the fourteen most common chronic complaints: chest pain, fatigue, dizziness, headache, edema, back pain, shortness of breath, insomnia, abdominal pain, numbness, impotence, weight loss, cough, and constipation. Kroenke found that patients who had three or more health conditions simultaneously, which had persisted for three months or more, had only one chance in six of getting well. The likelihood that conventional medical treatment would resolve the problem was less than 16 percent.

Unresolved Health Issues

In Kroenke's study of common chronic problems, 55 percent of the patients received symptomatic treatment, and this treatment was often ineffective. The conditions most likely to improve were those that had lasted less than four months in patients with a history of two or fewer symptoms, or whose symptoms turned out to have a specific cause. Among patients with vague, nonspecific, or difficult-to-treat complaints, such as chronic fatigue, frequent insomnia, or dizziness, only 39 percent reported relief from conventional therapies.

Although the study was performed back in 1989, in our experience, the findings are still valid. In fact, the problems seem to have magnified. The health care provided for these types of chronic conditions is often expensive and, in many cases, ineffective. It simply treats symptoms rather than getting at the underlying cause. We need to change the system. Integrative Medicine offers a solution. According to

Ralph Snyderman, M.D., Chancellor Emeritus, Duke University School of Medicine, "What we have now is a 'sick-care' system that is reactive to problems. The integrative approach flips the system on its head and puts the patient at the center, addressing not just symptoms, but the real causes of illness. It is care that is preventive, predictive, and personalized."

The Best of Medicine

Simply defined, Integrative Medicine provides the best of conventional medicine in tandem with the best of complementary therapies. It is a synergistic, real-world, and evidence-based approach to treatment.

We fully support the ethic described by Marcia Angell, M.D., former editor of the prestigious *New England Journal of Medicine*, who said, "There cannot be two kinds of medicine—conventional and alternative. There is only medicine that has been adequately tested and medicine that has not, medicine that works and medicine that may or may not work." However, complementary therapies are not easy to study in a controlled trial. It is difficult to perform sham acupuncture, for example, so that the results can be compared to similar patients who get real acupuncture. An integrative approach also often utilizes multiple less-invasive treatments simultaneously, making a study on this type of approach even more complicated.

The Goals of Integrative Medicine

As practitioners of Integrative Medicine, we aim for a new approach that emphasizes health and well-being. In Integrative Medicine, care is:

- **Personalized.** Health care customized to your genetics, body chemistry, stress level, and lifestyle.
- **Proactive.** An approach that involves you in your own care, focusing on practical action steps.
- **Preventive.** Treatment not only resolves current problems, but also reduces the risks of future health problems before they develop.
- **Patient-centered.** Treatment that includes you as the primary member of your health care team, acknowledging that you know your symptoms better than anyone does.
- **Empowering.** Providing you with an expanded range of tools that support your health and well-being, helping you to become more responsible for your health outcome.

Systems Biology and Your Health

Today, new technologies such as genomics, information technology, nanotechnology, bioinformatics, network biology, and translational research have given us a dramatically improved understanding of how we become ill. This new way of looking at the complex interactions in the human body is called systems biology.

Systems biology allows us to see that a number of major factors can contribute to the development of a specific disease in any given individual:

Social networks affect disease. Studies have shown that people with better social connections and support cope better than those who are isolated and lonely. These social connections may relate to family, partners or spouses, friends, peers, religious communities, or social groups. In general, financial, emotional, and even physical stresses tend to be cushioned if someone has a good support system. This tells

A Systems Biology Approach to Understanding Health and Disease

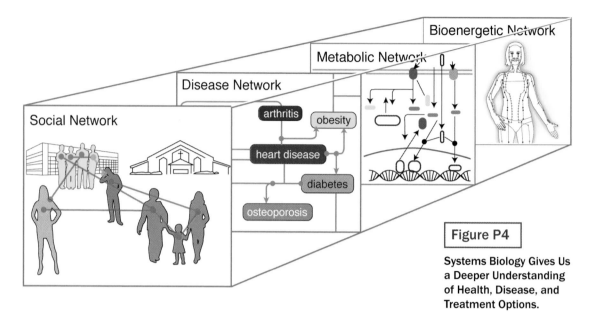

Figure P4

Systems Biology Gives Us a Deeper Understanding of Health, Disease, and Treatment Options.

us we can't view a patient as an isolated disease. We also need to view the person in the context of a social network, as this will influence how he or she will develop and express disease.

Diseases are linked to each other. Someone who is obese is more likely to develop heart disease, diabetes, and arthritis than someone who is not obese. These diseases are different, but they also tend to occur in tandem with one another. In medicine, such diseases are called comorbidities. When a patient has comorbidities, we find it is usually because their diseases share similar metabolic underpinnings.

Different diseases may share similar metabolic pathways. The chemical pathways that influence one disease may be simultaneously influencing another. A good example of this is inflammation. This low-grade fire in our bodies can simultaneously affect diseases such as coronary artery disease, arthritis, osteoporosis, Alzheimer's disease, and even cancer. The cells in our bodies constantly send chemical signals to each other. When we are inflamed, chemicals travel around our bodies, lighting fires in many

areas. That is why one metabolic dysfunction can result in many diseases. But herein also lies an opportunity to treat many diseases by using one approach that deals with the underlying problem.

Our bioenergetic networks affect our health. Traditional Chinese medicine has used the concept of bioenergetic networks for thousands of years. According to Chinese medicine, bioenergetic networks, also called meridian systems or biopsychotypes, affect the functioning of our metabolic pathways. By understanding the imbalances in these networks, it is possible to predict where disease will occur and simultaneously treat and prevent illness.

With a systems biology perspective, we can look at the myriad interacting internal and external factors that create health or disease. We can move away from the idea that disease will simply strike us as some misguided lightning bolt from the sky. We can learn to start affecting multiple aspects in multiple dimensions in order to both prevent and treat illness, as well as promote health.

Functional Medicine

Functional Medicine, a term coined by one of our mentors, Dr. Jeffrey Bland, explains how any disease is affected by multiple systems. Functional Medicine explains how external factors—stress, our community support, environmental toxins, diet, lifestyle, and exercise—interact with internal factors in our bodies. These include factors related to our genetic makeup, as well as, for example, our hormonal, immune and neurotransmitter balance, inflammation, gut health, and musculoskeletal health. Functional medicine is a modern, scientifically based approach, but many of its principles—especially the idea that we have multiple interacting and self-regulating systems—mirror the ideas of health and disease promoted by age-old principles of Chinese medicine and Ayurvedic (Indian) health care philosophies.

By looking at the body as a complex web of these interacting systems, we can view health as a dynamic balance between internal and external factors. We can understand that each person is biochemically and psychologically unique, responding in different ways to the many influences each one of us faces.

A Functional Medicine Explanation: How Internal and External Factors Influence Health and Disease

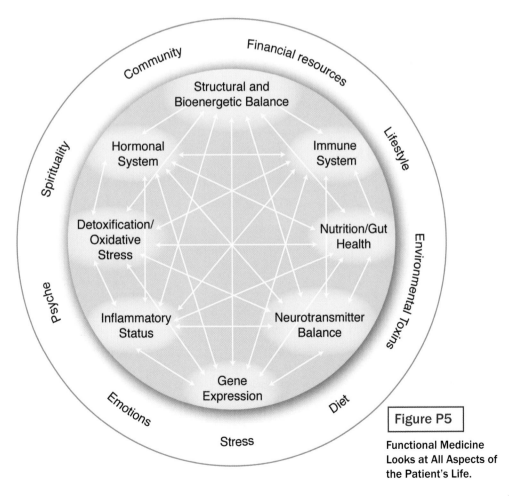

Figure P5

Functional Medicine Looks at All Aspects of the Patient's Life.

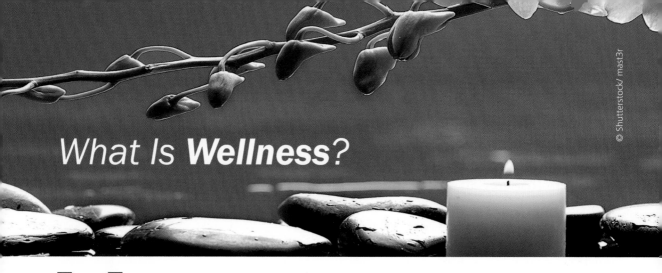

What Is **Wellness**?

Many people think of wellness as a blood test, Pap smear, mammogram, or colonoscopy that shows no problems. This is not wellness—these are merely tests that assist in the *early detection* of illness.

True wellness is the prevention of illness but also the promotion of vitality. This includes physical well-being, emotional stability, intel-lectual acuity, a sense of openness, and being able to embrace change. Wellness includes the ability to speak your own truth, a sense of intuition, and awareness of spiritual well-being. And wellness leads to healthy and appropriate aging. Although we have learned to equate aging with illness, this does not have to be the case.

Changing the Way We Think about Medicine

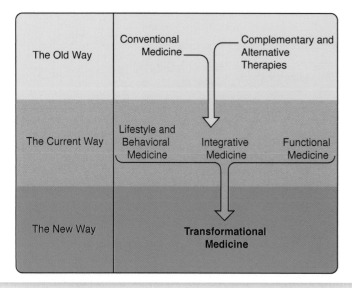

What's In A Name?

The Old Way	Conventional Medicine	Complementary and Alternative Therapies
The Current Way	Lifestyle and Behavioral Medicine	Integrative Medicine — Functional Medicine
The New Way		**Transformational Medicine**

| Figure P6 | The Development of Transformational Medicine. |

Often people seek out wellness by trying alternative therapies because of the focus these systems place on returning to an active state of well-being. In the old medical paradigm, physicians were resistant to alternative therapies, with the result being that patients either saw their conventional doctor or tried complementary or alternative therapies. The two approaches rarely coexisted—indeed, many patients never told their physicians about their use of complementary therapies. This has changed as the medical profession has become much more accepting of Integrative Medicine.

It is our opinion that medicine will and should continue to change.

18 PROLOGUE | *Expanding Your Medical Treatment Options*

New inventions, drugs, ideas, surgeries, and technologies will continue to advance the science of medicine. Genetic advances, biotechnology, and nanotechnology will be used to help our bodies heal in ways that we could never have imagined!

We also envision a new kind of medicine in which people will be asked to play a more active role in their own health care. What's more, we will be asked to recognize illness at a much earlier stage. As we each become more attuned to our health, we will be able to transform our health.

What we have learned using this approach is that when we affect multiple systems at the same time, we can accomplish three things at once—reduce the symptoms of illness, prevent future illness, and promote a feeling of health and vitality. This is what we call Transformational Medicine.

Transformational Medicine

In practicing both Integrative Medicine and Functional Medicine, we have learned to use the best of both complementary and conventional medicine to create a new state of vibrant health and well-being for our patients. We have come to realize that we all can move toward well-being by transforming our symptoms of dis-ease or dis-comfort into a new state of better health—and this is an approach we can each apply to our lives on a daily basis.

To transform your health, you need to see where you came from, assess where you are, and then make positive changes to influence where you are going.

Predisposition to illness. We all have a certain set of predispositions to illness. This may be due to our genes, a poor or toxic environment, emotional trauma, a dietary deficiency, or numerous other causes. This sets us on a course toward illness, whatever that illness may be. We call this course a trajectory.

Assessing your current health. To assess your current health, ask yourself if you have any symptoms of discomfort or disease. If you have a disease or health crisis, we would like you to see this as an opportunity for change, an inflection point.

Transforming your future health. We believe you can turn away from the illness trajectory and toward health.

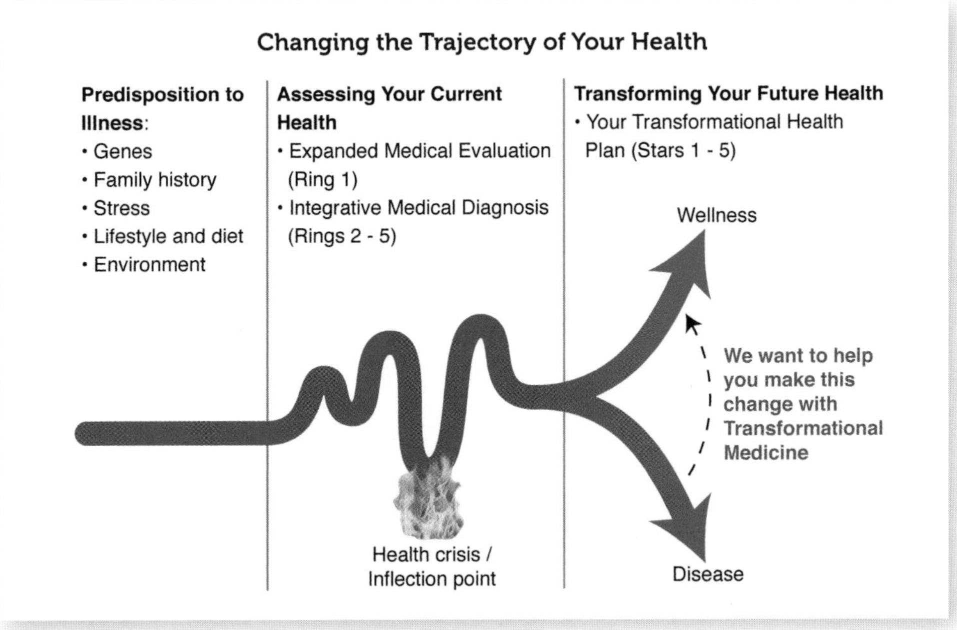

Changing the Trajectory of Your Health

Predisposition to Illness:
• Genes
• Family history
• Stress
• Lifestyle and diet
• Environment

Assessing Your Current Health
• Expanded Medical Evaluation (Ring 1)
• Integrative Medical Diagnosis (Rings 2 - 5)

Transforming Your Future Health
• Your Transformational Health Plan (Stars 1 - 5)

Wellness

We want to help you make this change with Transformational Medicine

Health crisis / Inflection point

Disease

Figure P7

Changing the Tragectory of Your Health

19

The Five Rings and the Five Stars—
a system of diagnosis and treatment in Transformational Medicine.

The Transformational Medicine Diagnosis

In Transformational Medicine, we think of your diagnosis as being made up of five linked rings.

Each Ring is a separate category that is both independent of and interdependent on the other rings. Together they help us understand the whole: the multifaceted, multidimensional being that is *you*, the person who wants to understand what is going on with your health.

We don't evaluate the environment as a separate ring, as it plays a role in each one.

The Five Rings we use to evaluate a patient are:

- **Ring 1:** Making an expanded medical diagnosis.
- **Ring 2:** Evaluating the effects of stress on the body.
- **Ring 3:** Evaluating imbalances in nutrition, immune function, metabolism, and body chemistry.
- **Ring 4:** Evaluating hormonal imbalances.
- **Ring 5:** Evaluating imbalances in body mechanics and bioenergy.

THE FIVE RINGS OF DIAGNOSIS

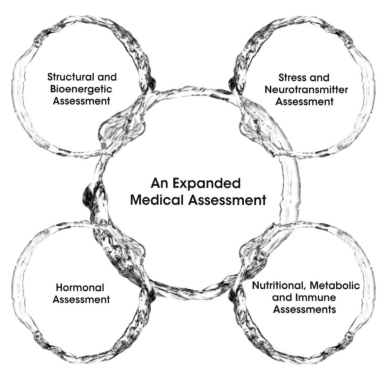

Structural and Bioenergetic Assessment

Stress and Neurotransmitter Assessment

An Expanded Medical Assessment

Hormonal Assessment

Nutritional, Metabolic and Immune Assessments

THE FIVE STARS OF TREATMENT

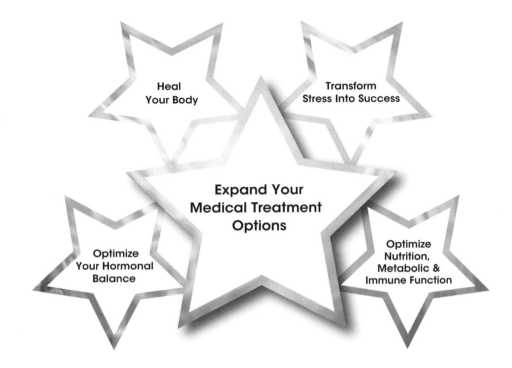

The Transformational Medicine Treatment Plan

Once we have used the Five Rings to assess your health and to diagnose problems, we use a system we call the Five Stars to create your Transformational Medicine Treatment plan. The Five Stars offer an interlinked approach to help you regain and optimize your health and well-being.

Transformational Medicine is an applied primary care approach that can be used to resolve many common medical problems. It doesn't replace the need for a primary care doctor, nor does it replace the need for a specialist. It augments both.

In Transformational Medicine, we spend time and effort on prevention and early intervention to reduce the burden of illness both now and in the future. Because our patients take a greater role in their own health care, they develop and expand a new sense of well-being. Our goal is for you to participate actively in your health care, to get well, and stay well.

The Five Stars of a Transformational Medicine Treatment Plan include:

- **Star 1:** Expanding your medical treatment options.

- **Star 2:** Transforming stress into success.

- **Star 3:** Optimizing nutrition and your metabolic and immune functions.

- **Star 4:** Optimizing your hormonal balance.

- **Star 5:** Healing your body.

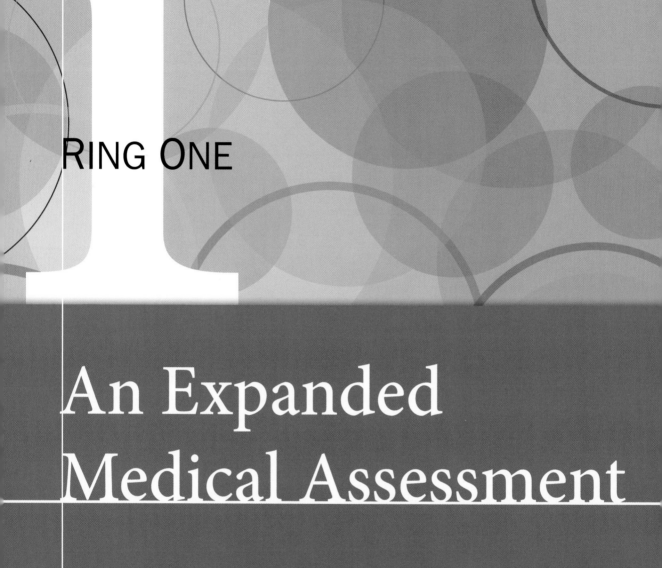

1

RING ONE

An Expanded
Medical Assessment

What to Do When You're Sick and **Where to Start if You Want to Get Healthy**

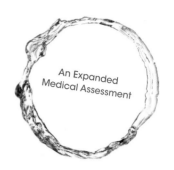

An Expanded Medical Assessment

Afull workup by a conventionally trained medical doctor remains the first and most important step in the diagnosis of medical problems. If you have a clear-cut issue that needs a specific test or treatment, we encourage you to see your primary care physician first. For example, if you have a bacterial infection, such as strep throat or pneumonia, or if you need an x-ray or a tetanus shot, or are due for preventive care such as a Pap smear, mammogram, or colonoscopy, your primary physician is the person who can take care of you or refer you to the right specialist or testing center.

But what if your chronic health problem doesn't improve, despite time and skillful standard treatment? This might be the time to seek out a physician who can delve further into the issue and help you resolve it. A slightly different approach to a health problem can lead you toward a transformational change.

What about those of you who are healthy but want to maintain your health or even achieve peak performance? We recommend following the steps we outline in order to tweak your body, mind, or metabolism to facilitate optimal health.

Begin with a Conventional Medical Workup

One of the primary reasons to have a yearly physical is to check your conventional health markers. How is your blood pressure? Are your glucose and cholesterol levels normal? Is your stool clear of blood? Abnormal markers indicate that your body isn't functioning properly, even if you feel reasonably well. The goal is to identify malfunctions in your system so normal functioning can be restored *before* you get sick. In matters of health, sooner is always better than later. It is much easier to intervene early on than it will be down the line when a disease has taken deeper root in your system.

Usually, when one of the health markers on your lab tests is abnormal, the problem isn't urgent—but it is important. Every time you restore balance to your body chemistry, you've lowered your risk of a more serious health problem. Sometimes, highly abnormal markers make further medical intervention or medication a necessary step. For instance, if you have very high triglycerides (tiny fat droplets in your blood), you're at an increased risk of an attack of pancreatitis. If your glucose levels are dangerously high, you likely have diabetes and need immediate treatment. Usually though, abnormal health markers simply tell us in which direction to point you in order to help you make a change.

If you feel healthy, but want to further optimize your health, we still recommend a conventional medical workup. Occasionally, this will uncover a medical issue, but in most cases your standard exam and lab work will all be normal. If that's the case, you can then move on to Rings 2 through 5 in order to really understand what you need to do to enhance your health and well-being. Stars 1 through 5 will give you practical advice on incorporating those ideas into your daily life. If you strive for peak performance in your life, this approach will help you attain it through optimized health and an improved ability to handle stress.

Desperate for a Diagnosis

Medical science puts us on a quest to pinpoint a single cause for an illness. Because of this, we've come to think that having a diagnosis is a necessary prerequisite for a cure. When there is no name for a set of symptoms, patients are concerned that they're not being taken seriously, or that a treatable cause is being missed.

A diagnosis alone, however, is often not enough. It tells us nothing about the cause of a person's symptoms. When a patient has a heart attack, for instance, we know what happened, but not why. The underlying cause may be very high cholesterol levels, high levels of inflammation due to gum disease, cocaine abuse, or any number of other reasons.

As physicians, we strongly support utilizing the best of scientific medicine to make a diagnosis. We will always do our best to find out what is happening by taking a thorough medical history, performing a physical examination, and using lab and radiological tests and even invasive testing, if necessary. However, there often comes a time when we realize that the best of medicine still can't explain what's going on. This is especially common when patients have had multiple symptoms for prolonged periods of time. At that point, we start looking under the hood to see what systems are malfunctioning.

When the Tests Are Normal, but You Don't Feel Normal

At times, you may simply feel "off" or "not yourself," yet you may not have a diagnosable illness. Often, your conventional lab markers are within the normal range, even though you don't feel well. Normal lab results don't necessarily mean good health. For instance, the common conventional blood tests for kidney function may not indicate a problem until your kidney

function is 50 percent compromised. Similarly, conventional liver function tests, such as aspartate transaminase (AST), may not indicate problems, such as cirrhosis, until liver disease is quite advanced.

If you don't feel well, we want to rule out a serious underlying condition, such as a tumor or a blocked artery. Most of the time, though, causes of common nonspecific medical complaints, such as fatigue, are difficult to pinpoint or treat. One reason for this is that medical tests aren't always sensitive enough to pick up causes of common symptoms. Good examples here are migraines and irritable bowel syndrome. In these cases, the patient may be completely debilitated by pain, yet the results of conventional testing are normal.

These are good examples of what we call *functional problems*. The patient's normal function has been disturbed, but there is no evidence of an illness or organic pathology, such as a brain tumor or inflammatory bowel disease. A functional disturbance such as a migraine may not progress to anything dangerous or life-threatening, but can severely impact a patient's daily life and well-being. On the other hand, it could be the start of a progressive path toward illness.

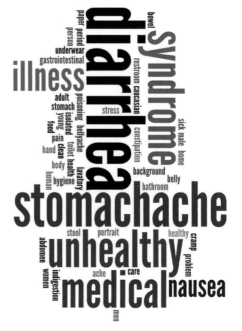

© Shutterstock/ mrfiza

Sleep Disorders: A Hidden Functional Problem

Sleep is extremely important to help the body regenerate, yet too often we find that our patients, even young children, don't get enough sleep. The cause could simply be too much to do or too many distractions, but often a sleep disorder is the problem.

Sleep disorders include:

- **Chronic insomnia**, where you have trouble more than a few times a week falling asleep or staying asleep.

- **Teeth grinding or clenching**, which can cause temporomandibular joint (TMJ) problems, headache, and tooth damage.

- **Sleep apnea**, or shallow breathing that causes loud snoring and frequent mini-awakenings from lack of oxygen throughout the night.

- **Restless legs syndrome**, which causes a crawling or "antsy" feeling in the legs and a powerful impulse to move the legs. This usually happens when the person is sitting or lying down and prevents restful sleep.

- **Narcolepsy**, a sleep disorder that causes trouble sleeping at night and periods of extreme daytime sleepiness.

Depression, irritability, memory and mood problems can all be associated with sleep disorders, as can unexplained chest pain, palpitations, shortness of breath, and fibromyalgia-like muscle soreness. Lack of sleep also raises your level of the stress hormone cortisol—and high cortisol levels are associated with weight gain, insulin resistance, and type 2 diabetes.

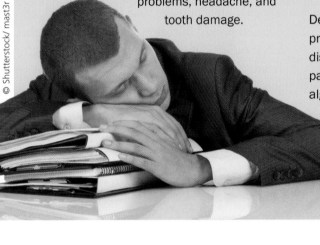

© Shutterstock/ mast3r

A Progressive Disturbance:
From Wellness to Illness

Many times, a patient comes to the doctor with a vague or ill-defined health complaint with no detectable cause. Some examples of this include:

- Fatigue
- Insomnia (sleeplessness)
- Moodiness, irritability, anxiety, and depression
- Lowered libido or impotence
- Pain
- Headaches
- Frequent infections
- Indigestion, heartburn, bloating, diarrhea, or constipation
- Weight gain or weight loss

Doctors often dismiss these symptoms as minor problems that may be psychosomatic or related to depression. In most cases, the physical exam and lab work are normal. However, this is where we believe that viewing symptoms in a different light can help reverse the course of illness, and even turn toward well-being. Learning to understand a problem as a disturbance of function can dramatically alter the way you look at it. Treating a sleep disorder, for instance, can significantly improve a person's life. Learning to understand that even what doctors label as psychosomatic disorders are really functional disorders can offer new and exciting ways to treat them.

When Do You Get Sick?

Getting sick is a process. Patients don't just suddenly develop chronic diseases, such as type 2 diabetes. At first, they develop what we call functional imbalances. These are small changes that begin to occur long before the patient has all the signs and symptoms that define a particular disease. Increased inflammation, oxidative damage, and altered immune function can start long before blood sugar problems rise to the level of type 2 diabetes, for example. We feel it is important to recognize these imbalances when we first see them, take them seriously, and correct them.

The earlier a condition is diagnosed, the greater the likelihood that it can be reversed, returning you to health.

Identifying Your Genetic Risks

To understand how we progress on the path from illness to wellness, we need to understand genetic makeup as well as the factors that affect how genes are expressed. In medical school, we were taught to think of genes as fixed and immutable, conferring upon us some inevitable disease. This is not the case. About 70 percent of our genes can be up- or down-regulated. In simple terms, they can be turned on or off. This is called altering gene expression. It turns out that our environment, our lifestyle, our emotional traumas, our diets, and numerous other factors affect our genes. All these factors together are called epigenetic factors. Think of your genes as your hardware and your epigenetic factors as your software. You know that good software can make your computer work much better. Similarly, a glitch in your software can shut down your computer.

Let's look at this example in real life. If many of your family members have type 2 diabetes, for instance, you are at greater risk for it as well. Why? Is it just your genes, or is it also the diet, lifestyle, and exercise habits you've learned from your family? You cannot change your genes, but you can modify the environment they are

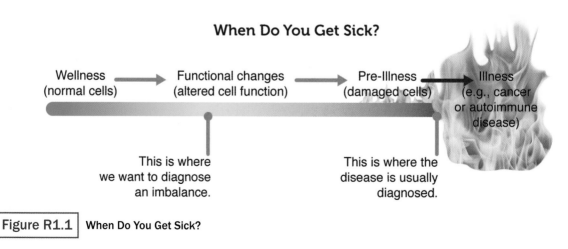

When Do You Get Sick?

Wellness (normal cells) → Functional changes (altered cell function) → Pre-Illness (damaged cells) → Illness (e.g., cancer or autoimmune disease)

This is where we want to diagnose an imbalance.

This is where the disease is usually diagnosed.

| Figure R1.1 | When Do You Get Sick?

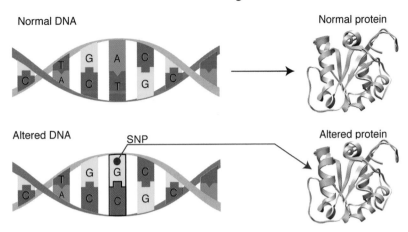

Understanding SNPs

Normal DNA

Normal protein

Altered DNA

SNP

Altered protein

Between any two individuals, there are many genetic differences. If even one base pair is different, which is known as a **Single-Nucleotide Polymorphism** (SNP), the DNA will code for a slightly different protein, which may have a different function.

Figure R1.2

Understanding SNPs

exposed to, thus changing your genetic expression. You can lose weight, eat a better diet, and exercise more. Making such changes is no guarantee against getting the disease, but it can prevent or delay it and make it easier to manage if it does happen.

We can get a general idea of your risk of illness from your family history. This alerts us to your risk for conditions such as diabetes, heart disease, Alzheimer's disease, and various types of cancers. It is now possible to study the entire human genome and know all your approximately thirty thousand genes. Each gene can have thousands of variations, however. The resultant permutations are diverse and make us all unique. Add to this that our genes are constantly being influenced by our lifestyle, diet, and environment. No wonder it is sometimes difficult to figure out what's going on!

Our genes are made up of DNA, which in turn is made up of bases called nucleotides. Sometimes genes can mutate because of a reaction to a virus or toxin, or for some other reason. The nucleotides can be switched, which causes a change in shape of the gene. These genetic variants are known as single nucleotide polymorphisms ("many shapes") or

Getting Around Genetic Glitches

An interesting example of a genetic glitch is a SNP called methylene-tetra-hydra-folate-reductase (MTHFR). This glitch affects an enzyme needed for the formation of the active form of folic acid, one of the B vitamins. People with a SNP for MTHFR may not be able to form enough active folic acid even if they consume generous amounts of green leafy vegetables (a good source of folic acid). Folic acid deficiency has been associated with neural tube defects in babies and Down syndrome, as well as anemia, arthritis, heart disease, strokes, certain cancers, and dementia. So, having a MTHFR SNP can predispose a person to any one of these diseases. However, if you know you have this SNP, you can add an activated folic acid supplement such as L-5-methyl tetrahydrofolate to your diet, which will help prevent later disease. By doing so, you circumvent your body's inability to properly activate the folic acid.

SNPs—called *snips* for short. The gene will then behave differently, churning out the incorrect protein or causing the body to react differently. SNPs can help explain why individuals respond differently to infections, chemicals, and toxins.

There are thousands of SNPs. Some common examples include:

- **E-Selectin (SELE) or endothelial leukocyte adhesion molecule-1.** If you have this SNP, you have "stickier" blood vessels and are at higher risk for developing blocked arteries.

- **Interleukin 6 (IL-6).** If you have inherited this SNP from both parents, you produce high amounts of this natural inflammatory chemical when you are stressed. This can result in inflammation, rapidly worsening osteoporosis, heart attacks, and severe pain.

- **ApoE4.** This SNP makes you more vulnerable to late-onset Alzheimer's disease and atherosclerosis (blocked arteries). People with ApoE4 are also more vulnerable to heavy metal toxicity.

- **Angiotensin I (AGT) and Angiotensin II Receptor-1 (AGTR1).** These SNPs deal with angiotensin, a hormone that plays a central role in regulating blood pressure as well as inflammation in the smooth muscles of blood vessels. People with these SNPs are more prone to hypertension, as well as diseases of small blood vessels such as those found in the kidneys, the heart or the brain. They will respond better to drugs that deal with angiotensin, such as angiotensin converting enzyme inhibitors (ACE inhibitors) or angiotensin receptor blockers (ARBs). Salt, as well as certain drugs such as oral contraceptives or estrogen replacement, will activate these SNPs. However, a diet high in fruit and vegetables, fish oils, magnesium, vitamin D, resveratrol (found in red wine), curcumin (turmeric), and a host of other factors will turn these SNPs off.

- **Weight control SNPs.** These help determine the best diet for you. Recent research has shown that knowing more about your body weight SNPs can help you decide if you will do best on a low-fat, low-carbohydrate, or "balanced" diet for weight control. (We'll discuss these diets more in Star 3.)

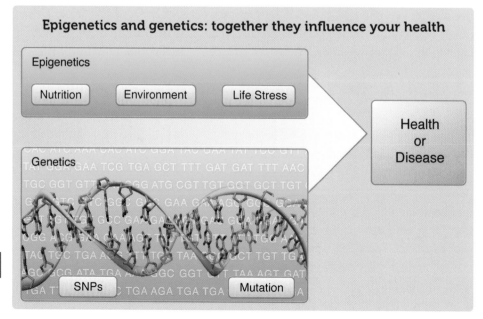

Figure R1.3

Epigenetics and Genetics

Interaction between genes and the environment

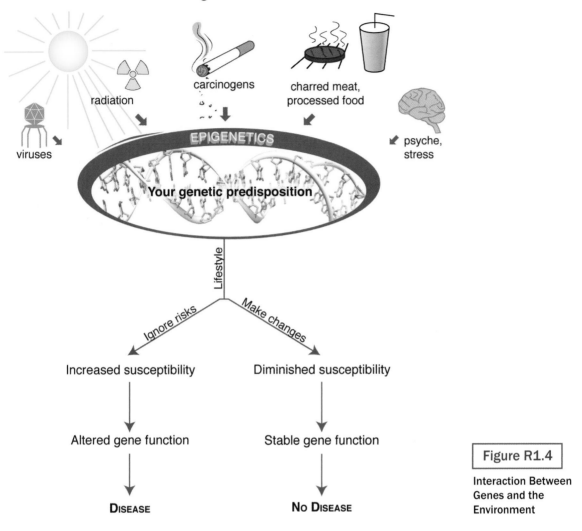

Figure R1.4

Interaction Between Genes and the Environment

SNPs don't necessarily imply something bad. GNB3 (guanine nucleotide-binding protein–3) is a SNP that causes elevated blood pressure and insulin resistance, but also creates greater resistance to hepatitis B and C and better responses to anti-HIV drugs and certain antihypertensive drugs.

Genomics is an evolving field, and new discoveries are being made all the time. Your risk of a genetic health problem isn't as simple as understanding one particular gene or having one particular SNP. For most of us, illness is a result of the interaction of multiple genes with multiple environmental factors. The science of nutrigenomics looks at the interaction of nutrition and genomics—in other words, how we eat and live can interact with our genes and our SNPs, switching them "on" or "off."

Epigenetics: How Diet, Lifestyle, and Environment Affect Our Genes

It's the old argument: nature versus nurture. Your genotype is your individual genetic makeup—your own personal instruction manual, or hardware, for your body. The genes you inherited are with you for your whole

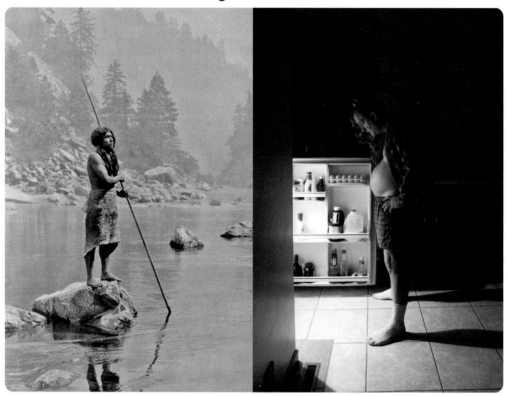

The Pima Indians have a high incidence of insulin resistance. This genetic trait once kept them alive on a hunter-gatherer's diet of protein and berries, but now they subsist primarily on refined foods, resulting in obesity and diabetes.

Figure R1.5	Pima Indians

life, but they don't necessarily determine your health. Your diet, lifestyle, and environment are the software and have a powerful effect on your genes. These factors can flip the genetic switch, either toward health or toward disease. You might have inherited the group of genes that predispose you to lung cancer, for example, but if you don't smoke and avoid the cigarette smoke of others, those genes are unlikely to be switched on. The study of how these factors influence your genes is called epigenetics.

The Pima Indians, who live in the Sonora Desert of southern Arizona, are a classic example of the interaction between genetics and epigenetics. This tribe has the highest rate of type 2 diabetes in the world—over half the adult population has the disease.

Why are the Pima Indians so susceptible to diabetes? For thousands of years, the Pimas lived in an environment that sometimes provided plenty of food and sometimes provided very little. Their genes adapted by allowing them to store body fat very efficiently during the good times in order to prevent starvation during the inevitable lean times. This is sometimes referred to as the "thrifty gene."

The Pima's genetic heritage hasn't changed over thousands of years, but their lifestyle has. For more than a century, the Pima Indians have lived on reservations. Instead of the hunter/gatherer diet of game, fruit, berries, and other foods, they now have a diet much higher in fat, refined carbohydrates, and processed foods.

In addition, they are far less active than their ancestors were. Their genes, which originally kept them alive by resisting starvation, now interact with their diet and lifestyle—their epigenetics—to produce a very high rate of obesity and diabetes.

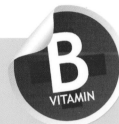

How the Diet of a Mother Affects Her Offspring

Agouti mice have a much higher incidence of obesity, diabetes and cancer than other mice, and are therefore frequently used as subjects in scientific studies. Typically these mice are fat, with a pale yellow coat.

A study compared the health of pregnant agouti mice fed two different diets. One group was fed a diet supplemented with folic acid, vitamin B12, choline, and betaine (vitamin B15), while the control group was fed a standard diet. Guess what happened? Rather than being fat and yellow, the offspring of the mice on the supplemented diet were slender, with brown coats, and had a much lower incidence of obesity, diabetes, and cancer. What's more, this protective effect persisted into the second generation.

So, it seems that a diet high in B vitamins protected the next two generations of mice. However, when the supplemental diet was stopped with the next generation, the protective effect wore off. Isn't it interesting how a simple change in the environmental exposure of the Agouti mice genes had such a profound impact on the health of the next generations?

Epigenetics in Action: The Agouti Mouse

Yellow agouti mice become obese and have a high risk of diabetes, cancer and shortened lifespan.

Brown agouti mice are thin, with a normal lifespan and reduced risk of diabetes and cancer.

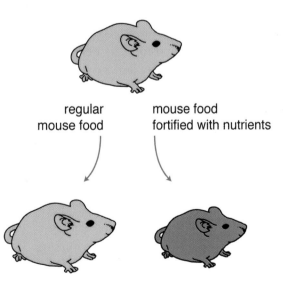

regular mouse food

mouse food fortified with nutrients

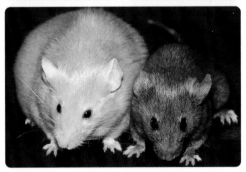

Photograph reproduced with permission from Environmental Health Perspectives: Weinhold B, Environ Health Perspect 114:4 (2006).

Figure R1.6 | Epigenetics in Action

Expanding Your Medical Options

If you have a health issue that has persisted three months or more and has not resolved despite conventional medical treatment, this might be the time to reconsider your approach. If you feel unwell much of the time or have a number of lingering health issues, now is the time to start thinking about taking a different approach. Alternatively, you may feel well, but want to do something simply to improve your health.

An Expanded History: The First Order of Personalized Medicine

You are not simply a "heart attack," a "back pain," or a "cancer." You are you, a unique individual, and you have a unique story your doctor needs to understand. The initial medical diagnosis is, in fact, only part of the story. *If we really want to find out what is going on, we need to get the whole story, or, as we like to say, the story behind the story!*

In order for us to better understand how you got sick, we need to be able to personalize your story:

- We need to know your risk for illness—your genetic predisposition, as well as the environmental, lifestyle, and genetic factors that placed you at risk.
- We want to know what your health was like before you got sick. Illness doesn't happen in a vacuum.
- We want to know what the precipitating factor or triggering cause of the illness is. This is the tipping point to illness. There are multiple factors that can be the "last straw" that cause us to get sick. The tipping points that make us get sick can include infections caused by viruses, bacteria, or even parasites, emotional stress, physical trauma such as a car accident, or major physical stressors such as surgery.

- We want to know what the mediators of the illness are—certain biochemicals, for example, can predispose you to sickness. If we understand this, we can design treatments to antidote the illness.

Why We Need the Whole Story

We can easily go for the quick medical fix. In fact, we should. This is why conventional diagnosis and treatment are so useful. However, if we miss the story behind the story, we lose the chance to harness the transformational opportunity of an illness. Every illness, no matter what it is, gives us a chance to reevaluate what we are doing and bring ourselves into balance in some way. If we simply go for the quick fix, we lose the chance to find and correct underlying problems that leave us vulnerable to recurrence. If we don't, the problems mount up, becoming cumulative in their ability to cause future problems. In functional medicine, these factors are called antecedent factors—they set us up for future illness. We need to know about your stress level, your nutritional, metabolic, and immune risk factors, how your hormones are doing, and whether you have any pain in your body.

Every time we get sick, that is feedback from our bodies. Consider the type of illness that stops us in our tracks—when we get it, we're usually very run down or stressed out. So rather than viewing illness as a bother, consider it a message with valuable information to be used to help us get better.

An Expanded Medical Workup

In a medical workup, lab tests are an invaluable aid to letting us know how you are. Sometimes a simple lab test may tell us all we need to know. If you're feeling fatigued and the lab test shows anemia, we can presume the anemia is associated with the fatigue, and then start investigating the cause of the anemia.

However, there are many times when someone may complain of fatigue yet have normal lab tests. This is where the systems approach we discussed previously can be so helpful. We can use functional lab tests to find out which system is malfunctioning.

Functional Lab Tests: Assessing Your Epigenetic Risk Factors

To discover what system or systems are malfunctioning, we can use conventional lab tests and also order additional tests from laboratories that specialize in functional medicine evaluations. We do this testing because often the magical, clear-cut diagnosis you have been looking for may not exist. Instead, you may have a complex problem involving a malfunction in one or more systems in your body. To heal, it may be necessary to look at all of these systems and consider how to improve the balance within each one. A systems approach can be especially helpful with chronic illness. By improving the functioning and balance of the major systems of the body, many patients find their symptoms just melt away!

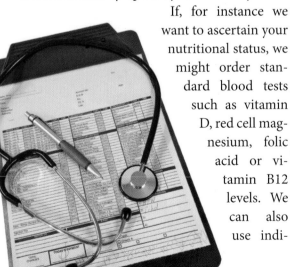

If, for instance we want to ascertain your nutritional status, we might order standard blood tests such as vitamin D, red cell magnesium, folic acid or vitamin B12 levels. We can also use indirect tests such as homocysteine, which can indicate a need for vitamins B6, B12 or folic acid, or methylmalonic acid (MMA) to help us understand if your body needs vitamin B12. We might order specific functional lab tests if we want to know if you are absorbing nutrients and have sufficient amino acid or protein building blocks to help you repair your body. We can also test further to see if you have enough of the good anti-inflammatory fats called omega-3 fatty acids. If we want to check to see if you are inflamed, we might use a conventional test called hs-CRP, or high sensitivity C-reactive protein. Or we could check chemicals called cytokines, such as interleukin-6 (IL-6) or TNF-α (tumor necrosis alpha), which further let us know about your inflammatory status. If we want to know if your body is "rusting," we could test markers that let us know about oxidative status.

Functional lab tests can be used to check stress-related problems, neurotransmitter imbalances, nutritional, metabolic, and immune problems, and subtle hormonal imbalances.

We can even check the length of small hairlike strands called telomeres, which sit atop your chromosomes. These, together with an enzyme called telomerase that governs their length, are related to your life span.

The list of these tests is extensive. As physicians, we need to constantly evaluate and balance the benefit of the information (including false-positive results) we will get from the results with the cost of the tests. This is similarly true if we decide to do further radiological testing, such as CT scans, MRIs, and ultrasounds.

Ultimately, we want to know where you are, what the causative factors are, and why you are in the situation you are in.

We call this a systems approach to lab testing. Using a systems approach, we are *not* trying to make a clinical diagnosis. We are looking for an imbalance in an underlying system, which we can then rectify. When we correct the imbalance, symptoms of illness often simply melt away.

Understanding a Diagnosis:
What It Means to Tease out a Story

> More important than knowing what kind of disease the patient has is knowing what kind of patient has the disease.
>
> – Sir William Osler
> 1849-1919

Sir William Osler

© University of Pennsylvania Archives

Let's start with a closer look at conventional Western medicine, which is highly effective in diagnosing and treating so many illnesses. We all want precision and accuracy, and that is what conventional medicine can usually deliver. Let's follow two stories that illustrate the ways acute illness is commonly approached by conventional medicine.

Sam's Story

Sam awoke with a sore throat. Two hours later, he started shivering as his temperature rose to 102.5 °F. Sam decided to go to work anyway, so he took two Tylenol tablets and headed out the door. At work, he began to feel even worse. By 5:00 p.m., he wasn't sure he even had enough strength to get home. At the urging of his wife, he called his family doctor, who fortunately had evening hours that day. Dr. Smith took a quick history from Sam and examined him, taking notice of his enlarged tonsils, which were coated with a thick, white discharge. A throat swab showed Sam was positive for strep throat. Dr. Smith gave Sam a prescription for penicillin. Less than 24 hours later, Sam was feeling much better, and two days after that, he hardly knew he had been ill.

Nila's Story

Nila was playing soccer when she felt a snap in her knee. It happened just as she planted her foot and began to pivot toward the oncoming ball. Within seconds, she dropped to the ground in agony, hardly able to move. Her knee was swelling rapidly, and she struggled to stop her tears from flowing. Before she knew it, the team trainer had arranged for her to be taken to the local emergency room. An MRI revealed a ruptured ACL (anterior cruciate ligament) and torn cartilage (medial meniscus). The orthopedic surgeon on call, a well-known sports physician, confirmed the diagnosis and scheduled her for surgery, assuring her that after rehab she would be playing soccer again within a few months.

Ah, the miracle of modern medicine! These stories are the ones we love to hear. We go to the doctor, and he fixes us. We feel better and go back to living our lives. But in the real world, these examples don't tell us the whole story.

Antecedent Factors

Let's take a closer look at Sam's situation. When Sam came down with strep throat, he had been under significant stress at work. Not only that, his relationship with his wife was at an all-time low. She had been depressed since the birth of their second child, less than a year after the first baby. Sam and his family had been living on fast food and take-outs. Their children, both infants, were frequently ill due to infections they picked up at day care. Sam was at a breaking point. And that is when he got sick.

Let's also look more closely at Nila. At first glance, it might appear that Nila just suffered from a mechanical injury. Simply put, the forces applied to twist her knee were greater than the strength of her ligament or cartilage. The result was that her tissues snapped under the shear force. However, Nila, too, was at a crossroads in her life. She loved playing soccer, mainly because it kept her weight down. She also forced herself to run five miles every day and worked out at the gym whenever she could. Given her academic schedule, that level of exertion left her vulnerable to a stress injury. Secretly, Nila also suffered from an eating disorder. No one noticed Nila slipping away from soccer parties into a bathroom so she could purge her french fries into the toilet. This had been going on for years.

Stress and the Mind-Body Connection

Both Sam's and Nila's stories illustrate the influence of psychological factors on the development of illness. In Sam's case, stress played a role. And a thorough history would have turned up the fact that Nila was upset that her boyfriend was not at the game. She was jealous about the time he had been spending with a pretty girl he worked with. In fact, that is what Nila was thinking about when she landed incorrectly on her foot and heard the snap. So mind-body factors played a role in her injury. Nila succumbed to thoughts of her boyfriend, and as a result, was not "totally in the moment." The lack of awareness of the position of her feet and knees, together with the weakened state of her knee tissue, were contributing factors to her injury.

Nutritional Deficiencies

We can argue that no matter what Nila had done, the shear force applied to her knee would have snapped the ligament. This is possibly true. But let's consider another way to assess her susceptibility to injury. Nila's frequent purging resulted in a low level of nutrients, particularly two essential amino acids found in protein (glycine and proline) that are necessary to maintain healthy ligaments. Other nutrients that help build muscle and joint strength are the B vitamins and vitamin C, as well as a host of cofactors. Nila's habit of purging seriously depleted these nutrients, leaving her vulnerable to injury.

Immune Function

In Sam's case, it is important to find out more about his poor diet. We also need to know about his stress, his long work hours, and the infections his children were bringing home from day care. These factors all affected his immunity. With a healthy immune system, Sam would probably not have come down with strep. But because his system was so vulnerable, he became sick.

Injury and Imbalances in the Body

The body's muscles are in a dynamic state of push and pull, or tensegrity (we will examine this in detail in Ring 5). In Nila's case, tight hamstrings and weak VMO muscle (the vastus medialis obliquus) on the upper inside of her knee could easily have contributed to her injury.

When Medical Tests Don't Tell the Whole Story

Isaac's Story

Isaac was a 54-year-old nonsmoker when he had his first heart attack. Overweight, with no family history of heart disease, Isaac was a successful representative for a pharmaceutical company. He often joked with the doctors he visited that his cholesterol and blood sugar levels were so good that he could ignore the fact that he was overweight. That's why he believed he could indulge in desserts as much as he liked. Then he would go home and exercise, certain that burning off the calories was a great way to take care of those extra custard donuts. One day, after returning from a run, he sat down to watch television. Fifteen minutes later, he was gasping for breath as he dialed 911, fighting waves of nausea and sweating as he slipped into a state of shock.

Six hours later, Isaac emerged from the cardiac catheterization lab. A coronary angiogram had shown almost complete occlusion of one of his coronary arteries. The cardiologist happily reported to Isaac that he had been able to dissolve the clot using a clot-busting drug, and that there was no residual damage to Isaac's heart muscle. The doctor had discovered a small kink in the artery which he said was just a "genetic variant." The clot had formed around the kink. To prevent future problems, the doctor placed a wire-like stent into the artery to stop it from closing up. Isaac went home from the hospital the next day.

Our patient Isaac is a miracle of modern medicine. He survived a serious heart attack because of prompt emergency treatment. But could Isaac's heart attack have been prevented? And what about his risk of another heart attack in the future?

Isaac thought that because his cholesterol levels and blood pressure were normal, because he had no family history of heart disease, and because he was a nonsmoker and exercised regularly, he was immune to a heart attack. He conveniently forgot that he was overweight, under a lot of stress, and had a poor diet. He also didn't know that he had risk factors that don't show up on routine lab tests. Isaac had two genetic variants that made him more vulnerable to blood clots. These two factors increased his risk—especially if his blood vessels were inflamed and he was under stress.

Isaac, although he didn't realize it, also had severe gum inflammation (gingivitis). The inflammation from his gum disease spilled over into his bloodstream, aggravating the tendency to form blood clots. The day he had his heart attack, the weather was sweltering hot. Isaac was in such a hurry to get out and jog off his calories that he overlooked both his usual prehydration drink and the electrolyte drink he usually took with him when he went running. When Isaac went for his run on a hot day without drinking anything, his predisposing genetic factors—inflammation and a tendency to develop blood clots—combined with dehydration to become the perfect storm for a heart attack. We call this final precipitating factor the tipping point.

The Tipping Point

The different physical stressors that toppled Isaac into an inflammatory cascade—one that resulted in a heart attack—were his tipping point.

Unfortunately, since conventional medicine is so focused on finding a singular cause for illness, doctors sometimes get caught up looking the one single thing, such as a virus or high cholesterol, that might have caused the illness. In reality, most illnesses are caused by a constellation of factors coming together.

Alex: A Wellness Patient Learns about His Health

Alex Young is a 48-year-old marketing executive who came to us not for treatment of an illness but because he wanted to feel better. He had recently completed his yearly physical with his primary care physician. Other than having mild seasonal allergies, his results were essentially normal. Even so, Alex had some persistent concerns. His back and his knees often ached. His lab tests were negative for any autoimmune disease, so his doctor suggested over-the-counter anti-inflammatories if he needed them.

Alex's blood pressure was 138/86, higher than his physician would like. Similarly, his cholesterol and triglyceride levels were a little elevated, and his fasting glucose level was just slightly above normal. To keep these slightly elevated numbers from getting worse, Alex's doctor told him to exercise and to cut the sugar, salt, and fat in his diet and repeat the tests in three months. Alex wondered how to do this. He already exercised three days a week at the gym, and when he wasn't out on business lunches or dinners, he felt he was pretty conscious of his diet. He was consistently trying to lose the extra fifteen pounds he had put on over the years.

Alex often felt bloated. Sometimes he would belch after a big meal, not to mention the flatulence he suffered when he went home. When the antacids his doctor suggested didn't help, the doctor thought this indicated mild irritable bowel syndrome.

Alex's parents were both in their seventies and essentially healthy. His father had both high cholesterol and high blood pressure, which were under control with medication. He also suffered from an enlarged prostate. His mother also had a small breast cancer removed when she was in her late sixties, but she was doing well, with no recurrence.

Despite his apparent career success, Alex was struggling with his life. Although he had worked for his boss for more than twenty years, he often felt like an intern. His boss treated his employees—Alex included—in ways that often left Alex fuming. And although he didn't admit it openly, his libido was waning, and there were times when he questioned if he still wanted to stay married.

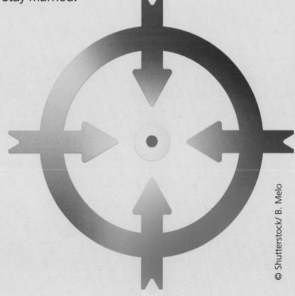

© Shutterstock/ B. Melo

Genetic Predispositions When Alex came to us with his list of minor but potentially serious health problems, we ran SNP tests to look at his genetic predispositions.

Alex had a number of SNPs that could lead to serious problems. He showed potential risks for hypertension (AGT, AGTR, and GNB). He had a definite predisposition to develop cholesterol-related problems (Apo E3/4) and problems metabolizing folic acid (MTHFR). He had a predisposition to form inflammatory chemicals called cytokines, especially when physically or emo-tionally stressed (IL-6). In addition, his SNPs for CYP1B1, CYP1A1, COMT, and GST all indicated potential problems with detoxification of estrogen, putting him at risk for prostate cancer. (His mother probably had similar genes, resulting in her breast cancer.)

Alex's routine physical examination was normal, but his genetic testing showed that he was heading toward illness—and his lifestyle wasn't helping. As you read through each Ring and Star, you will find out what Alex did to get well and stay well.

1

STAR ONE

How to Expand Your Medical Treatment Options

Taking Responsibility for Your Health:
Essential Lifestyle, Behavioral, and Exercise Techniques to Enhance Your Well-Being.

Expand Your Medical Treatment Options

We believe in patient education and empowerment. We want to help our patients make better decisions about their own health care. Our goal is to give patients a new way of looking at health and to provide them with expanded options for their care.

Transformational Medicine strives not only to cure illness and disease where possible, but also to achieve wholeness and health. We want you to do this in the safest, easiest, and most cost-effective manner.

Begin with a Conventional Medicine Approach

Just as we believe that a conventional assessment is the first place to start, we also think that conventional medicine is the most appropriate first line of action. We encourage patients to see their primary care or specialist physician when they have a clear-cut issue that needs a specific test or treatment. Conventional medicine is good if you have an acute illness, need surgery, or have an illness that is curable.

Good medical training allows practitioners to create what is called a differential diagnosis. For example, shoulder pain may originate in the shoulder, but it may also come from a herniated disc in the neck, from the heart (angina), or even from a gallbladder problem, and it is important to know if a pelvic mass is a fibroid

rather than ovarian cancer. Similarly, an experienced doctor can also look at a patient's lab work and differentiate between what is meaningful and what is not.

Expanding Medical Options

You may need to expand your medical options if:

- You feel you are being placed on more and more medications without seeing any improvement in your health.

- You are in chronic pain but surgery is not an option and medications aren't helping.

- You are feeling run down with no real medical explanation—you might be getting sick frequently without finding a good reason.

- You notice symptoms that your doctor can't explain. These symptoms include fatigue, muscle pain, joint pain, headaches, indigestion, bloating, difficulty thinking clearly, and weight gain.

- You have abnormal lab markers that don't fit any disease pattern.

- You are frustrated with conventional medicine's ability to deal with your illness.

- You want to improve your health by taking a personalized, proactive, and preventive approach.

Live well. Eat well. G
well. Walk well. Run
well. Love well. Live
well. Stretch well.
Dance well. Get well.

Taking the Next Step

By adding integrative medicine to your medical options, you can often find a way to develop a systems approach to healing. Doing so allows you to move outside the box of conventional medicine and draw on the knowledge of several disciplines to provide you with a range of solutions.

Using Integrative Medicine Therapies Wisely

The Institute of Medicine (IOM) is part of the National Academies, which includes the National Academy of Sciences (NAS) and the National Research Council (NRC). It serves as a nonprofit advisory organization to the government on matters relating to the nation's health. The recommendations of the NAS are considered authoritative. For example, the IOM sets the recommended daily allowances for vitamins, minerals, and other nutrients. In 2009, the IOM, together with the Bravewell Collaborative (a group of leading philanthropists working to improve health through the advancement of integrative medicine), hosted a summit conference called "Integrative Medicine and the Health of the Public." The report of the conference explains how integrative medicine can easily be incorporated by all medical specialties, professional disciplines, and health care systems. The report goes on to say how the adoption of the practices and principles of integrative medicine will transform health care, improve the health care system, reduce costs, and produce a healthier nation. The chart on page 42 is adapted from this report.

The first wealth is health.

– Ralph Waldo Emerson

Synergy Creates Transformation

Integrating therapies can result in a quantum leap in healing. By making a number of small but strategic changes, we can achieve a major effect. In treatment, we don't use only one approach; instead, we help our patients take a series of steps toward healing, sometimes very small steps in multiple areas. The results are synergistic. We approach treatment from the perspective of systems biology, a holistic view in which the "whole is greater than the sum of the individual parts." In this model, $1 + 1 + 1$ doesn't equal 3, it equals 6! The effect is more than you would expect.

The result of synergistic change is a quantum leap in your state of health. This is what we call transformation!

Now is a good time to start improving your health, whether you consider yourself healthy or are suffering from pain or illness. As we've said before, getting sick is a process, and getting better is a process, too. Remember, we don't just want the problem to go away; we want you to be able to use the problem to make your health and your life better.

Transformational medicine should lead to optimization of physical health, psychological transformation, and spiritual growth.

Current Medical Practice	Evolving to Integrative Practice
Health is most often considered to be the absence of disease.	Health is seen as a vital state of physical, mental, emotional, social, and spiritual wellbeing, which enables a person to be engaged in life.
The physician tends to act as the authority figure.	The physician acts as a partner in the patient's care.
The patient is encouraged to follow the physician's directions.	The empowered and informed patient is an integral part of the decision-making process.
The interventions are often directed only toward the treatment of a specific disease or trauma.	The interventions are designed to treat the illness as well as the whole person, addressing the physical, mental, emotional, social, and spiritual factors that influence health and disease.
A patient's stress level is not always taken into consideration or treated.	Patients are taught how to recognize, manage, and decrease stress.
A patient's dietary habits are largely ignored.	Patients are given nutritional counseling; food is understood to have a significant influence on health and disease.
Social determinants of health such as unemployment, abuse, neglect, and financial status are not always given full consideration.	Social determinants of health such as unemployment, abuse, neglect, and financial status are considered in the care.
Environmental influences are rarely addressed.	Environmental influences on health and healing are investigated, considered, and addressed in the care process.
Care is not always coordinated across providers.	Care is coordinated across providers.
Health plans are rarely created.	Each patient is given an individualized health plan based on his or her unique needs and circumstances.
Many decisions are based on the needs of the health care system.	Decisions are based on the needs of the patient.
Prevention and health promotion are not always practiced.	Prevention and health promotion are emphasized.
Only conventional interventions are considered.	The care makes use of all appropriate therapeutic approaches.

To Change Your Life,
Change Your L[...]

The best six doctors anywhere
And no one can deny it
Are sunshine, water, rest, and air
Exercise and diet.
These six will gladly you attend
If only you are willing
your mind they'll ease
your will they'll mend
And charge you not a shilling.

—**Nursery rhyme quoted by Wayne Fields,**
What the River Knows

While drug companies tout the magical benefit of the silver-bullet drugs to lower our blood pressure and cholesterol, we forget that simple changes in lifestyle may have much more far-reaching and profound effects on our health. In 2000, the World Health Organization published a ranking on the health of the world's nation. The United States ranked highest in expenditure per capita, but only thirty-sev[...] ing. Countries such as the [...] spend far less on health car[...] [...] the United States does, yet they rank higher on national healthcare scores. Is it their midday siesta, olive oil, community support, sunshine, or the need to walk rather than drive? What are the factors that make people healthy?

Our 24/7 lifestyle has brought us great benefits, but also potential for harm. Unless we become aware of what it is doing to us, we don't stand a chance. We may want to return to the good old days, yet there is one inescapable fact: We can't go back—we need to move forward.

We know that lifestyle is important; we experience it in our own lives. When we eat well, exercise, get enough sleep, and keep our stress level down, we feel better. But when things start to slip, sooner or later we're in trouble and our health suffers.

Clearly lifestyle is not the entire answer to illness. Yet without a healthy lifestyle, our ability to correct major health issues is severely limited. Coronary heart disease serves as an important example. State-of-the-art Western medicine is

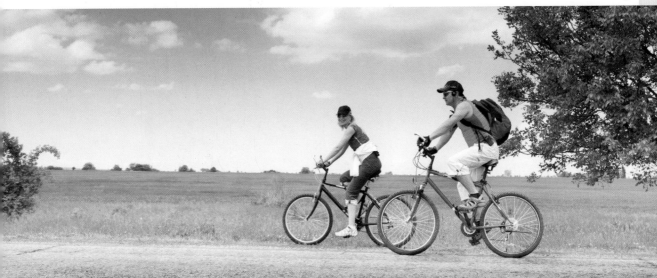

...y patient who has suffered a heart ...er such an event, doctors will refer ...patients for a dietary consultation and a ...rapeutic cardiac rehab exercise program. But why wait until you have a heart attack?

We want you to modify your lifestyle to enhance your health right now! Before you start justifying why you can't change, here are some practical suggestions:

Cultivate a Daily Healthy Lifestyle Routine

Most people resist change. The easiest way to steer your body toward a healthy lifestyle is to understand its basic components. Be open to inviting small changes into your life. Try new techniques, and keep those that resonate with you and improve your vitality. Create a schedule that allows you to achieve results with minimum stress or effort. In this way, you can restore a sense of rhythm into what can even seem like a chaotic lifestyle. It can help you remain centered and relaxed.

We recommend starting a daily healthy lifestyle program that includes both modern forms of exercise and ancient techniques, proven over centuries to have powerful effects on wellness. If you continue your practice on a daily basis, over the long term you will see major benefits.

The basic components we would like to suggest you include into your lifestyle include:

- Regular exercise
- Deep relaxation, including deep breathing, meditation, and restorative sleep
- A nutrient-rich diet (we will discuss this in more detail in Star 3 on page 121)

What else helps? Studies have shown that your health benefits from:

- Supportive relationships with family, friends, and community
- A meaningful purpose in your life and a sense of spiritual connection
- Avoiding environmental toxins where possible

From Intention to Action

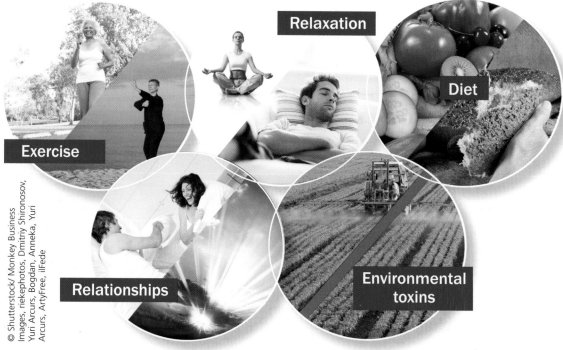

Relaxation

Diet

Exercise

Relationships

Environmental toxins

Forming your intention provides the first glimmer of change. Next, develop a strategy, a plan for success. Finally, you will want to tap into your self-discipline to put the strategy into practice. If you make the practice enjoyable, however, you will need less discipline. Make a decision right now to prioritize your health. Then choose a lifestyle that will reinforce this decision.

Go with the Flow, Stay in the Moment

The speed at which we go through life can create a resistance against which we must move. Sometimes minimal, and at other times huge, this friction is like an invisible brake, tugging at us, telling us to slow down. We need to learn to perceive both external cues from the environment, as well as internal cues from our minds and bodies. In many ways, life is like surfing. We need to enjoy the power of the wave when it is behind us, but relax if we hit a breaking swell.

If you fail to live each moment with appreciation, you may be missing the most profound source of both stress reduction and well-being. Most of us are so busy focusing on either the future or the past that we forget to simply be in the present. *We need to become a human being, not a human doing.*

Break the Couch Potato Habit

Regular exercise has been shown to prevent or treat anxiety and depression, hypertension, diabetes, heart disease, cancer, and osteoporosis. We all know we should exercise, yet many of us do not. In fact, those who do exercise tend to keep exercising, while those who are couch potatoes tend to remain so. These are habits we learn in childhood—and television, computers, and video games haven't helped. Our lifestyle doesn't help, either. We are too busy looking for the closest parking spot or other ways to avoid exerting ourselves.

People often ask us which type of exercise they should do. They want to know about jogging, cycling, gyms, personal trainers, yoga, tai chi, Pilates, mountain climbing, hiking, etc. What is best for you? The best exercise for you is exercise that you enjoy, whatever that might be. If you're having fun, if you're "playing," it's easier to continue doing it.

Exercise daily if possible and three to four days a week at a minimum. The Centers for Disease Control recommends at least 150 minutes of moderate-intensity exercise per week, as well as muscle-strengthening exercises on two or more days per week for adults aged 18 to 64. Exercise doesn't have to be done all at one time. Three walks of ten minutes each count as thirty minutes of exercise. Exercise doesn't have to be regimented or structured. Playing with a pet or child, taking a walk, or working in the garden may be as much fun and as much exercise as any class you can take. Walking from your parking space to the store counts as exercise. So does climbing stairs! Allow exercise to bring you into the present moment. Reading a book while walking on a treadmill only serves to further disconnect your mind from your body.

Exercise Slows Aging

Exercise is yet another way to affect epigenetics and help turn off aging. In a study published in the *Proceedings of the National Academy of Sciences,* researchers looked at mice that had been genetically programmed to age rapidly. Half the mice ran on a treadmill for forty-five minutes three times per week, while the control group did not. The exercising mice showed significant changes. They had full pelts of fur and retained brain volume, muscle mass and strength, normal testicle or ovary size, and normal heart function. The mice that did not exercise aged quickly, as they were genetically programmed to do, and died.

Does exercise work in humans to prolong

good health? It seems so, especially when humans combine different types of exercise.

Exercise Types

We generally divide exercise into four subtypes: aerobic, strength-training, balancing, and stretching. You need all four.

Aerobic exercise. Two of the benefits of this form of exercise are increased oxygen intake and increased heart rate. Benefits of aerobic exercise include improved fat metabolism, increased energy, better body composition, relief from stress and anxiety, reduced blood pressure, increased HDL (good cholesterol), enhanced mental performance and quality of sleep, and improved immune function.

Examples of aerobic exercise include brisk walking or long walks, jogging, cycling, Spinning™, Kranking™, swimming, exercising on an elliptical trainer, dance or dance fitness classes such as Zumba, and martial arts, such as karate and tai kwon do, among others.

Remember that while exercise has tremendous benefits, overexercising can cause problems too.

Aerobic or Anaerobic: Burning Fat or Building Muscle?

Typically, our bodies burn fat when we are exercising aerobically—doing exercise of relatively low intensity and long duration, such as walking briskly. During aerobic exercise, the body uses oxygen to generate energy, and burns fat. When we exercise anaerobically by doing high-intensity, short-duration activities, such as weight-training or sprinting, we starve our muscles of oxygen. This forces our muscles into a stressed state where they adapt by breaking down, then rebuilding as stronger muscles. It also builds up lactic acid, which can make muscles ache. You can figure out where you are on the aerobic/anaerobic exercise level by calculating your maximum heart rate, or MAX HR. Ideally, this is done by an exercise physiologist using sophisticated technology. If you have heart problems, this should be done by a cardiologist.

Estimating Your MAX HR

A common formula used to estimate your MAX HR is (220 — age) for males or (226 — age) for females. Although this is not precise, it is a good guideline to get you started. Aerobic exercise is when you exercise between 65 and 85 percent of your MAX HR. When your heart rate is over 85 percent of your MAX HR, you are exercising anaerobically.

An example: Estimating MAX HR for a 50-year-old male

1. **MAX HR** = 220 - 50 = 170 beats per minute.
2. **Aerobic exercise** = 65-85% of 220 = 110-145 beats per minute.
3. **Anaerobic exercise** = greater than 145 beats per minute.

Heart rate recovery

Once your exercise session is over, track your heart rate recovery time, or how quickly your heartbeat returns to your normal resting rate. Check your heart rate just after you stop exercising, and then check it again two minutes later. Subtract your resting heart rate from your exercise rate. Ideally, you want the difference between the two numbers to be between 25 and 50. The faster your heart rate slows down after exercise, the fitter you are. For example, you are fairly fit if your heart rate just after jogging half an hour is 140, and it has slowed to 115 two minutes later. Ideally, it will be under 100. If your heart rate drops less than 12 beats within two minutes, you need to see a cardiologist soon.

Strength training. Weightlifting exercises, strengthening yoga, or Pilates and Pilates-type exercises force your muscles to work and thus grow in strength and size. The benefit here is that muscle strength also increases the strength of your tendons, ligaments, and bones. This gives you an increase in power and muscular endurance. It also prevents osteoporosis (thinning bones) and improves your tone and body shape.

Balancing. Balancing exercises help the two sides of your brain communicate, simultaneously helping to synchronize the nervous system with the musculoskeletal system. Balancing exercises help you get a better sense of your joint position and help you avoid falls. Balance exercises, such as standing on one foot or walking heel to toe, can easily be part of your ex-ercise program. You can also try tai chi. Studies on elderly subjects who do tai chi show that they are less prone to falls than their peers. Yoga also improves balancing ability.

Stretching. Stretching is one of the gems of exercise. Stretching helps open up communication between muscle groups. Examples of beneficial approaches to stretching include basic stretching exercises, yoga, Pilates, and dance. Yoga effectively combines stretching with strengthening, breathing, and relaxation techniques, making it understandable why it is both therapeutic and popular. On the other hand, some people don't like yoga. Whether you are a fan or not, you should understand how basic stretches can improve your health. We have included a list of these in our Daily Regeneration Program at the end of this section.

Breathe Some Life into Your Day

We all know how to breathe—or so we think. When we're anxious, we tend to breathe more rapidly and use just the top part of the lungs. When we belly breathe, we do just the opposite, slowing our bodies down, returning them to the present.

Relaxation Breathing

Here is a simple way to use your breath to relax:
Sit comfortably in a chair—your spine erect, your eyes closed.

Pay attention to your breath. Do not try to change it. For one to two minutes, simply monitor how you are breathing. Is your breathing deep or shallow? Are you using your diaphragm (breathing from your abdomen) or just your upper chest? Simultaneously, pay attention to your thoughts without trying to change them.

After about two minutes of observing yourself, start belly breathing by using your diaphragm to breathe. To do this, push your tummy out as you breathe in. Then, as you breathe out, allow it to relax. Do this for about two minutes.

Close your eyes. Now, add your upper chest to your breathing technique. As you fill your

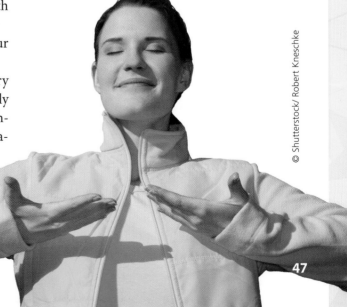

lungs, first push your tummy out; then, as you bring more air into your lungs, expand your chest.

As you breathe out, first let the air out of your upper chest. Finally, allow your tummy to draw in as you empty your belly breath.

Now, using this belly breath, count as you breathe in, hold, then breathe out. Start with four seconds in, four seconds hold, and four seconds out. As you breathe out, relax your body.

As you feel comfortable with this, increase to six seconds of each. And as you progress, build up to eight seconds of each.

The aim is not to get to eight seconds. The aim is to focus on your breath, relax, and return to the present. Progress slowly and comfortably.

After five minutes of doing your breathing technique, gently open your eyes.

Sit for a minute or two before returning to your day.

The Relaxation Response

Yogis and ascetics have claimed for thousands of years that the mind has an effect on the body. A meditative state appears to induce a condition of deep rest accompanied by a sense of restful alertness. In 2002, the *Harvard Gazette* published an article describing new research on how the mind can control the body under extreme conditions. Dr. Herbert Benson, an associate professor of medicine at the Harvard Medical School, had traveled to northern India to study the physiological effects of meditation and documented his findings.

In the study, Tibetan monks entered a state of deep meditation in a chilly room. As part of a demonstration, other monks placed sheets soaked in cold water (49 degrees F) over the meditators' shoulders. Instead of producing an extreme state of hypothermia, as would normally be expected under these circumstances, the opposite occurred. Steam began rising from the sheets, drying them in about an hour. This process was then repeated. Each monk was required to dry three sheets over a period of several hours. The experiment showed that the monks were able to profoundly influence their physiology through a state of deep meditation—they were able to lower their blood pressure and heart rate.

During subsequent visits to remote monasteries in the 1980s, Benson and his team studied monks living in the Himalaya Mountains who could raise the temperatures of their fingers and toes by as much as 17 degrees F. They also found monks who, by meditative techniques, could lower their metabolism 64 percent.

Dr. Benson also began studying the effects of transcendental meditation (TM), based on the internal repetition of a sound (mantra) during meditation. Studies on TM and other types of meditation have shown that this practice can induce a general state of deep rest. TM can have multiple benefits, usually due to normalization of hormonal, immune, psychological, and neurological systems. Blood pressure often normalizes, as well.

Based on his research, Benson developed a simple method for learning to achieve a state of deep relaxation. He first described how to do it in 1975 in his bestselling book, *The Relaxation Response.* You can read the book; or use the easy-to-follow instructions on page 49, which come from the Benson-Henry Institute for Mind-Body Medicine at Massachusetts General Hospital. Remember that deep relaxation takes some practice. Keep at it every day, and you'll probably feel you've made progress within a week; within a few weeks you'll probably be able to achieve deep relaxation quickly. This is an active approach, far more restorative than taking time to read a book or watch television. We need to allow the body to achieve a state of rest that is deeper than deep sleep, coupled with a sense of mental alertness.

The Relaxation Response appears to work at the level of our genes, counteracting cell damage due to chronic psychological stress, turning on protective responses while turning off cancer genes or oncogenes. This genetic regulatory effect was shown in a study by one of our Bravewell colleagues, Jeff Dusek, Ph.D., to occur within as little as eight weeks after initiating the Relaxation Response. The advantage was even more profound in those who were long-term meditators.

Mindfulness

No matter how bad things may be, we can choose to enjoy this very moment. The practice of becoming aware of the present moment is called mindfulness. Colors, textures, sounds, touch, and senses bring us back into the now. If we can sense, rather than think, we are forced into the present. Watch a dog, and see how it adapts to the moment. When dogs are sick, they lie in a cool place until they get better. When they are better, they get up and play. Time is not important to them. *Now* is important.

Yet how do we enjoy the now if strategy and planning are imperative to our success? Herein lies the essential paradox of stress management! The difference between us and dogs is that we can plan and strategize, yet if we spend our life doing it, we lose an essential component of happiness—the art of being in the present.

The Mindfulness-Based Stress Reduction (MBSR) program has been developed by Jon Kabat-Zinn, a well-known researcher and stress-reduction instructor at the University of Massachusetts Medical Center. His program is now taught in centers around the world as a tool to counteract stress. MBSR teaches its participants to be mindfully present. The immediate goal is not to reduce stress, but simply to increase awareness. The enhanced sense of relaxation that results is a by-product of the practice, rather than a goal. By becoming more mindful, you also learn to identify judgmental thoughts and release them. So whenever a negative thought arises, such as "I am a failure," you simply observe the thought and then return to the mindfulness practice and a state of deep relaxation. This distinction is important. Most of us have a habit of critical self-talk, which frequently echoes critical messages from childhood, buried deep in the unconscious. By becoming aware of these internalized judgments, we can gradually become desensitized to this type of thought, which may have been keeping us from living in the present. A good introduction to mindfulness is Jon Kabat-Zinn's book, *Wherever You Go, There You Are,* or *The Power of Now,* by Eckhart Tolle.

MBSR has been extensively studied. It appears to have a profound benefit on pain, mood

It is health that is real wealth and not pieces of gold and silver.

– Gandhi

disorders, and many other disease processes. An interesting study was done on the effect of MBSR on patients with psoriasis who were undergoing PUVA (psoralens plus ultra-violet light therapy). Patients who listened to guided meditation while receiving their ultraviolet light treatment healed at approximately four times the rate as the control group, who received just the light treatment. An eight-week course on MBSR has also been shown to change the structure of parts of the human brain that deal with memory, sense of self, empathy, and stress.

In summary, meditation and mind-body techniques can help you improve your physical health and become ever more present in your body and in your own life—and can help improve your psychological health.

Why Good Sleep Is Important

Do you ever wonder where you go when you sleep, or why we even need to sleep? Sleep is not only essential for physical rejuvenation; it also provides an opportunity for the memory to integrate information, as if file clerks were coming in on the night shift to file away the experiences of the day.

Sleep also appears to offer the body an opportunity for internal housekeeping. Research from the National Institutes of Health has found that immune chemicals rise as we drift off to sleep, recruiting immune cells to cruise the body and lowering bacteria levels throughout the system. Clearly, if we don't get enough sleep, we are much more prone to illness and accidents. In addition, lack of sleep raises the stress hormone cortisol, which can lead to weight gain and type 2 diabetes.

When you sleep, you move back and forth through various stages several times. As you fall asleep, you go into a light sleep, known as Stage

1 sleep, where you drift in and out of sleep. You then go through Stages 2 and 3, finally reaching Stage 4. Stages 3 and 4 are referred to as deep sleep, because this is where your body hardly moves. During deep sleep, you ordinarily generate the neurotransmitter serotonin. If you don't get enough deep sleep, you are thus more prone to depression, fibromyalgia, irritable bowel syndrome, premenstrual syndrome, migraines, and a host of other problems.

The next stage of sleep is a very important one called rapid eye movement (REM) sleep, where you dream. During this phase, your breathing speeds up, becoming irregular and shallow. Your eyelids jerk rapidly (hence the name "rapid eye movement"), and your limb muscles are temporarily paralyzed. Brain waves during this stage increase to levels experienced when you are awake. The heart rate increases, blood pressure rises, males de-

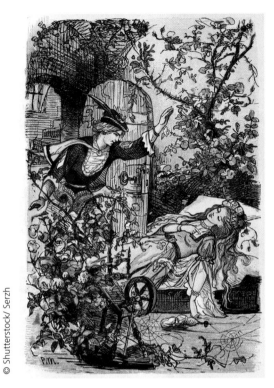

© Shutterstock/ Serzh

velop erections, and the body loses some ability to regulate its temperature.

REM sleep and dreaming appear to help us sort out our daily stressors. This is the time when the mind appears to process emotions, sort through memories, and help us cope with stress. A person deprived of REM sleep can suffer from mood and memory problems.

Over-the-counter sleep aids that contain diphenhydramine (Benadryl®) induce Stage 2 and 3, but not Stage 4 sleep, reducing your ability to regenerate serotonin. Utilizing these aids on a regular basis can therefore result in depression. There are other options for improving sleep. Herbs such as valerian root and supplements such as taurine, 4-amino-3-phenylbutyric acid and 5-Hydroxytryptophan are often extremely helpful. Drugs such as zolpidem (Ambien®) and trazodone maintain what is called normal sleep architecture, allowing a person to pass through all the different stages of sleep. However, these drugs are associated with side effects such as memory loss and dependency. Long-term use should be discussed with your physician.

A Healthy Sleep Cycle

Disrupted sleep or not enough sleep can result in feelings of fatigue and irritability, and can cause daytime sleepiness. It also raises stress hormone levels, which can cause a long list of health problems. Cultivating a healthy sleep cycle is crucial to overall health.

These are suggestions we make to our patients who have trouble getting restful sleep.

- Sleep only when sleepy. If you can't fall asleep within twenty minutes, get up and do something boring until you feel sleepy.

- Aim for a steady and regular bedtime.

- Avoid caffeine, alcohol, and heavy or spicy meals for four to six hours before bedtime.

- Exercise earlier in the day if you can. Avoid exercising after dinner.

- Create a nightly sleep ritual. A warm bath about ninety minutes before bedtime or a cup of herbal tea may serve as reminder to your body to calm down. Don't study hard, watch suspenseful television shows, or otherwise stimulate your mind, and then expect it to turn off suddenly. Read a relaxing book. Listen to music. Practice a relaxation technique.

- Use your bed for sleep and sex only. Avoid watching television in bed.

- Create a comfortable sleep environment, including a dark, quiet room, comfortable bedding, and a suitable temperature.

- Establish a day/night rhythm. Aim to get up and go to sleep at the same time each day.

- Get some sunlight exposure for at least fifteen minutes when you wake up.

- If you need to nap in the day, sleep less than one hour.

Alex learns to take charge of his life and his health

Alex decided he needed to take a more proactive and preventive approach to his health. He began to realize that his 48-year-old body was probably not going to behave like those "twenty pounds gone in one month" types of bodies he had seen on television. Anyway, he didn't like the high-intensity exercises he was doing. We switched Alex to a more sensible and effective exercise program. Each morning, he would wake up and do his gentle stretching routine, paying particular attention to his hamstring and ITB stretches. After this, he would do his breathing exercise for five minutes, then a relaxation response meditation for about twenty minutes. He found himself feeling centered and ready to cope with the day.

After a few weeks of following this routine, Alex decided he wanted to spend forty-five minutes to an hour doing aerobic exercise three to four times per week. He pulled his old bike out of the garage and discovered that he really enjoyed getting the childhood feeling of fun back as the wind whistled past him. His knees stopped hurting. Exercise wasn't a chore. His wife picked up on his enthusiasm and decided to join him. Before long, Alex had lost eight pounds—and he wasn't even trying!

Alex felt his health regenerating. Taking control of his health had given him a different outlook. Previously, he dreaded the idea of going for a medical checkup each year, only to find something else had gone downhill or wrong. Now, he was almost enthusiastic to check his blood pressure and lab results. He was pretty sure they would be changing.

Environmental Choices for Better Health

Unfortunately, our environment is filled with a soup of chemicals that may cause cancer and chronic illness. While we do not want to make you paranoid about this, we do want to educate you so that you become aware of potential hazards. Culprits include common cleaning agents and solvents used in paint thinners, paint, and grease removers, and in the dry cleaning industry. They have complicated names such as benzene, carbon tetrachloride, chloroform, dichloromethane (methylene chloride), tetrachloroethylene, and trichloroethylene.

Diesel exhaust particles, fibers such as asbestos or ceramic fibers, and fine particles and dust such as wood or silica dust that occur in industrial settings are associated with increased cancer risks. Unfortunately, just living in a city is a health risk for most of us.

There are things you can do to reduce your risk. Here are a few we suggest to our patients:

- If you smoke, try to quit. Where possible, avoid exposure to cigarette smoke (passive smoking).

- Limit your exposure to ultraviolet radiation. We believe that some sun is good for you, but that depends on your skin type. Fair-skinned people should have less sun exposure. Minimize your time in peak sunshine, usually between 10:00 a.m. and 4:00 p.m.

- Limit your exposure to ionizing radiation. Medical procedures such as CT scans and x-rays expose you to ionizing radiation. While these procedures are usually necessary and may be life-saving, excessive exposure can increase your risk of cancer. In some cases, an alternative testing option such as ultrasound may be possible. In other cases, repeat x-rays may not be necessary.

- Check radon levels in your house. Radon, found in the soil, is a naturally occurring radioactive gas. High levels are associated with lung cancer.

- Avoid deodorants and antiperspirants containing aluminum, which is potentially toxic.

- Cosmetics, nail polish, gels, hair dyes, and hair sprays can all contain hazardous chemicals that can be absorbed through the skin. Try to use products manufactured by environmentally responsible companies—check the website of the Environmental Working Group (www.ewg.org) for an up-to-date list.

- Avoid overusing antibacterial hand gels. While these products do kill bacteria, they can cause an emergence of super-bugs, or bacteria that are resistant to antibiotics. Simple soap and water works just as well most of the time.

- Limit dry cleaning where possible. Air out your dry-cleaned garments.

- Limit your exposure to electromagnetic field radiation. This includes living next to power plants, but we also suggest limiting the use of cell phones where possible. There is concern that cell phones may deliver too much radiation to the head. To prevent this, consider a speakerphone, an air tube headset, or even texting!

- Limit your exposure to pesticides and other chemicals in your food. We discuss this in more detail in Star 3 and Star 4.

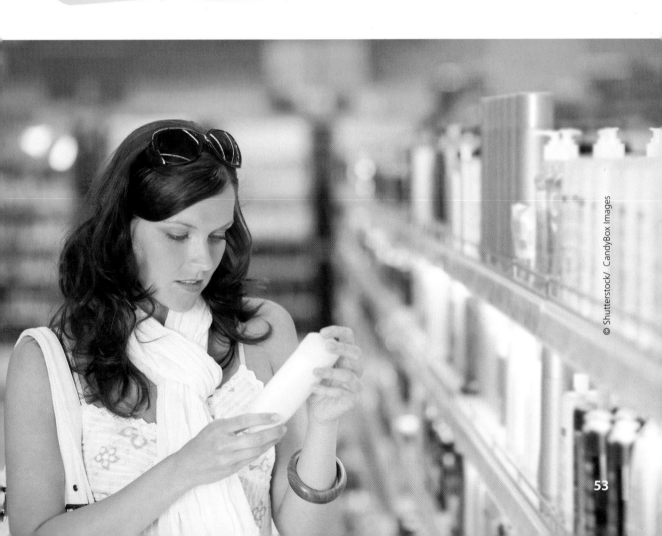

© Shutterstock/ CandyBox Images

A Simple Daily Regeneration Program

We recommend a simple daily regeneration program for our patients. It is easy to fit into your day, and we have seen its very powerful results. There are three basic parts:

1. A simple stretching routine, described below.

2. Vitality-enhancing breathing exercises, as described above on page 47.

3. A rejuvenating meditative technique, as described above on page 49.

Daily Stretches

Try these daily stretches and gentle exercises when you wake up.

Calf stretches

Hang off a step for two minutes. This helps alleviate and prevent foot pain, plantar fasciitis, and Achilles tendonitis.

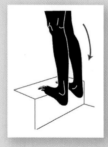

Hamstring stretches

Sitting on a bed, place one leg outstretched on the bed in front of you, and one foot on the floor. Bend forward and place one hand on either side of your knee. Be sure to bend from the hip and to feel the stretch in your hamstring (the muscles in the back of your thigh). If this causes pain to radiate down your leg, see your doctor—you may have a bulging disc in your lower back. Do not bounce. As you stretch, you will usually feel a slight "give" in your hamstring, allowing you to drop down a little farther. This usually happens once or twice in a two- to three-minute stretch. This helps alleviate and prevent back and neck problems.

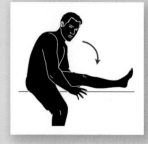

Tensor fascia lata/ Iliotibial Band (ITB) stretches

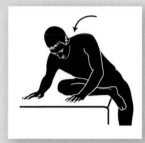

Sit on a bed. Fold your knee underneath you as seen on the diagram. Place one hand on either side of your knee and lean forward. You should feel a stretch in your buttock region and down the side of your leg. By moving left or right, you can intensify the stretch. Hold it where you feel the maximum stretch, and stay there for one to two minutes.

This helps alleviate and prevent pain on the outside of the hip (trochanteric bursitis), as well as pain on the outside of the knee (Iliotibial band syndrome).

Shoulder stretching

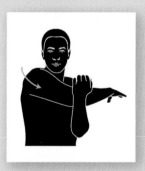

Bring one arm across your chest. Place the opposite wrist above your elbow and stretch the arm. You should feel the stretch at the back of your shoulder. Hold for ten to twenty seconds, then switch arms.

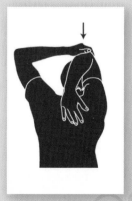

Lift both hands up above you. Drop one hand behind your neck. Grab your elbow with the opposite hand and push downward, feeling the stretch in your shoulder. Hold for ten to twenty seconds. Straighten both arms upward, and then repeat on opposite side.

These exercises help prevent rotator cuff syndrome, or shoulder tendonitis.

Neck exercises

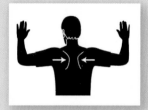

The *"Don't Shoot Me"* exercise helps prevent and treat neck problems. While sitting or standing, place your arms in the position shown in the diagram. Now, imagine there is a pencil placed vertically between your shoulder blades. Gentle squeeze your shoulder blades backward, as if you were trying to squeeze this pencil. Your upper shoulder (or trapezius) muscles should remain soft while you do this. Now bring your chin backward, as if you are making a double chin. Squeeze and hold for ten to twenty seconds. Repeat up to five to ten times. You will find this helps relieve neck pain, especially for those of us who are constantly in a neck-forward position, such as when typing, driving, or reading. During the day, if you get neck pain, simply squeeze your shoulder blades together and you will find that this can relieve your pain.

This helps alleviate and prevent neck arthritis and disc pain.

The "sniffing the armpit" exercise

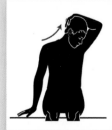

Turn your head to the right and place your right hand over your head, gently grabbing the back of your skull. Gently pull your nose toward your armpit. Stretch your opposite (left) hand toward the floor. Feel the stretch in the muscles at the back and side of the neck. Hold for twenty to thirty seconds. (If you feel pain radiating down your arm, stop and see your doctor: you may have a disc problem in your neck.) Now, turn your head to the left and repeat the exercise on the opposite side.

This helps alleviate and prevent neck and shoulder myofascial pain.

Gentle neck rolling

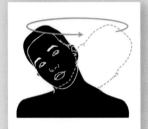

Gently roll your chin three times in one direction, and then three times in the opposite direction. It is quite common to hear mild crunching noises in your neck. However, if you feel at all uncomfortable or dizzy, stop this exercise.

This helps alleviate and prevent neck pain.

Forearm stretches

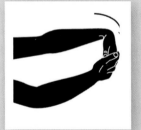

Hold your arm straight out in front of you. With the opposite hand, grab the top of your wrist and pull it down. (Your palm should be facing toward you.) Hold for twenty to thirty seconds. Then repeat on the opposite side.

This helps alleviate and prevent tennis elbow (lateral epicondylitis) pain.

Wrist stretches

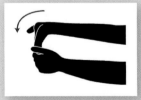

Hold your arm straight out in front of you. With the opposite hand, grab the top of your fingers and pull it down. (Your palm should now

be facing away from you.) Hold for twenty to thirty seconds. Then repeat on opposite side.

This helps alleviate and prevent golfer's elbow (medial epicondylitis) pain.

Abdominal exercises

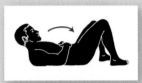

(*modified crunches*). Lie on your back, bend your knees, and place your hands on your abdomen. Then, bring your chin slowly up to your chest, while pushing your lower back flat against the floor (often called "tilting your pelvis"). Now, tighten your tummy (rectus abdominus) muscles by bringing your ribs down toward your pelvis. Hold for ten to twenty seconds. Keep breathing, even though you will feel your tummy muscles quiver when you do this. If this exercise hurts your back or neck, stop. Remember to keep breathing gently. Repeat five to ten times.

This helps to prevent and even treat low back pain.

Advanced abdominal exercise (sit-ups)

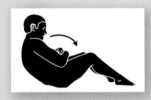

This starts off like the basic abdominal exercise, but you will slowly lift yourself into a sit-up. Keep your back arched in a C position, flattening your lower back and tightening your abdominal muscles. Then slowly lower yourself back, keeping your back in the forward C position. Exhale as you exert yourself. This means breathing out as you come up, and breathing in as you lower yourself down. If your back hurts, stop.

Is **Your** Transformational Health Plan Working?

How do you know if your transformational health plan is working?

You feel better.
Your pain and discomfort decrease and your sense of well-being improves.

Your markers change.
Disease markers such a high blood sugar go down. Health and longevity markers go up. Inflammation and oxidative stress markers fall. Weight, blood pressure, blood glucose, and cholesterol normalize.

Your health begins to improve.
As your markers normalize, your health issues are likely to decrease. By using a systems approach—rather than a silo approach—we find multiple problems simultaneously improve. The identical approach used to reverse cardiovascular disease can also reverse prostate cancer. This same approach will likely also improve diabetes, hypertension, arthritis, and osteoporosis. Changing your lifestyle can and will improve your health.

You gain resilience.
The diagnosis of any one illness can begin a calamitous downslide toward more illness. Physical pain in one area can herald pain in other areas. With the transformational medicine approach, you learn to bounce back. You learn how to manage your healing, creating further empowerment. A bump in the road does not have to lead to catastrophe.

Your vitality reawakens.
You should gain a new sense of vitality that can continue as you age. Your enjoyment of life, with fulfilling work, invigorating exercise, and a healthy sex life, can continue indefinitely. You can develop a joyful inner glow. Aging should be an achievement—not a complaint.

Live well. Eat well. Get well. Walk well. Run we
Love well. Live well. Stretch well. Dance well. G
well. Be well. Stay well. Breathe well. Stay well.
Sleep well. Think well. Love well. Relax well. Li

2

RING TWO

The Road to Illness

How **Stress and Lifestyle** Affect Your Trajectory toward Illness

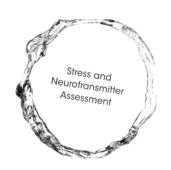

Stress and Neurotransmitter Assessment

The vast majority of our patients tell us the same story, in different forms. It is the story of how they got sick, and it always involves both physical and emotional stress. If you or someone you love has chronic illness, you'll want to give some thought to the stresses that may have contributed to that illness. Getting sick is a process, and reducing stress is often the first step in healing.

Three Patients: Different Scenarios with a Common Thread

We would like you to look at the pattern that emerges from three patient stories to see if your own experience has been similar.

Ana's Story

Ana lived what some might call an enchanted life. Married, three children, prosperous, she had a loving, happy family. The day she turned 40, she came home to devastating news: Her husband had been diagnosed with terminal, inoperable brain cancer. Determined to keep her family together, she became the perfect role model. As her husband's support system and lifeline, she was the one who took him to his radiation treatments and later to chemotherapy. She was there when he lost his hair. She was there for his treatment, there when the treatment failed, there when he developed recurrent pneumonia, and there when he eventually died.

About six months after her husband's death, Ana found her patience waning. She had put on some weight and was feeling testy and anxious much of the time. Her irritability caused screaming matches with her teenage daughter. After some counseling with her pastor, she realized that she was simply reeling from the stress of what had happened, so she resolved to pull herself together. She began attending exercise classes daily and went on a low-calorie diet. Over the next six months, she lost fifteen pounds, yet things weren't much better. She still felt exhausted. Her "subhuman" teenage daughter (as she called her) was hardly talking to her. At the suggestion of her friends, she had started dating again, but felt almost fraudulent doing so.

Then Ana began getting sick. Despite rounds of antibiotics for sore throats, bronchitis, and urinary tract infections, she still couldn't shake the infections. She became increasingly depressed. When she went back to the doctor, he ran a battery of tests. Eventually he made the diagnosis: autoimmune thyroiditis and depression.

Despite the optimum medical treatment for her thyroid condition and her depression, Ana continued to feel bad. That's when she came in to see us . . . .

Dominic's Story

Dominic was a successful businessman, a self-made man. He had come from a modest background but rose to become the CEO of a public company. As the oldest son of six children, Dominic doted on his mother. A widow after her husband died of a heart attack at age 35, Dominic's mom had worked three jobs to ensure that her children would have a good education. Dominic never forgot that.

A stellar example to his brothers and sisters, he had been a star athlete in high school, excelled in college, and was highly successful in business. Dominic continued to play a leading role in his family; he still looked out for his brothers and sisters and now employed almost all of them in his business.

Dominic first noticed his symptoms six weeks after his mom was diagnosed with ovarian cancer. That's when the backaches began. His back hurt so much that it would wake him up in the middle of the night. His joints hurt. His ability to concentrate at work suffered, first from the lack of sleep and then from the pain. His family complained that his sunny disposition had been replaced by grumpiness and suggested he see his doctor. At first, the doctor thought Dominic might have an autoimmune disease, but the lab work was negative. The MRIs and x-rays were also normal. A trial of a tranquilizer (alprazolam or Xanax®) only made him feel worse. A friend suggested he come to see us . . . .

Benita's Story

Benita still remembers her father's anger, his dark moods, and his drinking spells. Perhaps this all started when her mother died: she was only about 13 years old at the time. She remembers taking care of her father, trying her best to be "a good girl," cooking for him, mending his shirts—all the while trying to avoid his malicious, tirade-filled outbursts. She was never certain when there would be another outburst, so she developed a keen sense of perception, always on the alert to anticipate her father's moods. In a sense, she lost herself, never really learning to recognize her own needs and desires.

At age 17, it seemed as though all this was behind her. She had finally discovered what she truly wanted—a suave, handsome man who swept her off her feet. After a whirlwind courtship, she eloped at age 18 with the man of her dreams. Two babies followed in quick succession. The abuse started a short while later. At first, it was just emotional, but later it escalated and became physical, too. Initially, he only beat her when he was drunk, but soon it was all the time.

One day her husband simply vanished. Benita was left destitute, with two small children. They moved into a shelter until she could find a job. Eighteen months later, about the time she signed a lease on her first apartment, she found a lump in her breast. She was devastated when she heard her diagnosis: cancer of the right breast.

Luckily for Benita, her employer helped her through the dark days of surgery, radiation, and chemotherapy. Despite her remission from cancer, she never really felt good. She was tired all the time, listless and depressed, but antidepressants didn't help. She gained weight even though she was watching her diet. And now she needed medications for hypertension and high cholesterol. Her oncologist suggested she come to see us . . . .

Stress and Illness

The thread that ties these stories together is stress. It is a term that gets used a lot, but what does it really mean? We define stress as the body's response to physical, emotional, or mental demands. Our bodies handle stress by producing hormones that help us cope. When we're faced with a sudden danger—a close call in traffic, for instance—our bodies respond by releasing the hormone norepinephrine, which raises the heart rate and makes us more alert. Ordinarily, once the stressful situation is over, the body returns to normal. But what if the stress continues unabated? It is then that stress can start to affect health.

The Stress Curve

To understand how stress impacts your physical, emotional, and mental health, you need to know what a typical response to stress looks like. We call this the Stress Curve—check the diagram on page 63 to see what the curve looks like.

These three patients—examples of overextended and overworked individuals—are all suffering from extreme stress and burnout.

> Stress is like an iceberg. We can see one-eighth of it above, but what about what's below?
>
> — **Author Unknown**

This pattern was first described in the work of the pioneering physician and researcher Hans Selye, who, in the late 1930s and early 1940s, performed the initial studies on the stress syndrome, defined it, and then coined the term stress. His studies also looked at the effects of stress over time and at how we adapt to stress (described as the general adaptation syndrome).

Stress is a normal aspect of life. Initially, stress can be good for you. Selye called this eustress. Yet we now know that stress, left unmanaged, can lead to psychological problems and also to major physical problems, or what Selye called distress. Researchers have connected stress to almost every form of nonhereditary illness.

People respond to stress in unique ways. One person will thrive in a situation that causes another to crumble. However, we all have our breaking point. Once stress becomes chronic and overwhelming, almost all of us tend to experience a similar pattern of physical and emotional responses that reflect profound changes in our body chemistry.

What's more, stress tends to become both invasive and pervasive. When stress is chronic, you may get so depleted from it that you feel you no longer have the physical and emotional stamina to change the pattern. In other words, try as you might, you can't just pull yourself together anymore.

Going NUTS

According to stress researcher Dr. Sonia Lupien, a neuroscience researcher at the University of Montreal, life events likely to be stressful are usually those that drive us NUTS. That is, they are either new or novel

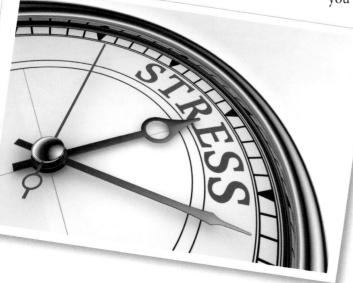

(N), unpredictable (U), threatening to our personality (T), or induce a sense (S) of loss of control. Each time we get stressed, and, in a sense, go a little bit NUTS, our bodies react by releasing hormones and other chemicals, readying us for the fight, flight, or freeze response.

Initially, the elevated levels of stress hormones can actually be beneficial and even invigorating. However, over the long term, the effects of the pressure and strain tend to be debilitating, chronic, and cumulative.

In the book *Why Zebras Don't Get Ulcers*, Stanford professor Robert Sapolsky affirms that wild animals are less likely to experience the type of stress induced by the constant worry and anxiety that plagues humans. In the animal kingdom, when confronted with the threat of an attack by a predator, the stress response enables an animal to either fight or run for its life. Both scenarios require an intense physical effort. In terms of body chemistry and the nervous system, the physical exertion of running or fighting completes the stress response. When the danger has passed, the animal returns to a baseline state, free of ongoing worry (until the next predator comes along).

Like animals, humans are genetically hardwired for experiencing cycles of acute stress. When stress is followed by intense physical activity, we are able to return naturally to baseline and a calmer state of mind. This sort of stress doesn't give us ulcers.

Stress can be habit-forming and even addicting. The pulsating adrenaline high we feel when we deal with acute stress may make us want to go back for more. Think of a roller coaster ride. You may scream while you're on it, but as soon as you get off, you start thinking, That was fun! Maybe I should do that again.

So, acute stress is fine, as long as you can deal with it and then return to your baseline low-stress level. But what happens when we are exposed to stress day in, day out, with nothing to help antidote it?

Stuck in the Stress Response

As we have seen from our three case studies, it is the constant, escalating, never-ending stress that can eventually make us sick. These patients were stuck in the stress response and couldn't see a way out.

Let's presume for a moment that you have a "normal" amount of stress in your life. We want to show here what happens when the demands of your life progressively increase your stress load, creating a scenario of chronic stress.

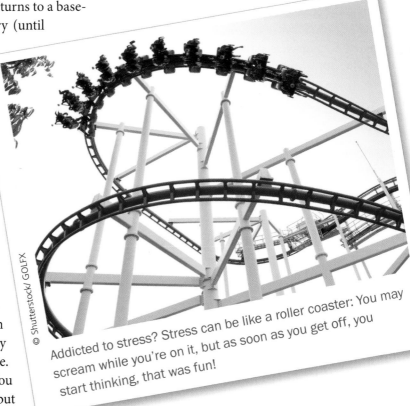

© Shutterstock/ GOLFX

Addicted to stress? Stress can be like a roller coaster: You may scream while you're on it, but as soon as you get off, you start thinking, that was fun!

Understanding the Stress Curve

The Exhilaration Aspect of the Stress Curve

Under initial mild or moderate stress, most of us typically respond well. If you're asked to complete a rush job with an urgent deadline or have to study for an exam, you can probably push yourself a little, respond to that stress, and meet the challenge. If it's an exciting opportunity, such as a new job, you'll probably even feel energized or exhilarated.

At this early stage, problems are simply challenges to be overcome. Stress is invigorating. This is the optimum response.

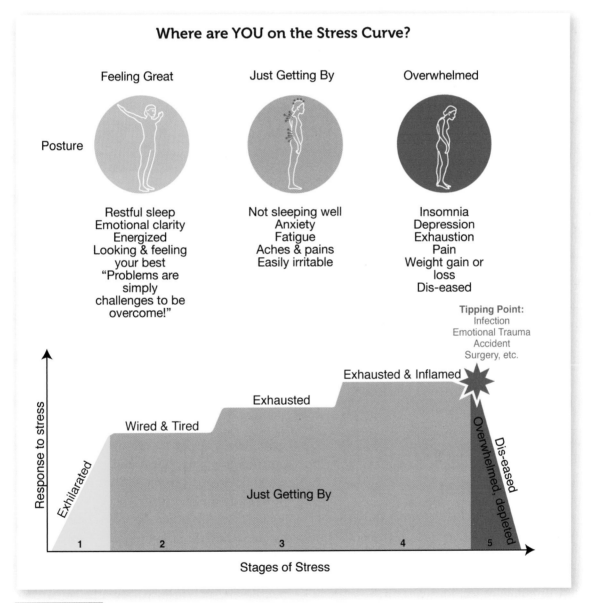

Where are YOU on the Stress Curve?

Feeling Great	Just Getting By	Overwhelmed
Restful sleep	Not sleeping well	Insomnia
Emotional clarity	Anxiety	Depression
Energized	Fatigue	Exhaustion
Looking & feeling your best	Aches & pains	Pain
"Problems are simply challenges to be overcome!"	Easily irritable	Weight gain or loss
		Dis-eased

Posture

Tipping Point:
Infection
Emotional Trauma
Accident
Surgery, etc.

Response to stress — Stages of Stress

Exhilarated — Wired & Tired — Exhausted — Exhausted & Inflamed — Overwhelmed, depleted — Dis-eased

Just Getting By

1 2 3 4 5

Figure R2.1 | The Stress Curve

Behind the Scenes in Stage 1: Invigorating Stress

Neurotransmitters are the natural brain chemicals that underlie our moods, emotions, and energy level. They are the natural stimulants that drive us and also play a major role in the stress response.

Some of the chemicals produced by our bodies serve as natural stimulants. That's how we're able to pull an all-nighter or get the driveway shoveled after the first big snow. When we feel invigorated, these natural stimulants have kicked in.

The chemicals in the brain that serve as accelerators to our mood and energy level are described as excitatory neurotransmitters. This chemistry—which includes epinephrine (also known as adrenaline) and norepinephrine (or noradrenaline)—comes into play when we're under stress and need to speed up our performance or respond to an emergency. Our bodies produce these natural stimulants to help us focus and give us the drive to respond to the task at hand. This same chemistry is present in all mammals and is evident whenever they are experiencing the "fight, flight, or freeze" response.

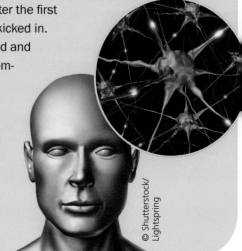

© Shutterstock/
Lightspring

When You Max Out on Stress: The "Stressed-and-Just-Getting-By" Phase of the Stress Curve

The stressed-and-just-getting-by phase comprises three progressive levels:

Stage 2: Wired and Tired

Stage 3: Exhausted

Stage 4: Exhausted and Inflamed

> It's not stress that kills us, it's our reaction to it.
>
> – Hans Selye

Stage 2

Wired and Tired

At what point does that sense of exhilaration become a drain? Let's say that the stress, the pressure, the long hours, and the deadlines continue day in and day out. You may be an emergency room nurse, a single parent working two (or three) jobs, a student preparing for a big exam, someone grappling with an addiction, the parent of a child with a chronic illness, or a caregiver for a family member with Alzheimer's. In these circumstances, you may be able to meet the demands of the tasks facing you, but eventually you will no longer respond as efficiently.

Your ability to keep adapting to stress diminishes as your stress response changes. Your adrenaline remains high, making you feel wired, while your cortisol begins to drop, making you feel tired. The stress curve flattens out, producing the stage we call "wired and tired."

At this point in the stress curve, you might begin to experience unpleasant or unnerving physical symptoms:

Emotional Feeling	Possible Physical Symptom
Feeling stressed	Developing aches and pains
Hypersensitive	Hyperactive
Irritable	Racing heartbeat at times
Tense	Elevated blood pressure
Anxious	Hot flashes or clammy sweats
Fatigued	Restless sleep, but at this stage, sleep is still restorative. With a good night's sleep, you feel ready to roar back into action.

Behind the Scenes in Stage 2: Wired and Tired

When we're wired and tired, our bodies are putting out too much of the stress hormone adrenaline—as well as exciting neurotransmitters such as glutamate, epinephrine, and norepinephrine. This causes a racy, yet anxious, feeling. When we are healthy, the stress hormone cortisol is high in the morning and then drops progressively during the day. Typically, we should have lots of energy in the morning, then run out of it at night so we can sleep. In this phase of the stress response, however, cortisol drops during the day, but then rises at night—so we feel tired in the day, but feel more alert and awake at night.

Over time, stress wears away at metabolic reserves, depletes vital nutrients, and puts a strain on different systems throughout the body. The body attempts to adapt. The mind tries to relax by secreting inhibitory or calming neurotransmitters such as GABA and serotonin—natural tranquilizers that act as brakes on a racing mind. At the same time, blood pressure, cholesterol, blood sugar, and triglycerides all continue to climb.

Stage 3

Exhausted

What happens when you feel you have to keep pushing despite the stress? What happens when you go past the wired and tired phase?

The body continues adapting to the chronic stress. To do so, it slows its metabolism, attempting to conserve energy. If you keep pressing on despite this, you move on to the next stage of stress. This stage is easy to recognize. We call it Exhaustion. As you become more depleted and move more deeply into the stress response, you become exhausted. Symptoms of exhaustion include:

- Extreme fatigue
- A sense of constantly dragging
- Weight gain or difficulty losing weight
- Feeling depressed, weak, worn down
- Libido suffers
- Cold hands and feet
- Menstrual irregularities
- Fertility issues (both men and women)
- Indigestion
- Recurrent infections
- Nonrestorative sleep (fatigue is no longer improved by a good night's sleep; you wake up tired rather than refreshed)

Stage 4

Exhausted and Inflamed

We are genetically hardwired to adapt to increased stress by turning on inflammation. If we were cavemen, this inflammatory cascade would help us repair wounds more quickly and resist infection. However, chronic stress and inflammation are different. When we reach the point of being exhausted and inflamed from chronic stress, health issues that are already present intensify. Asthma attacks become more frequent, migraines last a little longer, colitis may flare. Everything becomes a little worse as the body seems to catch on fire, figuratively speaking. With chronic inflammation, the immune system is overstressed, too, and as a result, we tend to get sick more often. We also have a sense of feeling progressively more out of sorts, or that something is vaguely wrong.

Depletion, infection, and inflammation are common at this point. Low serotonin is associated with an overreactive immune system and higher levels of inflammation throughout the body. When serotonin drops, we tend to get sick more easily. Infections, such as chronic si-

nusitis, may develop and then linger. The list of inflammatory conditions made worse by stress is seemingly endless: allergies, arthritis, asthma, autoimmune diseases, digestive disorders, eczema, hypertension, joint, shoulder and back problems, and spikes in cholesterol. Bruises, cuts, and other injuries tend to heal more slowly.

Whenever the immune system begins ramping up, inflammation levels increase throughout the body. The body is trying to defend itself—just as if it were fighting infection. This can trigger flare-ups of conditions such as arthritis and colitis (and just about any disorder that ends with "-itis").

Inflammation can affect any and all systems in the body. Increased inflammation is associated with:

- Aching joints
- Plaque and blockage inside arteries
- High blood pressure
- Certain cardiomyopathies (heart muscle problems)
- Worsening type 2 diabetes
- Diabetic complications
- Skin diseases, such as worsening psoriasis and eczema

- Worsening of asthma
- Chronic obstructive pulmonary disease (COPD)
- Worsening osteoporosis
- Allergy symptoms
- Heartburn or reflux (GERD)
- Colitis
- Cancer initiation or aggravation
- Neurological diseases such as Alzheimer's disease and Parkinson's disease

---

Behind the Scenes: Exhausted and Inflamed

What happens to your body when chronic stress leaves you exhausted and inflamed?

Stress hormones: Your cortisol levels remain low, so little of this hormone is available to dampen the inflammatory response. DHEA, your "well-being hormone," also drops. (We discuss this more in Ring 4.)

Inflammation: At this point, the ongoing stress sounds an alarm bell for your inflammatory system. Your body pours out chemicals called pro-inflammatory cytokines. This shift into a state of alarm is referred to as the "inflammatory cascade." Most cytokines are called interleukins, designated by the "IL-" moniker.

Pro-inflammatory cytokines, as the name suggests, promote inflammation and tend to rise during the exhausted and inflamed phase. Pro-inflammatory interleukins include: IL-1β, IL-2, IL-6, IL-8, IL-12, IL-17, interferon gamma (IFN-γ), and tumor necrosis factor alpha (TNF-α).

Anti-inflammatory cytokines tend to decrease during this phase. Anti-inflammatory interleukins include: IL-4, IL-5, IL-10, IL-13, and transforming growth factor beta (TGF-β).

Other cytokines called chemokines proliferate, as they try and help the body reduce infection and promote healing, often though by further inflammation. Chemokines include: Interleukin IL-8, monocyte chemotactic protein 1 (MCP-1), and macrophage inflammatory protein (MIP 1β).

Insulin Resistance and the Blood Sugar Blues: With increasing inflammation, the body becomes more insulin resistant, meaning the hormone insulin, which controls blood sugar, has trouble carrying blood sugar into the cells (we discuss this in more detail in Ring 4). This causes blood sugar highs and crashing lows. Often, we counter low energy with quick fixes—sugary snacks and junk food. Unfortunately, that just leads to more sugar highs and lows—more sugar cravings and more weight gain. Another vicious cycle.

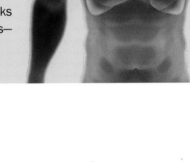

✸ The Tipping Point:
Total Exhaustion and the Final Straw

On the path to illness, exhaustion typically makes us more vulnerable. We may get sick more easily, have emotional crises and energy crashes, and be more susceptible to stress injuries and chronic health issues. When patients come to us with complex illnesses and a history of chronic stress and exhaustion, we trace back through their history to learn everything we can about the underlying cause(s) of their condition.

As physicians, we often find that after a long period of chronic stress, when yet another stressful event occurs in a patient's life, it becomes the final straw, pushing him or her over the edge of coping. They drop into the final phase of the stress response—they develop a disease. On the Stress Curve, we call this phase Overwhelmed and Depleted.

Patients often remark that they get sick just after the immediate stress abates. For example, they get a migraine on the weekend after a particularly intense work week. This is not unusual. The body is designed to cope with acute stress. A person may get shot in the leg during a heated battle, or injured in an important game. Because of the high circulating adrenaline, they might not feel pain until they get to the hospital and start calming down. When we see patients in the Overwhelmed and Depleted phase, they often ask us why they seemed to get sick just as life was getting easier. We tell them, it is not during the "war" that they should worry, but after it!

Almost any kind of stressful event can be-

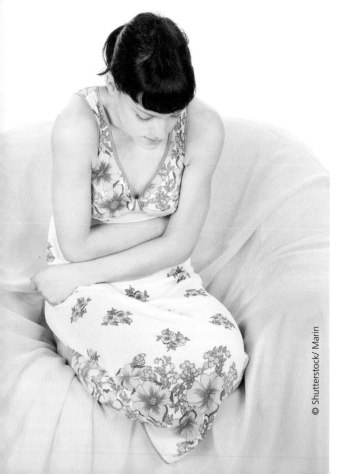

© Shutterstock/ Marin

come the final trigger for illness, particularly if it's intense enough. It could be a physical stress such as an accident, an infection, a surgery, or a toxic exposure in the workplace. It might be an emotional trauma, such as losing a job, a divorce, or the death of someone close. Sometimes a patient isn't overstressed, but the stress itself is huge. However, most times the final straw is a single event for a system that is already exhausted—a system that has been overcompensating for far too long. It is after this tipping point or triggering factor that patients can develop serious illnesses. The time from the stressful event until the time of illness can range from a matter of days to about eighteen months or even longer.

Unfortunately, society tends to misinterpret the cause of the disease. Health care providers tend to focus on the problem in front of them, viewing a single disorder as the cause and treating it alone. In reality, that particular illness or injury is simply the last straw. Our patients also tend to focus on one symptom or illness in their attempts to make sense of their lives. They may attribute their poor health to a viral infection that needs to be treated, or midlife hormonal changes. Unfortunately, the problem usually goes much deeper.

Such patients are suffering from a system-wide malfunction precipitated by a triggering event. A virus may seem to be the cause, for example, but it's not the foundation of the problem. Often the deeper issue is severe depletion as a result of chronic stress that has developed over a period of months or years.

Sometimes the final stressful event seems insignificant. This is because we become psychologically primed by previous stressors. A loss early in our lives that is repeated in some form later on can trigger intense emotional reactions. For example, your parents might have divorced when you were a child. You felt an intense sense of loss when your father moved out, but you got over it. Years later, though, when a beloved pet dies, that buried childhood sense of loss is triggered. You may seem to overreact emotionally and then become ill with something more serious within the next eighteen months.

This is similar to what occurs in post-traumatic stress disorder (PTSD), when people cope with an enormously stressful event and then become highly sensitized to reminders of that experience. They may survive a wartime situation and later overreact to any sound that reminds them of gunfire, for example.

In Benita's case, she felt abandoned at age 13 when her mother died. She coped reasonably well, but when her husband abandoned her years later, this triggered a sense of overwhelming loss that shut down her immune system and left her vulnerable to illness.

Stage 5

Overwhelmed and Depleted

In the final phase of stress, you feel overwhelmed and depleted. You're depressed, apathetic, and dis-eased. At this point, disease literally sets in. Many of our chronically stressed patients are diagnosed with cancer or autoimmune disorders such as lupus, rheumatoid arthritis, or multiple sclerosis, or struggle with emotional issues such as major depression. An experienced physician can diagnose any one of these illnesses without much trouble. However, many chronically stressed people develop complex symptoms that elude diagnosis.

Common symptoms in the Overwhelmed State include:

- Frequently feeling out of sorts or ill at ease
- Multiple symptoms not associated with any disease
- More than one disease
- Drastic weight gain or loss
- Depression, apathy, or hopelessness
- Feeling drained, emotionless
- Concentration becomes close to impossible
- Memory loss
- Dizziness, clammy sweats, or fever
- Rough skin and brittle nails
- Fertility problems
- Water retention (edema), puffiness
- Feeling lightheaded, especially when getting up or when exposed to increased heat, such as a sauna, a hot bath, or hot weather

Depletion: An Invisible Illness

If you are a patient whose system is in a state of overwhelm or exhaustion, you may go to the doctor and be diagnosed with an illness or with depression. However, in our experience, the majority of patients do not initially get any diagnosis at all. They may even even be told, "It's all in your head." Standard blood tests are usually normal, including a CBC (complete blood count), renal and electrolyte testing, and liver function tests. Thyroid tests may be borderline or minimally abnormal, showing some sluggishness in the thyroid gland, but nothing dramatic.

Let's go back to our three patients. Clearly the stress and the demands of their lives pushed them toward disease.

Ana's stress started when her husband became sick. The physiological and physical deficits caused by caring for her husband as he succumbed to cancer, paired with the continued stress of being a single parent, pushed her to the point where she was totally exhausted and overwhelmed. After that, she developed recurrent infections and was diagnosed with autoimmune thyroiditis (Graves' disease). She was probably genetically susceptible to this disease, but it took frequent infections from chronic stress to trigger the illness.

Dominic's stress started when his father died. He became a super-achiever, always on, always giving 100 percent. When his mother was diagnosed with a terminal illness, he quickly became exhausted on the stress curve—when you always give 100 percent, you have no reserves to fall back on. The possibility that his mother might die triggered memories of the stress associated with his father's death. Fortunately, Dominic had not yet gone into the final stage of exhaustion and overwhelm when he came to see us, so he recovered fairly quickly.

Benita's stress obviously started in childhood with her mother's death and her life with an abusive, alcoholic father. This stress depleted her at a young age. After she married, the stress of an abusive, alcoholic husband and his subsequent abandonment quickly pushed her into overwhelm, exhaustion, and then disease. At that point, another set of stressors wreaked havoc with her body: cancer, surgery, radiation, chemotherapy, and their aftermath. The resulting effect was even more dysfunction and illness.

> It is a lot harder to keep people well than it is to just get them over a sickness.
>
> – DeForest Clinton Jarvis

Scenes in Stage 5: Depleted and the Nervous System Out of Sync

Our autonomic nervous system is the part of our nervous system that runs our bodies on automatic pilot, regulating unconscious actions such as breathing and the beating of the heart—minute to minute, hour by hour, day in, day out. It consists of two parts: the sympathetic and parasympathetic nervous systems. The sympathetic nervous system controls our fight or flight responses. Under stress, the sympathetic nervous system makes our muscles tense up; our heart races and our blood pressure rises. The parasympathetic nervous system does just the opposite, activating our relaxation response, slowing our heart rate, lowering blood pressure, and aiding digestion. These two systems are designed to be a check and balance against each other. However, when we are under prolonged stress, our sympathetic nervous system stays turned on, effectively pushing us further along the Stress Curve.

By the time a patient becomes depleted and exhausted, the autonomic nervous system may become dysfunctional, resulting in a condition described as dysautonomia. Two forms of dysautonomia are neurally mediated hypotension (NMH) and postural orthostatic tachycardia syndrome (POTS). In NMH, a patient's blood pressure is normal when tested in the office, but often drops precipitously when he or she gets slightly overheated, such as after taking a hot bath or walking into a warm room while wearing a warm coat. The person feels exhausted and sweaty and can often faint. POTS syndrome is similar, although it results in a racing heart.

Understanding Cortisol and Stress

In a healthy person with a normal circadian rhythm, cortisol rises in the early morning and gradually decreases during the day. Ideally, we should pop out of bed after a good night's sleep, full of energy, then gradually run out of energy at night, allowing us to fall asleep easily and peacefully.

In the Wired and Tired phase, though, cortisol is low in the morning and starts rising in the late afternoon or evening. After feeling exhausted during the day, a person in this phase will go to bed at night but find it difficult to unwind and fall asleep.

In the Exhausted phase, the cortisol levels dip even further, remaining low for most of the day, consistent with feelings of exhaustion. By the time we get to the Exhausted and Inflamed Stage, our low cortisol levels can no longer combat any inflammation.

In the Overwhelmed and Depleted phase, the adrenal glands are no longer responsive to stress and produce very little cortisol. The cortisol levels tend to remain low and flat throughout the day. Along with this, neurotransmitters such as norepinephrine, epinephrine and serotonin bottom out, leaving people feeling apathetic and overwhelmed.

The important point here is that unless cortisol levels are extremely imbalanced, it is unlikely that a single test will pick up a problem. For this reason, we recommend four samples taken over the course of a day: upon wakening, at about 11 a.m., between 3:00 and 4:00 p.m., and finally before bed. Since measuring cortisol with blood tests this way would be expensive and cumbersome, we recommend saliva tests instead.

Are You Depressed?

Many of our patients feel depressed but refuse help, saying they just need to "pull themselves together." They feel embarrassed to speak to anyone about their sense of feeling overwhelmed. We want to assure you that this is nothing to feel embarrassed about. It is a physical condition. When your neurotransmitters are depleted, you cannot simply "pull yourself together."

The good news is that in most cases, depression can be easily treated.

According to the *Diagnostic and Statistical Manual of Mental Disorders*, fourth edition (better known as the DSM-IV), published by the American Psychiatric Association, a major depressive episode consists of at least two of the following symptoms:

- Depressed mood most of the day; feeling sad or empty, tearful
- Significant loss of interest or pleasure in activities that used to be enjoyable

- Significant weight loss (when not dieting) or weight gain; decrease or increase in appetite
- Difficulty sleeping or sleeping too much
- Agitation, or slowing down of thoughts, and reduction of physical movements
- Fatigue or loss of energy
- Feelings of worthlessness or inappropriate guilt
- Poor concentration or having difficulty making decisions
- Thinking about death or suicide

The level of depression is considered significant if the symptoms have occurred nearly every day for at least two weeks (clearly, some people struggle with depression for years before getting help). If you are suffering from any of these symptoms, don't feel embarrassed to talk to your physician about them.

Alex learns about stress

As a high-stress executive, Alex often found himself feeling wired and tired or even exhausted. At times, he wasn't sure if he was irritable with his wife and his boss, or if he was making them irritable. Salivary cortisol testing showed him to be in the Wired and Tired stage of the stress curve (check back to page 63 to see this diagram). His cortisol levels dipped in the day, especially after lunch, when he found himself the most tired, and then rose after dinner. Just when he hoped to flop into bed, Alex found himself quite wired and unable to get restful sleep. He also noticed that his joints ached the most when he was the most stressed.

Stress was switching on Alex's inflammatory genes. They were sending a message to his body to pour out inflammatory chemicals called cytokines. Alex's lifestyle was interacting with his genetic susceptibility to become inflamed. Inflammatory genes may once have helped his ancestors survive, but now they were making his knees and back hurt!

Alex continues to pursue Health and Wellness

UNDERSTANDING THE ROAD TO ILLNESS CAN HELP YOU ON YOUR ROAD TO RECOVERY AND TRANSFORMATION.

Understanding the Stress Curve gives you the ability to alter your trajectory toward illness. In Star 2 we will discuss techniques that will help to change your life by transforming stress into success.

All the evidence that we have indicates that it is reasonable to assume in practically every human being, and certainly in almost every newborn baby, that there is an active will toward health, an impulse toward growth, or toward the actualization.

– Abraham Maslow

How to Transform Stress into Success

Tools and Techniques to Help You Transform the Effects of Stress on Your Health and Your Life

Transform Stress into Success

Stress is a fact of daily life. Chronic stress is hard to avoid, but it isn't that hard to learn how to cope with it. You can learn to handle daily stress and stressful events—and you can learn how to be less reactive to old stresses. Moments of peak stress can become transformational moments, times when you make positive changes in your life.

Dealing with Stress

Stress is a challenge to the body, emotions, and mind. Dealing with it takes a toll, but if you have a good understanding of how stress affects you, you are better able to handle it. Based on our experience with our patients, we've learned some important lessons for coping with stress. Here are some tips:

Aim for a healthy lifestyle. Stress, by its very nature, counteracts a healthy lifestyle. Stress will push you to eat junk food, lose sleep, and set up a cascading wave of chemical damage that will flow throughout your body. In Star 1 we outlined some healthy lifestyle approaches that can become a welcome refuge against stress. In Star 2, we will give specific suggestions on how to tailor your lifestyle to antidote stress.

Mend the mind to mind the body. The mind is a powerful tool, yet it can be both helpful and harmful to you. Developing a different outlook can remarkably reshape your life and literally reformat your body chemistry. In Star 1, we suggested relaxation and meditation techniques that counter stress and promote well-being. In Star 2, we will give you specific techniques that will help you change your perspective.

Restore the body to revitalize the mind. Body chemistry can affect how we look, feel, and think. Learn to treat your body with the respect it deserves. When your body feels vital and alive, so do you. Here in Star 2, we offer suggestions to help your body develop a profound sense of vigor that will help carry you through tougher times. We discuss the use of healing therapies, adaptogenic herbs, and even medications. Always work with a physician who understands the benefits and side effects of the medications you are being prescribed. When working with a practitioner who prescribes nutritional supplements, work with someone who also understands that "natural" doesn't always mean good or safe. Supplements may have interactions with medications and can cause harm.

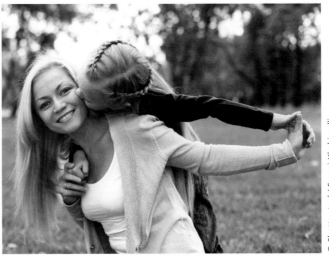

Techniques for Transforming Stress

Acute or sudden stress is different from chronic or long-term stress. We suggest you learn different ways to handle each of these.

Each episode of acute stress gives you an opportunity of choice. You can learn how to make decisions that will transform your health and your life.

To become whole again from chronic stress, though, you need to find ways to integrate deep rest and regeneration into your life. The goal is to move yourself back to the left side of the Stress Curve—to where you are Enthusiastic and Exhilarated once again.

Initially we discuss chronic stress. Later in the chapter, we will give you techniques to handle acute stress.

Healthy Lifestyle Habits to Reduce Ongoing Stress

Simplify your life. Learn how to say stop, and learn how to say no. When you feel yourself getting overwhelmed, it is usually OK to stop. Learn to take breaks. Getting away for a while is a good thing. It gives you a needed sense of perspective.

Manage your time. Make a priority list of what is important to you. Don't overcommit. Learn to recognize when you are biting off more than you can chew.

Listen to your body. Your body will know that you are stressed before you do. Become skilled at recognizing the familiar cues. Irritability, tightness and tension in your head, jaws, or shoulders, a gnawing feeling in the pit of your stomach may all be telling you that you are overdoing things.

Exercise in a manner that is beneficial to you is an important way to deal with stress, but it's important to be reasonable. Remember that running at midday without a shirt in a high-traffic area may count as exercise, but it probably isn't improving your health.

Develop healthy ways to dissipate stress. Volunteer work, an avocation, or a hobby can be excellent ways to deal with stress. Whether you are helping to repair a hiking trail or tutoring shelter kids after school, using your gifts to serve others adds another dimension to your life.

Use social connections. If you enjoy socializing in groups, stay connected with a religious organization, a self-help group, a support group, or the like. Even online social groups or disease-specific support groups can give you a sense of social identity. On the other hand, if you're energized by time spent one-on-one, tap those relationships to sustain you.

Avoid stimulants and eat well. Reduce the use of stimulants such as caffeine and nicotine. Reduce alcohol. Minimize junk foods; go for a nutrient-rich diet.

Take time every day just for yourself. Consider a relaxation or meditation technique for twenty minutes once or twice daily.

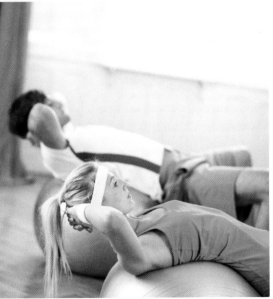

© Shutterstock/ Alliance

Mending the Mind and Minding the Body

Researchers at Ohio State University have recently shown how powerfully psychological stress can affect the immune system. Jan Kiecolt-Glaser is a professor of psychiatry and psychology at Ohio State University. Her husband, Ron Glaser, is a professor of internal medicine, molecular virology, immunology and medical genetics, and head of Ohio State's Institute for Behavioral Medicine Research.

They compared the rate of wound healing after a skin punch biopsy (a small incision that removes some tissue from the skin) in two groups: a "stressed group," consisting of caregivers to a spouse or family member with advanced Alzheimer's disease, and an "unstressed group." In the stressed group, wound healing took on average nine days longer. The study showed how much stress disrupts the immune system and makes us more vulnerable to infection and slower to heal. This finding has profound implications for medical care. If we can learn how to control or reduce stress, we can drastically affect how our bodies heal.

Mental Tips for Handling Stress

Stress has a major impact on emotions. The more stressed we feel, the more small things upset us and the more angry, anxious, or depressed we feel. We have learned a lot from our patients about mental tips that help them deal with their stress.

Journaling. Write down who or what is bothering you. Identify triggers: things that make you anxious, frustrated, or angry. As you do so, become aware of your own body's responses. Examine your physical reactions to thoughts and feelings that are stressful—rapid heartbeat, sweatiness, bowel habit changes—can all be part of this. Note how you're dealing with stress. Eating more? Smoking? Ruminating or obsessing? Hoarding? Then develop a problem-solving list.

Develop self-compassion. Imagine a small baby trying to walk. Each time she falls, you wouldn't deride her or tell her she's stupid. Learn to treat yourself with the same self-compassion you would a small child.

Be clear with other people. Make sure the people close to you understand your requests and intentions. We think that others understand what is going on inside our heads, but the truth is that they do not.

Change your perspective. Speaking to others may help you get a different point of view. Whether it is through a friend, pastor, counselor, or therapist, learn to see problems from another's point of view.

Work on balancing your emotions. If anger is your issue, learn to deal with it. When you feel frustrated, go work out rather than taking it out on anyone. Count to ten before you say something in a negative manner. Practice forgiveness. Practice mindfulness.

Express yourself differently. Learn to give "I feel . . ." rather than "You are . . ." messages. Learn to simply say, "I feel hurt when you . . ." or, "I feel angry when you . . ." This is a much better approach than saying, "You are a *#@**," which is judgmental and tends to make people defensive.

Express yourself factually. So often, we don't tell people when they are hurting our feelings. This is usually with people we like, as we don't want to offend them. However, there is a way to do this. Tell them accurately and factually what you are feeling and when it is occurring.

Laugh. Can you find humor in a situation? You might want to read *Anatomy of an Illness* by Norman Cousins, where he recounts how he overcame a chronic illness by watching comedies daily.

Develop resilience. Stress will always be part of our lives. Making ourselves more resilient to it is essential. Learn to bounce back.

Try to find meaning in your life. Can you feel gratitude for the experience you are going through, despite its hardship? What do you think you are here for? What are you learning? Where are you going?

Forgive transgressions against you. Forgiveness does not mean you have to like someone. It means learning to bear no resentment. Remember, if you harbor anger or resentment, it is you that suffers, not the person you are angry with!

Remain hopeful. Trust that you will be okay. This too shall pass! This is a learned behavior. Have faith.

Accept what life throws at you. Remember the phrase, "Lovingly and willingly accept all things."

Psychological Transformation

Each one of us is physically unique. Similarly, we are psychologically unique. Unfortunately, we may sense our uniqueness as a problem or an inadequacy—or even flip to the opposite side, where narcissistic qualities give us a false sense of greatness. Psychological transformation usually means discovering who you really are. It implies that you become more of your true self. Our true selves are usually stronger, kinder, and more loving than we believe. Yet our own psychological programming can hold us back from becoming our true selves. We may have been brought up in a family where either over- or underexpressing yourself emotionally might be considered inappropriate. Patients tell us how they were forced to grow out of sync with their own personality. A sensitive person may grow up in a macho family. An artist may grow up in a family, community, or time where his or her talents are devalued. We are vulnerable to having alien attributes imposed on us by families, teachers, communities, and even advertising media.

This leads to emotional miscues, or what we call mis-emotions. An example of a mis-emotion is laughing if you are scared, or crying if you are angry. Imagine you are the young child of an alcoholic, unhappy mother. One day you say to her, "Mommy, why are you so angry?" She glares at you, replying, "I'm not angry. Now go away." You decide that because she's an adult, she must be correct. She isn't angry. Therefore, your ability, at some core child-like level, to sense anger must be wrong. You start misinterpreting emotions, but missing emotional cues leads to further emotional misunderstandings. This can lead to becoming self-destructive and critical of ourselves, and disparaging of others.

Physical disease and psychological pain can force us to examine these traits. The threat of divorce may bring a couple into counseling. Similarly, a heart attack may force a person to examine underlying anger, resentment, or other emotions and behaviors.

> The greatest weapon against stress is our ability to choose one thought over another.
>
> —William James

A psychiatrist once told us he had a terrible relationship with his father. In fact, he had not spoken to his father for many years, until one day he was summoned to his father's hospital bed. His father had just been diagnosed with terminal pancreatic cancer. The psychiatrist knew that his father had only a few months to live. He also knew that he bore incredible anger toward his father. Although he taught his patients to deal with their own underlying anger, he had never done so himself. At the hospital, he paced up and down outside his father's room for hours, not knowing what to do. Finally, something inside him shifted. He walked into the room, feeling fully present, put his arms around his father, and told him he loved him. Bracing himself for rejection, he looked into his father's eyes. Instead of anger, they were filled with tears of happiness and love. His father responded by kissing him and telling him he loved him, too. Neither of them had ever said this to each other before.

What followed was even more remarkable. The two began to spend hours together every day. They went for walks together, held hands, and in tender times talked about their pain, fears, guilt, and sadness. They were able to forgive each other and transform this period into the most intense and loving period either had ever experienced. As the psychiatrist told us later, one of the most incredible parts of this story was the quality of life his father experienced after this. Instead of the expected three months of suffering, he lived nine wonderful months, finally succumbing peacefully in his sleep.

Transforming Toxic Emotions

To survive a bad situation, it is common to suppress a feeling or emotion. This feeling may resurface years later as a physical illness. By paying attention to your bodily sensations in times of stress, you can become aware of this link between suppressed emotional patterns and your physical reactions.

Psychologists know that if an illness serves as an unconscious strategy to cope with life, no amount of medicine alone is likely to heal the patient. Illness may reflect deep secret anguish, grief, shame, thwarted goals, or some other form of human pain. Ignoring the underlying block is like ignoring a large splinter. Healing is difficult until the obstruction has been gently removed so the wound can heal. If you feel that your emotions are out of control, we suggest seeking a mental health practitioner for help.

However, most of us have emotional issues for which we do not see a therapist. In Chinese medicine, physical feelings encompass a full spectrum of emotion, spanning the mirror opposites, or the yin and yang aspects of that emotion. Have you ever seen a baby girl that has just been fed a new food? She will sometimes shake with ecstatic apprehension. From the outside, when we look at her tremulousness, we can't be sure if she's happy or anxious. Later, she will give the label "happy" to the emotion that goes with the feeling of blissful tremulousness. Similarly, a two-year-old boy having a temper tantrum may not understand what it means to be "angry." He simply feels out of control, needing to explode, as tensions rise in his body. If we can help him understand how to better control his environment, and that he is experiencing an emotion of "anger," we can help him control both his behavior and the physical consequences in his body—being tense and uptight. These unresolved primordial emotions continue to have power over our behaviors well into adulthood.

By learning to become fully aware of our physical feelings, we can often learn to transform our emotions, to "flip" from the negative side of the emotional spectrum to the more positive side. This technique implies an "emotional aikido" of sorts, using the power of a negative emotion on itself. We can turn anger into power, fear into courage, worry into selflessness, anxiety into tranquility, and sadness into transcendence. This way, we become more of our true selves.

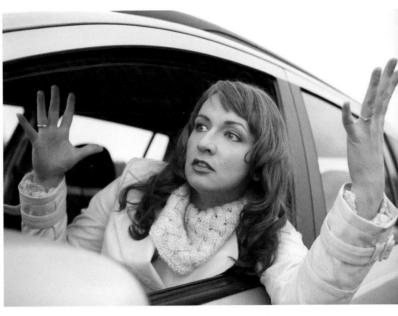

© Shutterstock/ Monika Wisniewska

Psychological transformation can therefore lead to new levels of psychological maturity with greater insight into and understanding of our own feelings and emotions. It calls for us to pay attention to our physical feelings.

We see patients transforming emotions every day. Let's look at some examples:

Betty's Story: Transforming Anger into Power

Betty first came to our center for acupuncture and massage for her fibromyalgia. It was clear to us that Betty felt angry all the time. Everything seemed to make her irritable. She couldn't remember when she wasn't seething with one grudge or another. We talked about her anger during one of her treatments. She had very good reasons to be angry. An abusive boss. A failed marriage. Problems with a teenage daughter. The reasons seemed endless. Betty felt like a victim of her own life. Then one day after a treatment, she had this insight: "I'm angry all the time, but I don't feel in charge of myself. I feel like a victim." We asked her to be aware of the anger and what happened when she got angry. Over the next few months, Betty's insights became more profound. She realized that when she became angry, her muscles would hurt more within the next twenty-four hours. She continued to come in for treatments for her pain.

A couple of months later, Betty sat down with one of our physicians and said simply, "My pain is much, much better. I began to realize that I could control my pain by deciding what I wanted to do with my anger. When I find myself getting angry, I simply sit with the feeling for a while, to try to get an overview of the situation I am in. I feel like I own this feeling of anger, and can then choose what to do with it. Putting it into my muscles is counterproductive. I just sit with it. Then, almost without doing anything, it changes. It dissolves. In its place I feel a sense of forgiveness, of control, of power."

Betty had learned the art of transforming an emotion. This is not therapy, simply a state of mindfulness about your emotions. By fully experiencing that emotion, the mind can be transported to the flip side of the emotion.

Here are a few epiphanies from some of our patients:

"I realized that I am so busy worrying because deep down I feel like people are judging me. I thought that if everything was perfect, then people would see me in a better light. But the reality is that I can never be perfect, and people don't really care anyway. I am worrying all the time about myself. If I ignore the self part of me, I stop worrying. I don't feel self-judged or self-pity. So now when I worry, I remind myself to be self-less, and then my worry-meter stops registering."

"I sank into this sense of sadness, which I feel as a pressure over my lungs. As I did, heaviness seemed to lift off me. This was followed by a sense of calmness or peace, something like I had never felt before. I feel connected to everyone and everything. I never want to get rid of my tendency to sadness. It is my gateway to connecting to the universe!"

Transforming a Toxic Emotional Environment

We need to learn to deal with our emotions. We need to learn to see when our emotions and feelings are changing the way we see the world, just like tinted glasses. However, we also need to recognize when we are living in a toxic emotional situation. We may have an abusive spouse, a rage-aholic parent, an offensive boss, or cruel friends.

Dealing with a toxic emotional environment means changing it. Leaving an abusive partner is difficult—you may well need help from a therapist, a lawyer, and even the police. Learning to stand up for yourself is an important survival tool. If you are struggling with this, don't feel embarrassed about seeking help. It may be the most important thing you ever do.

Spiritual Transformation

The goal of transformational medicine is optimization of physical health, psychological transformation, and spiritual growth. Whereas psychological transformation implies that we find a different way of viewing our selves, spiritual transformation implies a different way of viewing ourselves as part of the universe. Spiritual growth is a sense of understanding of how we fit into the universe. It is accompanied by greater love, more happiness, and less suffering.

In our quest to understand healing, we have had the privilege of treating or interviewing patients who have experienced "miraculous" healings. (Our definition of a miracle is a patient's response to an illness that defies all conventional medical expectations of their disease.) Many of these patients describe a profound connection with something greater than themselves. This may occur slowly or as a moment of clarity, in which a new insight or understanding is gained. These patients describe a sense of connectedness to their inner path that is not dependent on physical or material comforts. It becomes a source of inspiration and orientation as they rededicate their lives to the spiritual and tran-

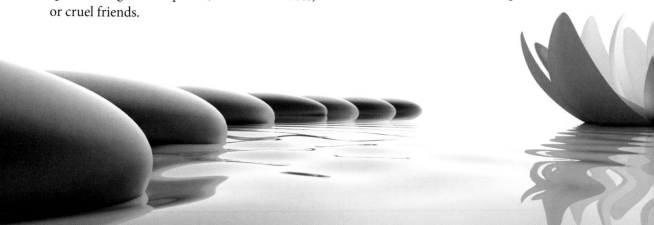

scendent nature of the universe. There seems to be a spontaneous shift. They are able to see life in a completely different way, with changes in thoughts, emotions, and behavior. They feel less suffering.

In our experience, patients often have similar experiences after acupuncture or energy healing treatments. Following these profound insights, they tend to reassign their priorities, establish new ones, or simply experience an enhanced state of well-being, love, and connectedness. This often comes as an unanticipated but pleasant surprise. (For example, a patient may not be expecting this if he comes in for treatment of knee pain.)

Sometimes patients become acutely aware of an inner struggle. Traditional Chinese medicine describes this as a discrepancy between mind and spirit. The spirit may want something different than the mind thinks it needs. Your family may have expected you to be a physician or a lawyer, yet you may have had a profound need to become something else, such as an artist or a writer. In this manner of thinking, discord between your mind and spirit may lead to an illness. Healing then involves uncovering and resolving these areas of discordance, allowing insight into ourselves and our lives. As this new awareness develops, an apparent burden of stress is easily resolved.

Unfortunately, many of us will only take a spiritual leap when we are faced with insurmountable odds. This may come with personal misfortune or even the diagnosis of a terminal illness. No matter what, spiritual growth helps us learn how to cope and bounce back from a stressful situation. This enhances our resilience.

Personal Growth Is a Journey

Both psychological and spiritual transformation require constant work. We may grow in leaps and bounds at times, or remain stagnant for prolonged periods. As with everything, we can choose how we want to work on ourselves.

Restoring the Body to Revitalize the Mind

All emotional and spiritual states have their physical counterparts. Functional MRIs of the brain show different areas lighting up with alterations in mood. Neurotransmitters in our brains relate to how we feel. Low serotonin levels, for example, result in anxiety and depression. Similarly, people in spiritual states of ecstasy, as well as drug-induced highs, have been shown to have huge outpourings of serotonin as well as another neurotransmitter called anandamide (n-arachidonoylethanolamine) or "the bliss chemical." Your physiology will mirror your psychological state. What if we help your physiology to feel better? We encourage you to learn how to help your body make more feel-good chemicals.

Medicines that Affect the Mind

Over the past thirty years, the use of antidepressants has increased significantly. The reason for this is because the development of selective serotonin reuptake inhibitors (SSRIs) have allowed for a relatively safe way to treat depression with fewer side effects than older classes of antidepressants. SSRIs such as fluoxetine (Prozac®), sertraline (Zoloft®), and escitalopram (Lexapro®) mainly increase serotonin levels. These led the way to drugs such as venlafaxine (Effexor®) and duloxetene (Cymbalta®), which mainly increase serotonin and norepinephrine levels. Other drugs, such as bupropion (Wellbutrin®), primarily affect dopamine levels.

Drugs can help people feel better. Certain drugs can also make patients feel worse. Beta-blockers such as propranolol, acne drugs such as isotretinoin (Accutane®), birth control pills, and even statin drugs can cause depression. So if you're feeling depressed, fatigued, achy, or anything unusual, always ask your physician or your pharmacist if the drug could be aggravating your problem.

We are always amazed at how different doctors treat the same condition, depending on their viewpoints. A perimenopausal woman complaining of depression and hot flashes may receive estrogen from her gynecologist, but antidepressants from her primary care doctor or psychiatrist. Both work. Why? Estrogen has an effect on serotonin, and SSRI drugs have an effect on both depression and hot flashes.

Drugs and psychotherapy are not the only way to help patients feel better. Besides teaching coping skills and lifestyle changing behaviors, we also find that correcting underlying functional imbalances can help overcome feelings of depression.

Supplements for Stress

In our experience, it is difficult to overcome chronic depression without supporting adrenal function and reducing inflammation. Patients suffering from depression are often also chronically stressed. Simply put, their adrenal glands are shot. We can support the adrenals by using adaptogenic herbs to increase the body's resistance to stress and trauma, helping to balance the endocrine and immune systems and maintain a state of balance within the body. Adaptogenic herbs tend to tone down hyperfunction-

> Clouds come floating into my life, no longer to carry rain or usher storm, but to add color to my sunset sky.
>
> – Rabindranath Tagore

ing systems, while improving systems that are functioning at too low a level.

Adaptogenic herbs have been used safely for centuries in various cultures. They go by names such as restorative herbs, chi tonics, rasayanas, and rejuvenating herbs. Some examples of adaptogenic herbs are American ginseng, Siberian ginseng, Asian ginseng (*Panax ginseng*), Indian ginseng (also called ashwaganda and withania), and *Rhodiola rosea* root extract.

Nutritional supplements can also be helpful for coping with stress. Nutritionists often advise taking more B vitamins during stress. Magnesium and zinc supplements are also often recommended.

Adrenal recovery can be supported with amino acids, such as L-methionine, L-histidine, and N-acetyltyrosine. Neurotransmitter function also can be improved with nutritional supplements. Amino acids, such as 5-hydroxytryptophan, suntheanine (L-theanine), and taurine, all help increase serotonin levels. Levels of the neurotransmitter dopamine can be elevated with vicia faba bean extract and N-acetylcysteine (NAC). NAC also increases glutathione, a powerful antioxidant and main driver of the body's toxin-neutralizing system.

We suggest that you work with a qualified health practitioner who understands when and how to use herbal and nutritional products. These products are not regulated by the FDA, and their quality may vary. For one particular herb, one company may use the root, while another may use the bark or the flower. Some companies maintain pharmaceu-

© Shutterstock/ PePI

tical-like quality, while others have pills that don't degrade well or even contain contaminants. In addition, supplements and even vitamins may have drug interactions.

Treating the Body to Heal the Mind

Treating the body with integrative therapies is often an excellent way to help deal with stress. Numerous physical modalities, also known as bodywork, help both mind and body. These include acupuncture, massage therapy, energy healing techniques, Feldenkrais therapy, Alexander therapy, Rolfing, yoga, and tai chi.

Practitioners of acupuncture have claimed for thousands of years that acupuncture needles affect both the mind and the body. Part of this is easy to explain. Acupuncture changes the blood flow in the brain. It also raises endorphins in the central nervous system, which makes us feel a little euphoric. This is what causes a runner's high, also called an endorphin rush. The philosophy of acupuncture goes deeper than endorphin changes, however. It connects the body and the emotions in a body-mind link we frequently see. Louise's case is a perfect example of how the mind and body connect.

Louise's Story: Carrying the World on Her Shoulders

Louise is a 45-year-old woman who came to see us with pain in her right scapula (shoulder blade) region. It had been present for almost eighteen months. She had seen her family doctor, as well as two orthopedic surgeons without any success. X-rays and MRIs were normal. A trial of physical therapy and anti-inflammatories had hardly helped. She seemed quite despondent.

Examining her, it became obvious that she had a trigger point—a small, painful knot in her infraspinatus (lower part of shoulder blade) muscle. We injected the point with some local anesthetic, and within a minute her pain was gone. The next week, Louise returned. After a few days of being pain-free, her shoulder ache had returned with a vengeance. We noticed that the path of the pain ran along the small intestine meridian. In acupuncture, this is a line that runs from the neck into the shoulder blade and down the arm into the pinky. We asked if she wanted to try acupuncture for the pain, just to see if it would help. Acupuncture

did work. The pain stayed away for a few more days, but returned again.

At her next visit, it became clear that her pain was not staying away. We explained to her that in acupuncture theory, the small intestine meridian sifts the "pure from the impure," helping digestion both physically and emotionally. (This aspect of acupuncture is discussed in more detail in Ring and Star 5.) We asked her if she thought she was having a difficult time digesting her emotions. The wording seemed to trigger something quite deep inside her. She lowered her head, beginning to weep, and then sobbed uncontrollably. We let her cry for a few minutes and then asked her what was troubling her. It was only then that she began to tell us about her abusive, alcoholic boyfriend.

The acupuncture treatment worked on many levels. It worked so well, in fact, that Louise went home, confronted her boyfriend, and told him to leave. With the resolution of her problem, her shoulder pain stayed away forever.

Transforming Chronic Stress

In this chapter, we want to help you learn how to transform chronic stress. First, you need to decide where you are on the Stress Curve. Check the chart of the Stress Response Curve on this page. (Check back to Ring 2 if you are having trouble deciding.) Your aim should be to get to the left side—the Exhilarated section—where stress is invigorating. Let's look at how you can do this.

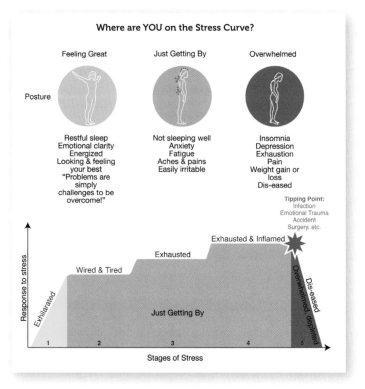

Where are YOU on the Stress Curve?

Feeling Great	Just Getting By	Overwhelmed

Posture

Restful sleep	Not sleeping well	Insomnia
Emotional clarity	Anxiety	Depression
Energized	Fatigue	Exhaustion
Looking & feeling	Aches & pains	Pain
your best	Easily irritable	Weight gain or
"Problems are		loss
simply		Dis-eased
challenges to be		
overcome!"		

Tipping Point:
Infection
Emotional Trauma
Accident
Surgery, etc.

Response to stress / Stages of Stress

Exhilarated · Wired & Tired · Exhausted · Exhausted & Inflamed · Just Getting By · Overwhelmed, depleted · Dis-eased

1   2   3   4   5

Stage 1

Riding the Wave of Exhilarating Stress

In general, exhilarating or invigorating stress is the positive side of the stress response. We may have an exciting challenge in our lives—a new job, graduate school, or another child in the family. We are usually energized, motivated, and excited by these changes. At times like this, it's important not to neglect yourself. Recognize that you can only sustain this level of effort for so long before you move to the right on the curve. Maintain a sense of balance and control over your life. Develop a strategy for the long term.

Stage 2

Transforming the "Wired and Tired"

You know you have pushed too hard when you find yourself on the Wired and Tired part of the curve. Fortunately, you can usually reverse these early changes, quickly and easily.

We always suggest that you start by examining your life. We do not suggest making big changes—in fact, just the opposite. A much more effective approach is to make small but meaningful changes to address the major cause(s) of the stress. If tension or a toxic relationship is driving the stress, now is the time to deal with it. You want to address the cause of your stress before it results in burnout.

Lifestyle. Maintain a healthy lifestyle and keep your daily healthy lifestyle routine going (see Star 1). This is where exercise, especially aerobic exercise, can help burn off the extra adrenaline you are carrying around. Breath work will help you simultaneously revitalize and relax your body.

Body chemistry. Consider supplements and/or adaptogenic herbs to prevent depletion. We often use a blend of Chinese herbs. These include rehmannia root *(Rehmannia glutinosa)*, schisandra fruit *(Schisandra chinensis)*, jujube fruit *(Zizyphus spinosa)*, dong quai root *(Angelica sinensis)*, Chinese asparagus root *(Asparagus cochinchinensis)*, scrophularia root *(Scrophularia ningpoensis)*, Asian ginseng root *(Panax*

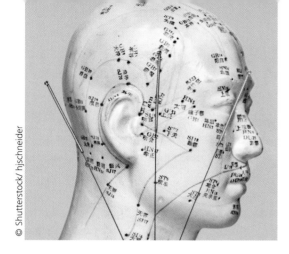
© Shutterstock/ hjschneider

ginseng), Chinese salvia root *(Salvia miltior-rhiza)*, poria fungus *(Wolfiporia cocos)*, polygala root *(Polygala tenuifolia)*, and platycodon root *(Platycodon grandiflorum)*. Other options include American ginseng, Siberian ginseng or eleutherococcus, ashwaganda or Indian ginseng, astragalus, passion flower, rhodiola, valerian, skullcap and magnolia bark, and many others.

Additional nutritional supplements. These include vitamin C, zinc, and B vitamins. If you are under a lot of stress, you may need up to 200 mg of vitamin B6 (pyridoxine) daily, or even up to 1500 mg of vitamin B5 (pantothenic acid) daily. These vitamins help you metabolize stress hormones. Phosphatidylserine, L-theanine, and GABA can also be helpful for reducing anxiety and helping you relax.

Healing therapies. Acupuncture, energy healing, and massage or other bodywork can be instrumental in helping you reduce bodily tension and achieve restorative sleep. The effects of one session can last for several weeks. These therapies promote deep relaxation and balance that sense of being wired by balancing stress hormones and calming your nervous system.

Stage 3

Transforming Fatigue and Exhaustion

The sense of exhaustion we are referring to here isn't temporary fatigue. It is a state of deep de-pletion that occurs over a period of months or even years. Over the long term, it is usually not one single factor that wears us down and results in exhaustion. Ask yourself if the stress is occurring too often. Is it too much, or lasting too long? You can tolerate high levels of stress for a time, but consider setting a limit. Apply the same rule of thumb for psychological stress that you would for a physical health problem. Any condition that persists longer than three months is considered chronic. If the condition, whether physical or psychological, isn't improving, or if it keeps coming back, seek professional help.

Lifestyle. To optimize your quality of life, despite the challenges you are facing, put yourself first. This is really a time to say "*no*" and "*stop.*" At this stage, you definitely need to take more time for self-care, to look after yourself. Take ten to twenty minutes three to four times a day to meditate and relax. Exercise, but gently. *Aim to do only about 60 percent of what you think you should do.* In other words, take it easy on yourself. If you feel tired when you exercise, cut down even further. This is also a good time to reduce stimulants, such as chocolate and caffeine, especially after noon. Avoid junk food and cut out alcohol. Find other ways to support your energy. Consider nutritional supplements and adaptogenic herbal supplements.

Body chemistry. To help your body cope, consider adaptogenic herbal supplements. We suggest slightly different ones to those when you are "wired and tired;" American ginseng, Siberian ginseng or eleutherococcus, ashwaganda or Indian ginseng, astragalus, schizandra, rhodiola, and licorice are helpful. (Licorice can raise blood pressure, so avoid it if you have hypertension.) We routinely suggest a combination of cordyceps mycelium extract *(Paecilomyces hepiali)*, Asian ginseng root extract *(Panax ginseng)*, and rhodiola root extract *(Rhodiola rosea)* to our patients at this point.

Consider additional nutritional supplements.

These are similar to when you are "wired and tired," and include Vitamin C, zinc, and B vitamins. You may need up to 200 mg of vitamin B6 (pyridoxine) daily, or even up to 1500 mg of vitamin B5 (pantothenic acid) daily. Phosphatidylserine, GABA, and L-theanine can all be helpful here.

Healing therapies. Once again, healing therapies can have a profound effect in transforming your health. We will discuss these in depth in Star 5.

Transforming Exhaustion and Inflammation

In the exhaustion and inflammation stage of the Stress Curve, your body is screaming at you. It's saying, "Help, I'm on fire!" Pay attention to your diet, mood, and lifestyle. At this point, we suggest following the same steps you would during the Exhausted phase. In addition, add in these steps:

Lifestyle. Make sure you are addressing insulin resistance, which can be caused by high cortisol levels. (We will discuss this crucial issue in detail in Star 4.) Ensure your diet is high in anti-inflammatory foods (see Star 3). Continue to exercise gently. Aim for 60 to 80 percent of what you think you can do.

Mind-body techniques. At this point, the Relaxation Response becomes all-important. Learn to do this twice daily for ten to thirty minutes each time (check back to page 49 for a guide to learning the Relaxation Response).

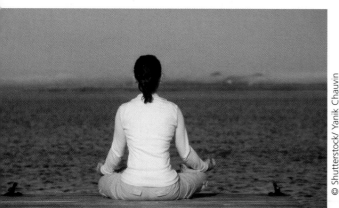

Body chemistry. If you are depressed, consider an antidepressant or nutritional supplements such as 5-HTP (5 hydroxytryptophan) to help increase serotonin. Higher levels of serotonin will also help reduce inflammation.

Nutritional anti-inflammatories. These include mercury-free fish oils, iso-alpha acids from hops (e.g., Kaprex by Metagenics), turmeric (curcumin) with added pepper extract for improved absorption, bee propolis extracts with caffeic acid phenethyl ester (CAPE), and supplements containing *Boswellia serrata* extract. There are many other anti-inflammatory supplements. Work with an experienced nutritionist or integrative medicine physician to find the supplements that are best for you.

Anti-inflammatory medical foods. These are powders containing amino acids and supplements that can be used as a meal replacement. Examples are UltraInflamX® PLUS 360 by Metagenics and Inflammacore by Orthomolecular Products.

Healing therapies. These become an even more important part of your journey toward a return to health. (We discuss them more in Star 5.)

Transforming Depletion and Overwhelm

If you are depleted and overwhelmed because you're all the way at the right side of the Stress Curve, chances are good you're also ill. What can you do to speed your recovery?

Lifestyle. At this point, you definitely need to be under the care of a physician. Everything we stated earlier about lifestyle becomes even more important. Once again, follow the steps outlined earlier in this chapter on how to deal with everyday stress. Only restorative exercise should be done at this phase. In other words, do not overexert yourself at the gym. You might think you need to get stronger to get past this phase, but what your body really needs is rest. Gentle yoga, tai chi, or chi gong exercises are all very helpful.

Body chemistry. If you are very depressed, you may need an antidepressant. You might need testing and treatment for neurally mediated hypotension. Your thyroid may be sluggish. If this is the case, your TSH (thyroid stimulating hormone) will be raised, but other thyroid hormones will be normal.

Nutritional supplements. Rosemary leaf extract, selenium, zinc, bladderwrack (kelp), and iodine can all help correct thyroid problems. To help with the fatigue, we use a combination of licorice root extract, withania (or ashwaganda), rehmannia, and Chinese yam extract. Licorice can make your blood pressure go up and should not be used if you already have high blood pressure. Most people who are depleted and overwhelmed have low blood pressure, however.

Healing therapies. This is where we have found healing therapies to have an irreplaceable role in your recovery. We have not found any conventional medical treatments that can do for you what integrative therapies offer. We have found that therapies such as acupuncture, energy healing, ACE^{SM} (acupuncture, chiropractic, and energy healing) treatments, and FSM (frequency specific microcurrent) work well to restore normal function by restoring adrenal and thyroid function, balancing the autonomic and immune systems, and reducing inflammation. These are discussed in more detail in Star 5.

Learning to Transform Acute Stress

In Chinese calligraphy, the symbol for a crisis is made up of two different symbols, one meaning "danger," and the other "opportunity." A health crisis is no different. We call this a Transformational Moment. Russell's story is a great example of how a Transformational Moment can change your health and your life.

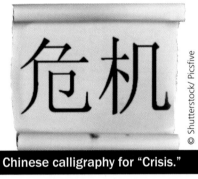

© Shutterstock/ Picsfive

Chinese calligraphy for "Crisis."

Russell's Story: Dealing with Transformational Stress

As far back as I can remember, I have been well. When I was 55, my wife persuaded me go for a physical. No big deal, until I got the call from the doctor's office saying that my PSA (prostate specific antigen) test was raised. It was 6.4, and it should be less than 4. I was told to see a urologist to have my prostate gland checked.

The urologist was nice enough, saying that he needed to do an ultrasound and biopsy as soon as possible. The PSA could go up for reasons other than cancer, but the biopsy result would let us know. So I waited with bated breath for the result.

The doctor was very clear when he gave me the result. "Cancer." "A milder form." "Gleason stage 4." He gave me a few options: a radical prostatectomy or radiation seeds. Possibly hormonal treatment later on, giving me a male menopause. "Frankly," he said, "if it were me I would have the prostatectomy [prostate removal]. You're young, and that way it will be out!" He reviewed the side effects: possible impotence [not being able to have an erection] and incontinence [loss of bladder control.] When we discussed a second opinion, he answered curtly, "Any doctor worth anything will tell you what I told you."

I struggled very hard to keep a sense of self-control, trying to understand what he was saying. I was trembling as I tried to take notes. My mind was racing. I was thinking about the way the words "impotence" and "incontinence" kept coming up. "I am a healthy person," I wanted to say. "You don't understand."

I was pretty upset by all this—none of the options seemed acceptable. I began researching prostate cancer on my own. Based on what I learned, I realized that although it made sense on one level to remove the cancer surgically and be done with it, there wasn't a consensus that this was really the best approach. Something deep inside me said I could wait and watch. In fact, many urologists were advocating this approach, called "active surveillance." I could feel myself regaining control of my emotions. Instead of feeling passive and stupid each time I saw the doctor, I was starting to feel smart and empowered. It was a huge turning point in my life. I began to see a urologist who felt perfectly comfortable with us both watching the progress, or lack of it.

A friend gave me a book to read by Dr. Dean Ornish, *The Spectrum*, in which he details stories of patients who reversed their prostate cancers using lifestyle, dietary, and meditative approaches. I had nutrigenomic testing, which showed that my genes have a proclivity toward making toxic estrogen by-products—the by-products that are associated with prostate cancer. So now I follow a very healthy, predominantly vegetarian diet. I drink pomegranate juice daily and take a bunch of supplements that have already altered my estrogen by-product profile. Three months after starting the program, my PSA level is now down from 6.4 to 1.9. What's more, I feel better than I have in the last twenty years!

When I was first diagnosed with prostate cancer, my wife talked me into an acupuncture treatment. I remember the doctor said something about low kidney chi, but I didn't really care. I had the acupuncture treatment and fell into a deep sleep.

Later that day I felt as though I had unlocked some sensation in my kidney areas. They both had this sense of warmth around them. For the first time, I could actually feel this sense of panic and fear about cancer, yet I also felt oddly detached, as if it were no longer controlling me. I just sat on the couch, seeing my life in front of me. I didn't move or think, just sinking into this sensation of warmth in my back. Then almost without noticing it, my vantage point changed. I suddenly realized that I could cope. I would be OK. I felt as if I was in this peaceful, prayerful state. Fear and panic had somehow transformed into courage. It was as if the huge wave of shock that hit me was moving on. The water was now still. And out of its depths, courage had arisen. That courage has remained with me constantly, but a funny thing has happened. I don't feel fear-less. I still feel fear. But every time I feel fear and panic, I just sit with the emotion, and it transforms itself. It is as if I still need the fear in order to gain courage!

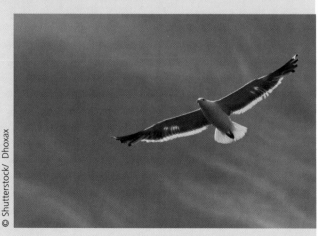

© Shutterstock/ Dhoxax

Transformational Moments

Sometimes in life, we come to the proverbial crossroads, a place where we need to make a choice. We can go one way or the other, but not stay the same. The problem needn't be one that concerns your health directly. It could be something that relates to work, relationships, finances, or some aspect of your life that suddenly careens out of control. We are suddenly faced with Transformational Moments.

Sometimes Transformational Moments occur when we are listening to music, meditating, walking, or doing some activity when the thinking mind is essentially switched off. However, at other times, these moments occur when we feel overwhelmed.

A wonderful teacher once said to us, "Inherent in every problem is the solution. Inherent in every stressful situation is the energy required to overcome and transcend this same situation."

We do not choose Transformational Moments. Generally, they happen to us. They force us to think and look outside the box. By definition, there is no obvious solution, so we are forced to find a different way.

Seize the **Transformational Moment**

We have seen many patients harness the power of shock and stress and use it to recover and bounce back to a new and better level of being. Here are some tips for seizing your Transformational Moment:

1. When you hit a Transformational Moment, become aware of your emotions and feelings. Do not judge what you are feeling or try to label it.

2. Pay attention to your senses. Transformational Moments can allow you to achieve a new state of being. Observe your sensations, smells, tastes, sights, and sounds.

3. Surrender to this feeling. Learn to sink into it.

4. Learn to transform the emotion. Remember that e-motion = energy in motion.

(This is very different from wallowing in it.)

5. Allow yourself to transcend logic. You may feel confused at first, but insight will develop.

6. Adding healing therapies such as acupuncture and energy healing can help you attain this new state of awareness.

7. Faith and prayer are profoundly valuable for some in times of peak stress.

8. Remember, a Transformational Moment is a process. It is time-independent—it may occur in seconds or even take months to years.

9. If you are not succeeding, not coping, or feeling out of control, seek professional help.

well. Eat well. Get well. Walk well. Run well. well. Live well. Stretch well. Dance well. Get Be well. Stay well. Breathe well. Stay well. well. Think well. Love well. Relax well. Live

Alex Learns to Transform His Viewpoint

Alex continues to pursue Health and Wellness

As Alex exercised every day, he found his perspective changing slightly. He seemed to approach life from a more upbeat perspective. The runner's high (or cycler's high in his case) he was getting from his regular exercise and meditation seemed to carry into his day. As he explained to us, "Ever have those days when parking places appear just as you arrive at them—when everything seems to unfold in front of you just as it should? I'm feeling more and more of those!"

One day, Alex saw his boss berating a young new intern. He felt his blood boil. Normally, he would have swallowed his anger, but he followed his boss into his office, closing the door gently behind him. He asked his boss to sit down, and then quietly started articulating his feelings. He explained that he was a long-term, loyal employee, but that as a person, he found it difficult to cope with his boss's outbursts. He felt a need to protect the younger employees and that was why he was there that day in the office. His boss initially fumed, sputtering with indignation, but Alex kept reiterating his need to make sure that what he did was best for the business. Eventually his boss calmed down, looked Alex in the eye and said, "You're right. I wish you said this to me ten years ago." That day became the turning point for Alex. No longer an underling, he became a trusted confidant and ultimately a vice president in the company.

Alex started bouncing out of bed each morning with renewed vigor, looking forward to each day on the job. His job was now an exhilarating challenge and no longer a chore. He remembered what it was like to be on the left side of the stress curve. Alex had successfully transformed stress into success!

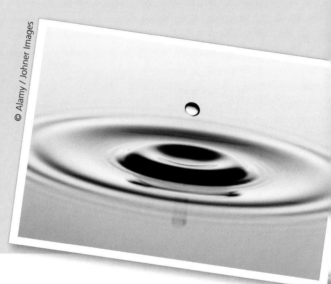

© Alamy / Johner Images

When we change our daily lives—the way we think, speak and act—we change the world.

– Thich Nhat Hanh

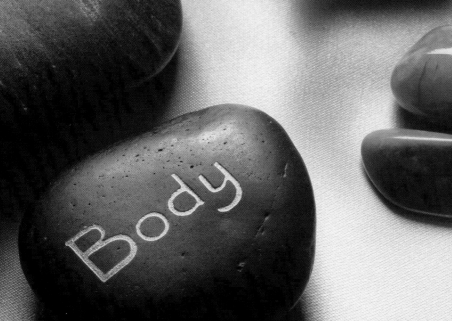

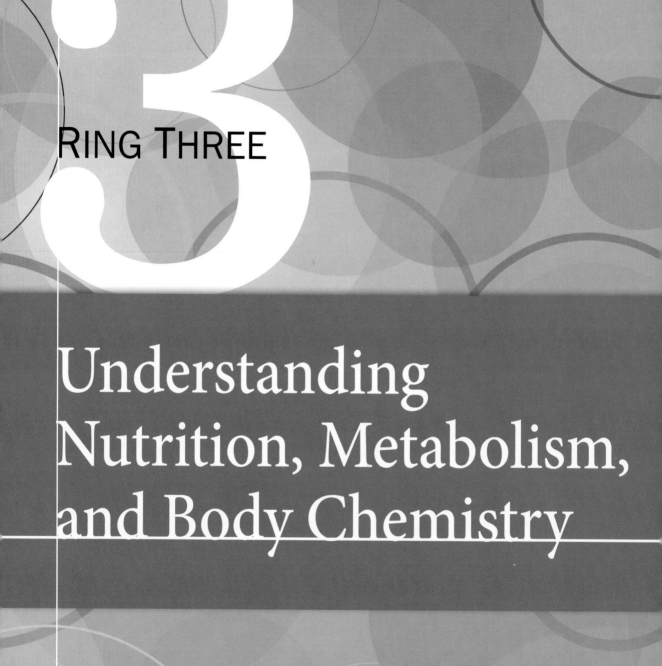

RING THREE

Understanding Nutrition, Metabolism, and Body Chemistry

How Your Genetics, Your Food, Your Environment, and Your Lifestyle Interact to Affect How You Look, Feel, and Function

Metabolic and Immune Assessment

Your genes, your food, and your lifestyle influence each other. Nutrition (what we eat), metabolism (how our bodies process what we eat), and our immune systems (how our bodies react to the environment) affect how our genes work and vice versa. Knowing how well these processes are working, and making changes if needed, is important for your long-term well-being.

Do You Know What You're Eating?

Many millennia ago, our hunter-gatherer ancestors lived on game and whatever they could gather, such as berries. Skip ahead to 9,000 years ago. That puts us in Jericho, where archeologists have found signs of the first large-scale farming and a dietary shift to grains. Now fast forward to 150 years ago. It's the Industrial Revolution, and machines are on the scene, creating a factory-based culture that has changed everything from how we work to what we eat. Suddenly it's not just royalty and the rich who have access to sugar and white flour.

Over the past century, our palates have grown more and more accustomed to an array of highly artificial, chemicalized, manufactured foods, flavors, and nutrients. Food manufacturers have helped this process along by creating foods that are high in fat, salt, and sugar, the three primal tastes our bodies crave. At the same time, we are bombarded with messages from our doctors and others about the importance of eating less fat, less salt, less sugar, and fewer calories.

The food manufacturers are clearly winning this battle. The shape of Americans has changed more in the past twenty years than it did in the past two centuries. Today 65 percent of all Americans are overweight or obese, and one in four Americans has diabetes. Another 57 million are at risk of developing this devastating chronic disease. Why is this happening?

Why We Can't Stop Eating

Recently, we sat at a midwestern airport watching people wolf down burgers and fries—others were gobbling down jelly doughnuts, hardly taking a breath between bites. It would have been easy to assume they are just gluttons, with no self-discipline. But is this really true? They may not have the self-discipline they wish for, but they're also actually victims of addiction to the sugar, salt, and fat in the fast food

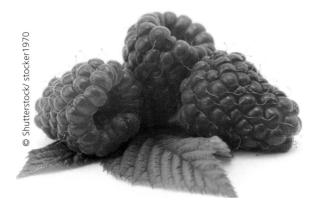

© Shutterstock/ stocker1970

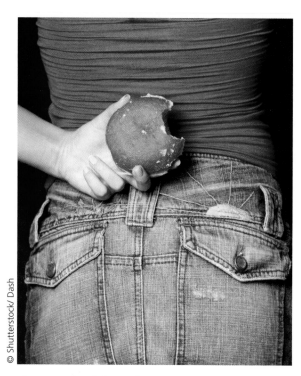

found that those who were given a drop of sugar water stopped crying far sooner than those who received no sugar. Studies of rats show that they will stand on electrified pads and withstand recurrent shocks in order to keep eating sugary foods. The key point here is that from the day we are born, we are hardwired with a preference for sweets. Throughout our lives, sweets remain the ultimate comfort food. It's no wonder we can't stop eating junk food.

We Are Getting Fatter

Obesity, prediabetes, and diabetes are among the fastest growing, most important health issues of our time. We are in the midst of a global pandemic. While industrialized nations are clearly at the epicenter of this trend, other countries are affected as well. In the Marshall Islands, a tiny nation in the middle of the Pacific Ocean, one in three women and one in four men now have diabetes. About 22 percent of the population of Saudi Arabia now has diabetes. These issues matter. Diabetes increases the risk for strokes and cancers and doubles the risk of heart disease. Of every three people with diabetes, two will die of heart disease or a stroke. The cost of treating diabetes and its associated complications is already huge and gets more so all the time as the population ages and gets fatter. How did we get to this diabetes epidemic?

they eat. And this is happening to entire populations worldwide, not just in this country, but also in Europe, Asia, and Africa.

Many studies have shown that sugar, salt, and fat all have addictive properties. So guess what ingredients food companies like to add to our foods? They know exactly what makes us gulp down their products. The crunchy textures, tantalizing aromas, and foods that seem to melt in our mouths—they are an irresistible invitation to the next bite. Food marketers manipulate our sensual drives and survival instincts to make us want to buy their products.

On an instinctive level, we still see food for what it is: a basic survival need. So while addiction to food should not be a problem, our addiction to the salt, sugar, and fat, which are contained in processed food, is making us fat and sick.

Sugar may be the most addictive food of all, and the preference for sugar appears to be hardwired directly into our survival instincts. One study of newborns who were receiving a tiny pinprick to test their blood

The most effective approach to stopping any epidemic is to trace the problem back to its source. We have already conquered diseases such as smallpox, yellow fever, and polio. We have controlled childhood infections, such as measles, mumps, and diphtheria, that used to strike terror in every parent's heart.

But this new epidemic is different. It reflects a conflict between our genetic hardwiring and our lifestyle. Our hardwiring is our genes, and our genes haven't really changed in the past few thousand years. Unfortunately, the software that interacts with the hardware is changing rapidly. So what is our software? It includes lifestyle, diet, exercise, stress levels, and toxins in our environment. The results aren't always pretty.

Our Profoundly Altered Diet

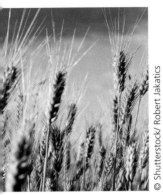

© Shutterstock/ Robert Jakatics

The short version of this story is that our genes, which haven't changed for many thousands of years, are dealing with a whole new environment. We still walk around with essentially the same genetic instructions as our ancient hunter and gatherer ancestors. Their diet was the essence of simplicity—berries, nuts, seeds, and other edible plants, as well as fish, birds, and game. Everything that could be consumed was eaten, so parts that we discard today were consumed at every meal, including husks and seeds, which contain fiber. Organ meats, high in trace minerals and other vital nutrients, were also routinely eaten. This provided a diet high in complex nutrients. Our ancestors also had to work hard to get enough calories and rarely were able to overeat.

Our bodies are still genetically programmed to eat these kinds of complex foods. Today, however, we eat foods that have been profoundly al-

> *Your body is a temple, not a drive-through.*
>
> **– Author Unknown**

tered. Foods are often heavily processed and are high in sugar, simple starches, salt, and fats—and devoid of nutrients. Our crops are often genetically modified and grown in soil depleted of minerals and other organic factors. Our grains are milled, discarding the nutritious seed and the fibrous hull, leaving only a simple starch. Food is often canned or frozen in a factory and eaten months later.

Devitalized refined sugars and starches are unfortunately standard in the Western diet and are becoming more prevalent in the rest of the world. Most people now take these nutrient-depleted, unhealthy foods for granted. Prime examples include bottled fruit juice, most boxed cereals and pancakes, cookies, and potato chips. To restore flavor, most food is laced with sugar, salt, and fat. Manufacturers add chemical flavorings and preservatives. The outcome is something we refer to with author Michael Pollan's term, "edible food-like substances." These "new to nature" chemicals serve to confuse our epigenetic signals, sending messages that our body's genes don't know how to deal with. Is this causing a rise of chronic illness in our society? We think so!

Diabetes: A Disease that Affects Rich and Poor Alike

We saw firsthand the effects of diet when we were medical residents in the hospitals of South Africa in the 1970s. At that time, because of the scourge of apartheid, there were two separate hospital systems—one for whites and one for blacks. Although these facilities were geographically separated by only a few miles, the disease patterns we saw in these different hospitals were worlds apart.

The majority of patients in the white hospitals presented with Western diseases of affluence: heart attacks, strokes, and diabetes. In the black hospitals, patients were admitted for diseases of malnutrition, infectious illness, and chronic tuberculosis. That led us to wonder to what extent these diseases were related to diet and lifestyle. It was extremely rare to see a black person with coronary artery disease. While we were in medical school, when a black patient came into the hospital with chest pains, it was never a heart attack. It simply did not happen. This was soon to change.

As the black population in South Africa began adopting a sedentary Western lifestyle and eating a diet of Western refined food, they began to develop the same diseases as the white population. Their rates of heart disease, strokes, diabetes, and cancer all increased.

Similar patterns have become appar-

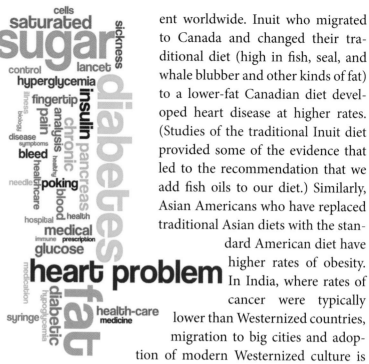

ent worldwide. Inuit who migrated to Canada and changed their traditional diet (high in fish, seal, and whale blubber and other kinds of fat) to a lower-fat Canadian diet developed heart disease at higher rates. (Studies of the traditional Inuit diet provided some of the evidence that led to the recommendation that we add fish oils to our diet.) Similarly, Asian Americans who have replaced traditional Asian diets with the standard American diet have higher rates of obesity. In India, where rates of cancer were typically lower than Westernized countries, migration to big cities and adoption of modern Westernized culture is causing a trend in higher rates of cancer.

Metabolism and the
Hidden Causes of Illness

Your metabolism is the ongoing set of chemical reactions that happen in your body to keep you alive. Your metabolism is what keeps your heart beating, your lungs breathing, your brain thinking, and your body repair functions operating normally. These processes allow us to grow, mend injuries, and recover from illness. They essentially comprise every aspect of the body's function. This is the miracle of nourishment—the process by which what we eat becomes part of our cells and tissues. Metabolism provides the energy for our bodies. It is essential for every breath and every move we make.

We view metabolism as the leverage point for improving the health of our patients. The key is to identify imbalances during the pre-illness phase, before the damage is done, because

once the disease process deepens, it becomes much more difficult to reverse. Functional and conventional lab tests provide the lens through which we can actually see how the body is functioning; in this way, we can monitor metabolism and body chemistry to determine which systems are out of balance. With this functional approach, we can devise a strategy to restore normal function at the earliest opportunity.

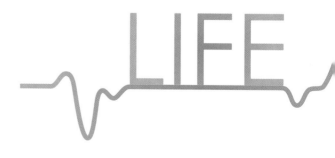

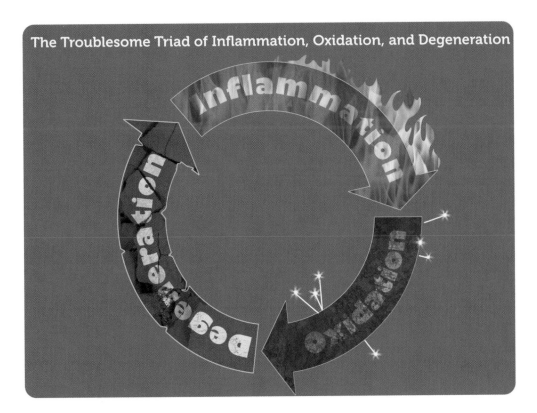

The **Troublesome Triad** of Inflammation, Oxidation, and Degeneration

Inflammation: The Body on Fire

To understand the ravages of aging and disease, let's look at the body's response to injury or infection. In both of these cases, the immune system responds by ramping up the process of inflammation. Signs of inflammation include redness, swelling, pain, and fever or heat. When you develop a fever during a viral or bacterial illness, your body is turning on its defense mechanisms. That is also the case with swelling, redness, pain, and warmth when you sprain your ankle or cut yourself. In most cases, inflammation is a sign that the body's immune system is working efficiently to defend itself against foreign invaders.

When inflammation is chronic, however, it can be damaging to the body. This is because the inflammatory response releases many natural chemicals that affect the whole body. If you're getting over a cold, which most people do in a few days, the inflammatory response doesn't have much of a long-term impact. But if you have a chronic illness such as gum disease or are under chronic stress, your whole body is constantly exposed to those inflammatory substances. That's when painful chronic conditions such as aching joints, as well as ulcers, colitis, asthma, and eczema, can develop. We now know that inflammation is also associated with many other major diseases, such as heart disease, cancer, and neurological disorders such as Alzheimer's disease.

Autoimmune conditions, such as multiple sclerosis and thyroid disease, are a different aspect of this process. With autoimmune illnesses, the immune function goes haywire, and the body seems to be raging out of control, attacking itself rather than the foreign molecules.

97

Inflammation and Infection: The Inflammatory Cascade

Acute inflammation is usually a good thing when it is associated with any type of injury or infection. Once the immune system recognizes an infection, the body begins producing chemicals called cytokines that signal a state of red alert. As the call goes out, these messenger chemicals course through the bloodstream, recruiting infection fighters and launching an immune artillery. This shift to a state of emergency is referred to as the inflammatory cascade.

Our body always tries to maintain harmony. So, if there is an on switch for acute inflammation, there is also an off switch to put out the fire. This process is also performed by cytokines. Some cytokines drive (upregulate) inflammation; others switch off (or downregulate) the inflammatory process, putting out the fire.

Lingering Inflammation

Chronic inflammation acts like a simmering fire that burns in our bodies, stimulating a cascade of chemical reactions that can destroy cells and compromise tissues over time. Inflammation can occur locally, in one area, or throughout the body. When inflammation occurs within a specific area or organ, it is described with a term ending in the Latin suffix "-itis." For instance, gastritis refers to inflamed gastric tissue in the stomach. Localized inflammation can lead to further disease. As an example, we know that at least 40 percent of stomach cancer is associated with the chronic inflammation caused by gastric ulcers.

Inflammation can also occur throughout the entire body. Systemic, low-grade inflammation can, over time, result in widespread disease. Coronary artery disease and stroke were once thought to be linked primarily to high cholesterol, but new studies show that inflammation within the arteries can have as great an impact on blocked arteries as that of elevated cholesterol. Chronic inflammation has also been associated with cancer, Alzheimer's disease and neurological disorders, insulin resistance and diabetes, and asthma and allergies.

Because chronic inflammation can have a devastating effect on the body, it is important to understand what triggers it.

Here are some of the **causes of chronic inflammation:**

- Genetic tendencies to develop inflammation
- Impaired digestion and detoxification processes
- Autoimmune diseases
- Chronic infections such as gingivitis (gum disease)
- Chronic stress (as we discussed in Ring 2)
- Poor diet
- Smoking
- High blood sugar
- Medications—for example, birth control pills can aggravate inflammation in certain women

All of these factors keep your body from switching off the inflammatory process. Instead, your cells are constantly exposed to inflammatory cytokines and other damaging natural chemicals. In the long run, these factors cause chronic diseases.

Dietary Causes of Chronic Inflammation

Research over the past few decades has linked chronic inflammation to impaired function of many metabolic processes, including digestion and detoxification. When these metabolic systems aren't working correctly, the end result can be chronic inflammation.

When diagnosing an illness caused by

chronic inflammation, we often start by looking at what the patient is eating. Unfortunately, the Standard American Diet is filled with foods that cause inflammation. Saturated fats, trans fats, and high sugar in the diet cause higher blood levels of an inflammatory chemical called arachidonic acid. (Many nonsteroidal anti-inflammatory drugs, such as aspirin and ibuprofen, work by counteracting this chemical.) Processed foods, junk foods, lunch meats, hot dogs, and sausages are filled with chemicals such as nitrates that promote chronic inflammation and disease. In addition, many people have antibodies to certain foods that can aggravate a chronically inflamed state.

Good Fats, Bad Fats

We hear the low-fat message so often that we forget our bodies need dietary fat—the good kind, that is. Good fats include the omega-3 fatty acids from fish oil, flax seeds, and nuts, which tend to be anti-inflammatory. The oleic acid in olive oil, as well as the monounsaturated fats in avocados are also good fats.

Bad fats on the other hand are saturated fats (found in meat and dairy), and foods high in pro-inflammatory omega-6 fatty acids. (These are found in highly processed foods, trans-fats and heavily processed vegetable oils such as corn oil.) Not surprisingly, fast food, junk food, and prepared foods such as frozen meals are high in omega-6 fatty acids.

The ratio of omega-3 to omega-6 fats can play an important role in driving inflammation. Today, our diet tends to have a predominance of omega-6 fats. For example, thirty years ago, most eggs had a ratio of omega-3 to omega-6 of 1:6. Now that ratio is more like 1:15, or more! The "same" egg is more pro-inflammatory because the chicken's feed has changed, and the chicken is stressed, cooped up in a cage with lights constantly turned on. Similarly, our highly processed diet can trigger chronic inflammation in our own bodies. (In Star 3, we suggest antidotes to this problem.)

Inflammation and Weight Gain

Weight gain plays a role in system-wide inflammation, especially if it collects around the belly (resulting in the so-called apple shape.) We used to think of fat as inert tissue that just stored excess calories, but it is actually fairly active. Among other things, fat tissue produces inflammatory cytokines. This inflammatory effect tends to increase the propensity to gain weight, which then creates further inflammation. It's a vicious cycle. This cycle leads to many problems we see today that occur in clusters, such as type 2 diabetes and Alzheimer's disease (sometimes now even referred to as type 3 diabetes) or cholesterol problems and coronary artery disease.

Lab Tests for Inflammation

We can easily test for your level of inflammation. One way to measure inflammation is to use conventional blood tests for a marker known as high-sensitivity C-reactive protein, or hs-CRP. This is a nonspecific test—it tells us that a patient is inflamed, but not why. An indirect way to test for inflammation is to look at the patient's omega-3 index by testing the ratio of omega-3 to omega-6 fatty acids in the blood. Newer tests are becoming available to test for cytokine abnormalities. By measuring these, we can see which part of the immune system is being activated. Then we can work backward and figure out why.

Oxidative Stress: The Body Rusting

Another of the primary contributors to aging and illness is oxidative stress, which might be described as the body rusting. If you leave your car outside, unprotected and exposed to the elements, patches of rust can develop. Leave it out long enough, and the rust will eat into the structure and eventually corrode it. Similarly, our own bodies can "rust" due to internal oxidation reactions. When cells burn glucose for fuel—oxidize it—by-products are produced, just as a car produces exhaust fumes from the gas it burns. In the human body, the exhaust fumes from oxidation are called free radicals. Free radicals act like chemical terrorists, making random attacks on cell membranes and other tissues, aging our bodies and causing chronic illness and even cancer as they do so.

Free radicals are natural by-products of fighting infection or of chronic inflammation. They also occur with any kind of extreme exposure, such as overexposure to sunlight or ultraviolet rays or by the exertion of extreme sports, such as marathons and triathlons. Oxidative stress also results from exposure to chemicals, including food additives, pesticides, and preser-

> *He who takes medicine and neglects his diet wastes the skill of his doctors.*
>
> – Chinese proverb

vatives, as well as organic and chemical toxins that have been found in the tap water of many major cities. In general, chronic stress increases oxidative stress on the body.

The good news is that the body can turn off oxidative stress. Again, a lot of this has to do with our genes. Some of us have SNPs (genetic variants) that affect our oxidative stress, making us either prone to excessive oxidation or even resistant to it.

Fortunately, because free radicals are a normal part of metabolism, the body is well equipped to handle them. The human body has plenty of antioxidant chemicals, such as glutathione and vitamin C, that are designed to corral the free radicals and neutralize them before they can do much damage. At the same time, just as inflammation can be beneficial, so can oxidation, especially when the body is defending against bacteria, toxins, chemicals, or cancerous cells. For example, when fighting off viruses, the immune system uses oxygen as a form of chemical warfare to blow up these microbes.

Once again, the body has an elegant system of checks and balances. So, while oxidation can be useful to the body, there are times when the body's antioxidant mechanisms can't keep up with all the free radicals due to poor diet, illness, vitamin deficiencies, or other factors. It is during these times that oxidative stress is not held in check, and we can develop degeneration, cancer and chronic illness.

Degeneration

Our own experience living in different cultures around the world has shown us that aging and degeneration do not have to go together. People who eat a traditional, nonprocessed diet, main-

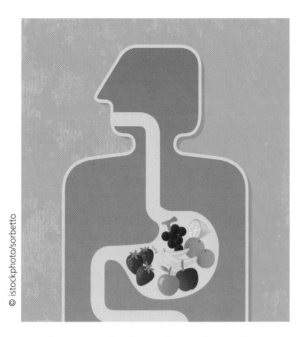

© istockphoto/sorbetto

an assembly line that breaks down food, converts it into useable nutrients, and disposes of the spent food as waste. This system is the source of all your nourishment and all the nutrients you have available for repair due to injury, illness, or aging. This miraculous system is also one of the major sources of your physical energy.

Maldigestion and Malabsorption

In order to assimilate the necessary nutrients from our food, we first need to digest it, and then absorb it. An inability to do so is called maldigestion and then malabsorption. When these problems first arise, they cause burping, heartburn, and bloating. Ultimately, they can make us get sick, because they keep us from having the necessary nutrients to help us regenerate and heal. Let's look at this process in a little more depth.

Stomach Acid

Mundane, underappreciated, even maligned, the hydrochloric acid (HCl) that is produced in the stomach begins the digestive process for everything we eat. Without it, we have trouble digesting food properly.

Malfunction. Although criticized as a cause of indigestion, stomach acid is actually one of the secrets of good digestion. Stomach acid is necessary to break down food to release its nutrients, particularly proteins essential for muscle repair and minerals essential for strong bones. This acid also destroys invading bacteria and other bad bugs.

Yet to watch the television ads, you might think that everyone in our society has an excess of stomach acid. We are implored to take various antacids or acid-blocking medications to stop heartburn, burping, and a host of related maladies. Although it is true that these medications have been miraculous in curing peptic ulcers and severe gastroesophageal reflux disease

tain low stress levels, and are physically active tend to age more slowly, retaining their youthful appearance and good joint health. They go gray later in life (sometimes decades later), and their skin retains its natural resilience. They also experience fewer degenerative diseases, such as heart attacks, strokes, and cancer, compared with their counterparts of a similar age and income level in industrial societies. This phenomenon is documented by author Dan Buettner in his book *The Blue Zones.* Buettner looked at places in the world where higher percentages of people enjoy remarkably long, full lives and tried to pin down what makes them different.

What we all want to know is how we can do this too. How can we lower inflammation and oxidative stress? How can we learn to balance our metabolic processes so that we make ourselves more resilient to illness and more likely to age well? Let's look at some other parts of your metabolism.

Digestive Function and Elusive Illness

Digestive health is one of the least appreciated factors in our ability to repair and restore our bodies. The gastrointestinal (GI) tract serves as

(GERD), chronic overuse can cause medical complications.

In general, stomach acid should keep the stomach pH low, meaning acidic. When you don't have enough stomach acid, the pH rises, the stomach becomes less acidic, and bacteria such as *H. pylori* (the culprit behind many stomach ulcers), aren't killed or kept in check by the acid. Instead, they're able to grow and can cause damage to the stomach lining, leading to inflammation. When the mucosal lining of the stomach is damaged, it's exposed to stomach acid, which results in heartburn—a burning sensation in the upper abdomen, just where the ribs come together. The acid can regurgitate (reflux) up into the esophagus, producing a burning pain behind the breastbone. If reflux becomes severe enough, it can even send stomach acid up into the throat, causing a sore throat. In extreme cases, the acid can spill into the voice box area, causing hoarseness, and even into the lungs, causing coughing and wheezing and making asthma worse. This is why drugs that switch off stomach acid are so effective in relieving these types of symptoms. Remember, however, that relieving these symptoms will not treat the underlying bacterial overgrowth. That usually needs to be addressed with antibiotics and acid-inhibiting drugs.

Paradoxically, it is often just as important to address the underlying issue of insufficient stomach acid. This may create a sense of indigestion, because it creates a sense of fullness after a meal that won't go away. Many of our patients come to us believing they have excess stomach acid, when in fact they have too little. They try antacids to no effect. In these cases, a single capsule of HCl from the health-food store can alleviate all the patient's symptoms of burping and belching.

Ultimately, it remains important to address the damaged stomach lining. We discuss an approach to this in Star 3.

Digestive Enzymes

Enzymes are another underappreciated aspect of the body's magic. Basically, they are catalysts—chemicals that make things happen faster. Digestive enzymes are necessary to further digest foods as they pass from the stomach into the small intestine. These enzymes include proteases, which digest protein, carbohydrases such as amylase, which digest starches, and lipase, which digests fat.

Low digestive enzyme levels typically cause symptoms of bloating and gas. When lipases are deficient, fat does not digest well. This can cause extremely foul-smelling stools that float and are difficult to flush. Some of our patients lack sufficient digestive enzymes. Sometimes a lack of digestive enzymes can be the result of significant digestive illness, such as a pancreatic disorder. However, in other cases, it is simply due to a deficiency of zinc, a mineral that is necessary to help the tiny microvilli (tiny projecting "fingers" in the small intestine) regenerate. Digestive enzymes are found on the microvilli, so sometimes zinc replenishment can have a profound effect on maldigestion.

Testing for maldigestion and malabsorption from a lack of digestive enzymes is often cumbersome and difficult. It is often simpler to try a digestive enzyme supplement to see if this helps. However, if the supplement works, it is still important to find out why the enzymes are low.

Malabsorption and Amino Acid Imbalances

Amino acids are the building blocks of protein—and your body needs plenty of them to build the many thousands of proteins that are hormones, neurotransmitters, enzymes, and other crucial body chemicals. Amino acids are also necessary for building tissues and making repairs. We have found that a surprising number of people have amino acid imbalances or deficiencies. When the missing nutrients are provided, the body can rebalance and symptoms usually resolve naturally.

Testing for amino acid imbalances can be done with simple blood or urine tests at laboratories that specialize in functional testing.

Vitamin and Mineral Deficiencies

Vitamin deficiencies can be caused by insufficient intake, decreased absorption, or in some cases an overgrowth of bowel bacteria (dysbiosis). If a deficiency is severe, the patient may have an illness such as pellagra, caused by a deficiency of the B vitamin niacin. In our overfed society, true deficiency diseases are rare, but minor deficiencies may cause nonspecific symptoms such as mental fogginess, irritability, skin rashes, and fatigue. Since minor deficiencies can be difficult to diagnose, we call this subclinical dysfunction.

In Africa, we unfortunately saw vitamin deficiencies such as pellagra and beriberi from severe deficiencies of B vitamins, and we saw rickets caused by severe vitamin D deficiency. In Western society, we sometimes see a form of dementia in older people caused by vitamin B12 deficiency, but we are more likely to see subclinical deficiencies—aches and pains or seasonal affective disorder—that may relate to vitamin D deficiency.

Mineral deficiencies can also have a pro-

found impact on our health. Magnesium deficiency can cause muscle spasms, neurological symptoms, aggravate insulin resistance, and even increase the risk of irregular heart rhythm or heart failure. Zinc deficiency can cause hair loss and skin, immune and digestive problems. It is also associated with loss of smell, taste, eyesight, and memory.

Testing for vitamin and mineral deficiencies. In our experience, we have found the best way to test for vitamin and mineral deficiencies is with a combination of conventional and functional lab tests. If you are interested in this type of testing, we recommend you see someone who has expertise in this area.

Friendly Flora— Your Inner Garden

The world inside your digestive tract is like an inner garden. Within this environment you have more than one hundred trillion bacteria that help perform all the different functions of digestion. That's more bacteria in your intestines than you have cells in your body. Our internal flora isn't just a minor player in our metabolism. It's an entire ecosystem within the body, with the potential to be a thriving garden or a toxic wasteland. These bacteria, or flora, are made up of thousands of different types, including many that are beneficial and some that are harmful. When the good guys are in control, they keep down the bad guys and we thrive. Proper digestion is almost impossible without healthy flora. These beneficial bacteria also manufacture vitamins, fight off the bad guys (pathogenic bacteria, parasites, and candida or yeast), combat allergies, and help manage the immune system. If the bad guys take over, we begin to develop problems. This imbalance is called *dysbiosis.*

Symptoms of dysbiosis. Bacterial imbalance or dysbiosis can cause bloating, indigestion, poor absorption of nutrients, and lack of nourish-

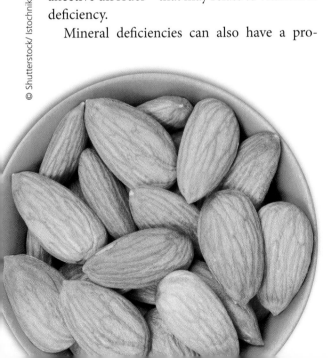

© Shutterstock/ Istochnik

ment (malnutrition). Dysbiosis can also play a role in allergies, ulcers, autoimmune reactions, and illnesses such as irritable bowel syndrome (IBS)—with bloating, gas, diarrhea, or constipation. Recent studies in mice also show that dysbiosis can result in obesity.

Malfunction. Children who grow up in Third World countries, where sanitation and hygiene are poor, tend to have a much lower incidence of allergies, Crohn's disease, and irritable bowel syndrome. Researchers now believe that this may be due to the growth of good bacteria in their digestive tracts. They are exposed to many pathogens early in life, which exercises their immune systems and lets them recognize bad bacteria for what they are and respond appropriately.

In adults, antibiotic overuse, medications such as anti-inflammatories and birth control pills, poor diet, and excessive alcohol use can all adversely affect the ratio of good bacteria to bad bacteria in our intestines, often with resultant excessive yeast overgrowth as well.

Antidoting dysbiosis. Americans have become more attuned to their intestinal flora, and, like many Europeans, now consume a range of sophisticated yogurts, kefirs, and probiotic products (foods and supplements that contain good bacteria). These foods and supplements are the perfect example of a functional approach to metabolism. This is just the start, though. Adding just a *probiotic* (good bacteria) is like throwing grass seed on a yard and expecting a good outcome with-

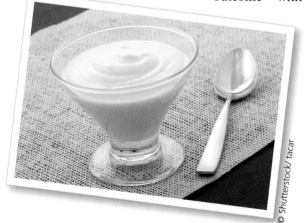

out understanding when to water, when to apply weed killer (medications or supplements to kill the bad bacteria) and when to apply fertilizers. The fertilizers we refer to here are substances such as fructo-oligosaccharides (FOS) which help the good bacteria grow. These fertilizing agents are called *prebiotics*. As you can see, addressing dysbiosis can be a complex issue. It is important to work with a health care practitioner who is well versed in this subject.

Food Sensitivities and Gut Hyperpermeability (Leaky Gut Syndrome)

In order to absorb our food, we start breaking it down in the mouth as we chew and mix it with saliva and then in the stomach with acid. Digestion continues with the addition of enzymes by our digestive tract, and then the action of the flora on our food. But the final step in digestion is the absorption of the microscopic food particles as they diffuse into our bloodstream through the tiny junctions or pores between the cells that line our intestines. From there, these particles are transported to the liver for further processing before they are sent out to the cells to finally be used as fuel.

When looking for the steps in the process where function breaks down, permeability turns out to be a major piece of the puzzle. Normally, the pores in our gut allow only small molecules to pass through. However, if the body is under stress, these pores can expand and open too wide, allowing larger molecules that haven't been completely broken down to pass through and enter the bloodstream. Increased gut permeability can happen under a lot of different circumstances: infection, intense physical stress, shock, surgery, injury, or food poisoning are all common examples. It can also occur with excessive alcohol consumption, radiation therapy, excessive simple sugar consumption, anti-inflammatory medications, nutrient deficiencies, premature birth, and whole food exposure before the age of four months.

When the pores in the lining of the GI tract open too wide for whatever reason, the result is called altered intestinal permeability, hyperpermeability, or, most commonly, leaky gut syndrome. This process can be compared to the way the pores in your skin expand and open wider when you take a hot shower.

In the gut, open pores are a bit of a disaster. When leaky gut syndrome happens, large molecules of food are released directly into the bloodstream. The digestive tract's immune system, also called gut associated lymphoid tissue (GALT), quickly responds to these oversized molecules. The immune system reacts as if these foods were invaders (antigens) and may launch an attack—even if the molecules are just food, innocent bystanders so to speak. In other words, the immune system falsely assumes that the foods are the molecules that are making the body sick and pours out antibodies to these foods, creating an immune and inflammatory response.

Malfunction. Leaky gut syndrome is both a cause of food sensitivity and is also triggered by reactions to food. Once you're sensitized to certain foods, you'll release antibodies every time you eat these foods. Removing the offending foods may help reduce symptoms, but you won't get better until you do something to heal the altered intestinal permeability.

It is very important to differentiate between food allergies and food sensitivities. An example of a food allergy is when someone eats an oyster or shellfish, then almost immediately starts struggling to breathe as their throat swells shut. Food sensitivities can occur hours to days after eating a food and usually aren't as dramatic. This is because they have different mechanisms. Food allergies are the result of IgE antibodies (think "E" for emergency) interacting with a protein in the food, while food sensitivities are usually the result of IgG (think "G" for gradual) antibodies reacting with food.

Symptoms of Gut Hyperpermeability, or "Leaky Gut Syndrome"

Gut hyperpermeability, or leaky gut syndrome, can lead to exaggerated antibody reactions to certain foods, also called food sensitivity. This altered immune response can be a contributing factor to a broad range of apparently unrelated conditions:

- Arthritis, auto-immune problems and fibromyalgia
- Chronic fatigue syndrome and multiple chemical sensitivities
- Cognitive malfunction, from brain fog to exacerbation of attention deficit disorder and autism
- Digestive disorders, such as inflammatory bowel disease (IBD), irritable bowel syndrome (IBS), malnutrition, and compromised liver function
- Food allergies and sensitivities
- Skin conditions, including acne, dermatitis, eczema, psoriasis, and urticaria (hives)

Eat well. Get well. Walk well. Run well. Love well. Live well. Stretch well. Dance well. Get well. Be well. Stay well. Breathe well. Stay

The Case of the Mysterious Rash

In her 50s, Kamiko developed a strange rash that would come and go. The rash started after a sinus infection and a period of prolonged stress and was originally attributed to the antibiotics she was taking. She saw multiple dermatologists and allergists to no avail. Skin tests for allergies were not helpful. Neither were antihistamine medications. Her bowel movements had also changed. She suffered from alternating constipation and diarrhea, severe flatulence, and abdominal cramping. She also complained of a "brain fog" that would come over her at times. A gastroenterologist had done a colonoscopy, which was normal. Tests for celiac disease were negative. He diagnosed Kamiko with irritable bowel syndrome (IBS). Unfortunately, the usual medications for IBS didn't help. That was when she came to us, frustrated and itchy.

IgG food sensitivity tests revealed high antibody levels to almonds and cashews. In her attempts to stay healthy, she had been eating almond or cashew butter daily. Removal of these foods from her diet resulted in a complete cure of her rash. In Star 3 we will discuss how we successfully treated her IBS.

Symptoms. Unlike true food allergies, which can be immediate and life-threatening, food sensitivities are less immediate and less dangerous. The response can be delayed as much as twenty-four or even thirty-six hours, so we may feel ill and not know why. For instance, if we develop a headache on a Wednesday, we may not connect our throbbing head with the wheat in the sandwich we ate for lunch on Monday.

Symptoms from food sensitivity can take the form of a headache, bloating, difficulty losing weight, irritable bowel syndrome (IBS), or rash. However, food sensitivities have also been linked to many other conditions, including allergies, asthma, bedwetting, canker sores, constipation, chronic bladder infections, eczema, psoriasis, urticaria, IBD, joint pain, migraines, palpitations, spontaneous bruising, and ulcers. These sensitivities have also been associated with serous otitis media (fluid in the middle ear).

Malfunction. Many foods and food additives can be related to food intolerances. Here are some to look out for:

- Chemicals like MSG (a flavor enhancer), dyes and food colorings, and sulfites (preservatives found in wine and dried fruit).

- Lactose intolerance related to a deficiency in the enzyme lactase, so that the sugar in dairy products, lactose, cannot be digested properly. This can result in pain, bloating, and gas when dairy products such as milk are consumed.

- Fructose sensitivity, the difficulty absorbing fructose, a sugar found in fruit and high-fructose corn syrup. The symptoms are similar to those of IBS and lactose intolerance.

- Nightshade sensitivity from plants in the nightshade family, including tomatoes, eggplants, bell peppers, chili peppers, potatoes, goji berries, and tamarillos, can cause a flare of arthritic symptoms in certain people.

- Wheat intolerance. Not the same as wheat allergy or celiac disease, wheat sensitivity can result in any of the symptoms we have discussed in this section.

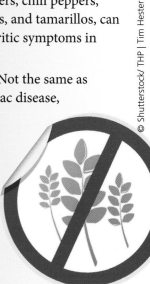

WHEAT FREE

The **body detoxifies** through the liver, kidneys, gut, skin and lungs. In this section we discuss the **liver**.

Your detoxification systems play an important role in your metabolism, reducing your risk of chronic illness by clearing your body of toxins.

Detoxification is another misunderstood aspect of health. Although toxins are removed from the body through the kidneys, colon, skin, and lungs, primary detoxification occurs in the liver, where toxins are broken down or degraded. When the liver's detoxification system is fully functional, it filters out many types of toxins recognized by the body as potentially harmful. This process disposes of toxins from our environment such as chemicals and drugs foreign to the body, which are known as *xenobiotics*. We are exposed to toxins in tap water, pesticides, herbicides, food additives, vehicle and industrial emissions, prescription, nonprescription and recreational drugs as well as through occupational exposure. Toxins also occur naturally within the body as by-products of metabolism, and include our own hormones, which also need to be detoxified and excreted.

Symptoms of poor detoxification.

We may consume the best nutrition in the world, but if our body's self-cleaning detoxification systems aren't working, toxins can build up and put us at risk for illness. These symptoms of impaired detoxification are usually nonspecific but include the following:

- Exaggerated or altered response to medications.
- Increasing sensitivity to medications or chemical exposure.
- Increasing sensitivity to odors.
- Multiple food sensitivities.
- Chronic fatigue and muscle pain. In fact, many patients with fibromyalgia suffer from impaired detoxification.
- Impaired cognition, including memory problems, confusion.
- Unusual tingling and numbness patterns.
- A tendency to dysautonomia (see Ring 2).
- Recurrent ankle edema (swelling) for no obvious reason.
- Hives, dry skin.
- Recurrent illness.
- A tendency to bloating and weight gain even though you watch your diet.

If you are suffering from some of these symptoms, a history of exposure to potentially toxic chemicals at home or work may be a clue to look further. You might be suffering from an overload of toxins. These may include pesticides, herbicides, and many petrochemicals found in yard chemicals, dry cleaning agents, and car exhaust fumes. If you have a significant number of amalgam fillings, or have had synthetic materials put in your body such as implants or prosthetics, see if your symptoms started within two years of having these procedures done. If you are on multiple medications, these may be interfering with your body's detoxification systems.

Malfunction. Our detoxification processes are vulnerable to overload for a few reasons. Some of us have SNPs in our detoxification genes that simply make our detoxification processes slower than average. In our experience, patients who have a number of these SNPs are hypersensitive to alcohol, drugs, and chemicals. They simply take longer to get rid of them. They may feel woozy from a small amount of alcohol or develop side effects on a regular dose of medication.

Our detoxification systems may malfunction due to exposure to a wide range of chemicals in our environment and even our food. For example, certain drugs, herbicides, pesticides, and even charred meats can interfere with our ability to detoxify. When our detoxifying systems are not working well, they create reactive intermediate products—by-products of detoxification that are not fully broken down. They are highly toxic to our DNA, and may contribute to creating chronic disease, premature aging, and some forms of cancer.

Many foods can help our detoxification processes. These are mainly vegetables and fruits (starting to sound familiar?). The best detoxing foods are cruciferous vegetables such as broccoli (which is superb), cauliflower, broccoli-rabe, brussels sprouts, kale, cabbage, collard greens, kohlrabi, mustard greens, rutabaga, turnips, arugula, radish, wasabi, Chinese cabbage, bok choy, and watercress. Also helpful for detoxification are artichokes, onions, shallots, garlic, green tea, and even fresh coffee. Much of the population does not eat enough of these foods, making them vulnerable to self-pollution.

Heavy metals and detoxification. Metals such as mercury and lead can have a deleterious effect on detoxification systems, with an eventual impact on the health of cells and tissues. Although heavy metals aren't usually toxic when present in the body at low doses, the accumulation of multiple toxins in low doses can be harmful. Studies on rats showed a hundredfold increase in toxicity when mercury and lead in low doses were combined.

The same amplification of toxicity is likely to be true of exposure to multiple toxins from the environment. A low dose of a single toxin has little or no effect on most of us. It is the combination of multiple toxins in low doses that finally overwhelms our systems. Young children and the frail elderly generally have less resilience to the impact of multiple toxins. Children have immature detoxification systems, and the elderly may have systems that are compromised by both the deterioration of aging and a lifetime of cumulative toxic exposure.

We may be exposed to heavy metals through eating fish that is tainted with mercury (usually bigger fish such as shark, swordfish, farm-raised salmon, tilefish, mackerel, grouper, sea bass, and tuna), mercury-containing products, mercury-emitting coal plants, and leaking mercury amalgam dental fillings. Lead exposure from lead paint used in houses built prior to 1977 may also be a source of exposure. Many products imported from China have been tainted with lead or cadmium. Aluminum exposure may be due to aluminum-containing underarm deodorants, antacids, and pots and pans.

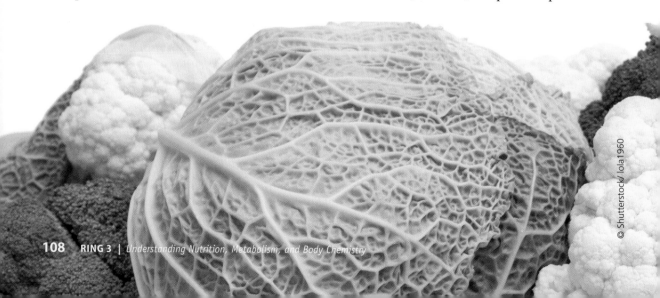

© Shutterstock/ lola1960

How Your Body **Detoxifies**

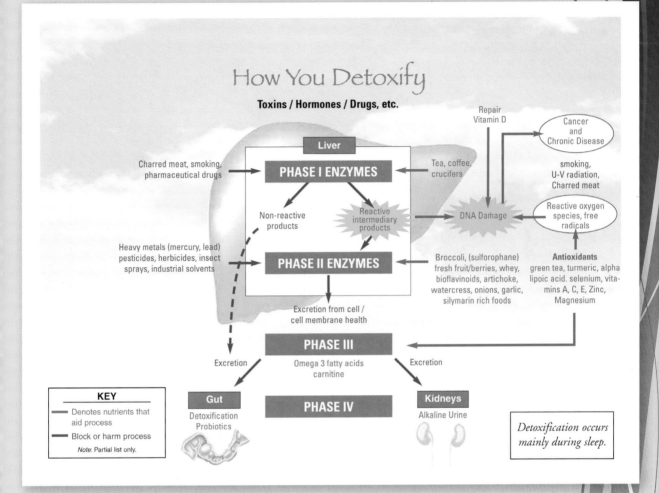

Figure R3.1 **How You Detoxify**

Initial detoxification occurs in the liver, where environmental toxins, many drugs and even hormones go through the steps of a detoxification pathway referred to as Phase I; the cytochrome P450 enzyme system is crucial for making the pathways work efficiently. After going through Phase I, many toxins are neutralized and are then excreted through the gut into the feces. A positive balance of good bacteria in the gut makes this part of the detoxification process move smoothly. Other neutralized toxins are expelled through the kidney into the urine. Toxins that cannot be neutralized just by the Phase I system pass through the Phase II enzyme system and then pass out of the body through the feces or urine.

Phase I.

Phase I enzymes are supported by substances such as green tea, fresh coffee, and cruciferous vegetables (e.g., broccoli, cauliflower, brussels sprouts, kale, cabbage, and bok choy). SNPs in Phase I enzymes can affect how well we detoxify. These SNPs affect what are known as the cytochrome P450 (or CYP) pathways. SNPs such as CYP1B1, CYP2A6, CYP2C9, and CYP2C19 help detoxify medications. Certain drugs and foods can interfere with these SNPs and thus create potential problems in the body by interfering with phase 1 detoxification. Examples include antifungal medications such as ketoconazole (Nizoral®), itraconazole (Sporanox®), antibiotics such as erythromycin or ciprofloxacin, acid reducers such as omeprazole (Prilosec®) and cimetidine (Tagamet®), and foods such as grapefruit juice.

Phase II.

If a particular xenobiotic, metabolic by-product, drug, or foreign chemical is not adequately broken down by the Phase I system, it is called a reactive intermediary product, which can actually be more toxic than the original substance. Reactive intermediary products can cause DNA damage; over time, they may even cause cancer or chronic disease. Adequate levels of vitamin D and antioxidants can provide crucial protection against DNA damage from reactive intermediary products.

To remove the reactive intermediary products, your liver passes them through a second series of processes, the Phase II enzyme system, to neutralize them and then excrete them through the gut or kidneys. Phase II detoxification includes glucuronidation through Glutathione S-Transferase (GST); methylation via catechol-O-methyltransferase (COMT); acetylation via N-acetyltransferase (NAT); and oxidative protection via superoxide dismutase (SOD). SNPs on these pathways can cause further problems with detoxification.

During Phase II detoxification, enzyme systems can be supported by beneficial factors found in cruciferous vegetables, garlic and onions, artichokes, and whey. Once again, genetic SNPs may cause the system to detoxify at a faster or slower rate than normal. In fact, research has shown that the rate of detoxification can vary as much as thirty-five–fold from one person to the next.

Phase III.

The next part of detoxification occurs via cell membranes all over the body. Although it is not officially called this, we refer to this aspect of detoxification as Phase III. Cell membranes are composed of fats. An inadequate amount of healthy fats in the diet can result in brittle and inflexible cell membranes with limited capacity to take in nutrients or expel wastes. As a result, toxins may become trapped inside the body's cells. Poor detoxification has been implicated in cancer and a myriad of other diseases—another reason good fats are so important in our diet.

Phase IV.

In Phase IV detoxification, neutralized toxins are excreted through the gut or the kidneys. In the GI tract, the disposal of toxins is facilitated by a positive balance of good bacteria. In the kidneys, the urine must be somewhat alkaline for improved excretability. Beneficial flora and a slightly alkaline balance in the body both have implications for the importance of diet in supporting healthy detoxification.

In Ring 1 we discussed a systems approach to diagnosis. We reviewed how we can see a patient's genetic predispositions to an illness by assessing his or her family history and SNPs. In Ring 2 we discussed the impact of stress on the body. In Ring 3 we start to look at the factors affecting a patient's epigenetics.

In other words, we want to evaluate the effect of diet, lifestyle and environmental factors that ultimately affect gene expression. We want to evaluate imbalances early on in processes, that left unchecked, will ultimately cause illness. To do this, we again use a systems approach. We assess each system and see if and where it is malfunctioning. We do this by evaluating factors such as nutritional depletion, inflammation, oxidative stress, gut dysfunction, immune dysfunction, and so on.

Understanding system-wide dysfunction is extremely helpful. Often, even if there is no medical or clinical diagnosis, we find that when we support these systems using diet, nutrition, lifestyle changes, stress reduction, supplements, and medications, symptoms of illness simply melt away. In Star 3 we will discuss ways to make this happen.

Alex Learns About His Metabolism

Alex continues to pursue Health and Wellness

Conventional lab testing showed that Alex had low vitamin D levels—not surprising, because Alex worked such long hours that he was rarely outdoors during daylight hours. Functional lab testing also revealed he was low on omega-3 and omega-9 fatty acids, dietary fats that are important for their anti-inflammatory action. In addition, functional lab testing showed a high need for folic acid, in addition to a high homocysteine level. Homocysteine is an amino acid naturally produced by the body, and elevated levels are associated with an increased risk of atherosclerosis, heart attack, stroke, blood clots, and possibly even Alzheimer's disease. The body needs folic acid to break down homocysteine. Because Alex has the MTHFR SNP, he cannot activate enough folic acid from his diet in order to reduce his homocysteine level. (In other words, he was not methylating well.) Alex had other problems too. A test of his hs-CRP level showed that Alex had higher than normal levels of inflammation, while other functional tests showed a high level of oxidative stress. A functional stool test showed that Alex wasn't digesting his food properly. He had a marked dysbiosis, or imbalance between good and bad bacteria in his gut.

Although Alex was outwardly "healthy," we were able to show him some of the hidden problems that could eventually cause illness. When we explained all this to Alex, he nodded. Deep down, he said, he could feel himself "aging and rusting away." No wonder Alex was feeling the way he did. What he needed now was a way to deal with his problems.

3

STAR THREE

How to Optimize Your Nutrition and Your Metabolism

- **Personalize Your Diet and Nutrition to Interact Optimally with Your Genes**

- **Use Supplements Effectively to Optimize Your Metabolism**

- **Improve Your Immune Function**

- **Balance Your Body Chemistry**

Did you ever think that changing your diet might save your life? You might be nodding your head if you thought about someone who was starving or someone living completely on fast food.
But what about you? You may say, "I am eating a good diet!"
What if you changed your diet? Would it make a difference?

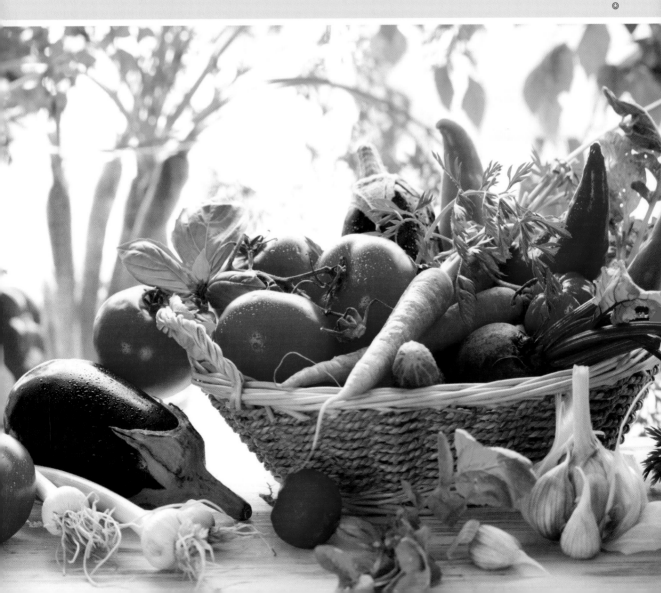

Growing Healthier with Every Bite

I n one paradigm-shifting study published in 2001, patients who had experienced a heart attack were put on either a low-fat diet recommended by the American Heart Association (AHA) or a Mediterranean diet. The AHA diet is essentially standard American fare, with minimal fat intake. A typical Mediterranean diet emphasizes fresh vegetables and fruits and includes whole grains and lentils, with olive oil, fish, and meat in moderation. The researchers found that patients on the Mediterranean diet did so much better than those on the AHA diet that they stopped the study early, feeling it was unethical to deprive half the subjects of the more efficacious diet. The AHA changed their recommendations after this experiment. The study was eye-opening for many of us interested in nutrition. Food can have a profound impact on our health.

It Doesn't Matter When You Start

Improving your diet at any age can help. Another important study in 2004 found that introducing a Mediterranean diet to seniors between the ages of 70 and 77 resulted in a 50 percent reduction in disease risk, including heart disease, along with a significant reduction in arthritis and other health problems.

If you could take a pill to reduce your risk of degenerative disease by 50 percent, wouldn't you be rushing to get it? You might even be willing to pay an exorbitant amount of money for it. So why not make basic, inexpensive changes in your diet to achieve this type of result?

The first step is changing your concept of food. When you eat, you are marinating your cells in nutrients. Your choice of nutrients has a profound affects on your body chemistry, often within minutes. Long-term consumption of the wrong foods can result in inflammation, oxidation, and degeneration—the terrible trio we talked about in Ring 3.

Eating Mindfully

Brian Wansink, Ph.D., professor of marketing and nutritional science at Cornell University, has spent a lifetime studying the cues of what makes us overeat. In *Mindless Eating: Why We Eat More Than We Think*, he describes his ingenious and often funny experiments that show how all of us are influenced by the way food is packaged and presented. In one experiment, called the "bottomless soup bowl," subjects were served soup in a bowl that kept on filling up through a pipe attached at the bottom of the soup bowl as the soup was eaten. Guess what happened? The people just kept on eating, because their internal "full" register never switched off. Food companies have been quick to realize how much our food intake can be manipulated by labels, smells, environment, textures (such as crunchiness), and a host of other factors. We get supersized, indulged, and overstuffed by a variety of manipulative behaviors. As much as we like to think of ourselves as being conscious of our food intake, most of us rarely are.

Eating while you drive, watch television, or read removes awareness of the act of eating. Interestingly, it is your brain that sets the digestive machinery in process. This happens in response to the look, smell, and texture of foods, which then triggers a cascade of acids, enzymes, and digestive processes that help you assimilate food.

It is important to become aware of *how* you eat as much as *how much* you eat. Immerse yourself in the moment as you savor each bite. Really take notice of what your food looks like—as well as its aroma, flavor and texture. Slow down. In our fast paced world, its easy to overlook the importance of the ritual and pleasure of mindful eating.

Optimize Nutrition, Metabolic and Immune Function

Diet and Lifestyle Go Together

In *Thrive: Find Happiness the Blue Zones Way*, Dan Buettner describes areas of the world where people commonly live active lives past the age of 100. He calls these Blue Zones. The areas he studied were Sardinia, Italy; the islands of Okinawa, Japan; Loma Linda, California (a Seventh Day Adventist community); the Nicoya Peninsula in Costa Rica; and the island of Ikaria in Greece. On Ikaria, almost a third of the population lives into their 90s. According to Buettner, Ikarians have about 20 percent lower rates of cancer, 50 percent lower rates of heart disease than people in industrial countries, and almost no dementia. Buettner discusses the common features he found in the Blue Zones. They are:

- Emphasis on the importance of family and social engagement
- Not smoking
- A plant-based diet derived mainly from fresh vegetables and legumes
- Frequent, moderate physical activity

Finding the Right Diet

In modern Westernized countries, we have an almost unlimited supply of food. We are no longer confined to eating local, seasonal foods. The good news is that this gives us a wonderful choice of nutrients. The bad news is that sometimes the choices are overwhelming. Let's look at what makes a good, nutritionally rich diet.

A Nutritionally Dense Diet

The idea of a universal daily allowance of various nutrients for everyone is currently being reconsidered by the nutritional research community. It is clear that some people require far more of certain nutrients than others, due to both genetic factors and the demands of lifestyle. It is also clear that diets that are nutritionally dense are much healthier than diets that are highly refined and depleted of vital nutrients. "White" means stripped of nutrients. White bread, white rice, and semolina pasta all have had the fiber and vitamin-filled bran removed from the grain. "Enriched" implies an attempt to reintroduce those same nutrients back into the food—but it is never as good as the original, and it costs more. Why eat enriched or processed foods that are still lacking important

Why You Should Eat Your Broccoli?

Broccoli has natural cancer-fighting chemicals called sulforophanes, so tangible they can be measured in a lab. The broccoli plant does not make sulforophanes to prevent its own cancer–it uses them to defend against attacking insects and repair damage. When broccoli is stressed by inclement weather and having to fight off bugs, it automatically increases the amount of sulforophane it produces. Placing broccoli in a refrigerator also stresses it. Therefore, both organically grown broccoli and refrigerated broccoli have higher amounts of sulforophanes than does broccoli grown in a cushy environment and then frozen. These cancer-fighters also become most available to our bodies when broccoli is steamed or blanched for just one to two minutes. The broccoli that has no cancer-fighting chemicals is the kind left in a steamer for hours on end (unfortunately, like the overcooked kind often found in a hospital cafeteria).

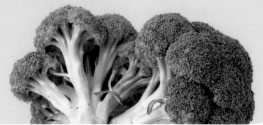

© Shutterstock/ Nattika

nutrients such as fiber when you can eat the original whole grains and get all the natural nutrition they contain?

The soil in which the food is grown affects the nutrient concentration of that food. In addition, how foods are ripened, transported, prepared, and cooked are important factors. All of these can affect the nutritional value of a food. Whole Foods Market, the worlds largest retailer of organic foods has adopted the use of the Aggregate Nutritional Density Index (ANDI) to better help shoppers understand nutritional density. For more information on the nutritional density of your foods, go to www.eatrightamerica.com/andi-superfoods.

Low Glycemic Load Foods

The glycemic index (GI) is a way of rating how a carbohydrate-containing food (one that is sugary or starchy) affects your blood sugar, (also known as your blood glucose.) A spoonful of refined white sugar has a GI rank of 100, because the sugar hits your bloodstream almost immediately. By comparison, a serving of baked sweet potato has a GI rank of only 44, while a raw carrot has a rank of 16. Broccoli and just about all other green vegetables have a GI rank of zero—these foods have no impact on your blood sugar. The same is true for nuts. Foods that rapidly convert to sugar have a high rating on the index (above 70), while those with a low GI (below 55) release sugar slowly.

The glycemic index turns out to be a key leverage point for improving health. Whenever blood sugar spikes from eating a high-carbohydrate food, the pancreas must produce more of the hormone insulin to carry away the excess blood sugar. This is a form of wear and tear that puts us at risk for diabetes. What's more, each time insulin pulls blood sugar levels down to a normal range, it achieves this by storing that sugar in our cells, usually somewhere around the waistline. We can avoid this roller coaster scenario by consuming more low-glycemic and moderate-glycemic index foods, which minimize the need for insulin.

The glycemic load (GL) is an even more accurate indicator of the overall impact of carbohydrates on our blood sugar and insulin levels. The GL of a food is calculated by combining both the quality and quantity of starch or carbohydrate it contains in a serving. It is a fairly accurate way to predict the blood glucose impact of a serving of food. A GL of above 20 is high, whereas 10 or less is low. Typically, the GI is similar to the GL, but not always. Take carrots, for example: a raw carrot has a low GI rank of 16 but a very low GL of 2. The reason is that although a carrot has sugar in it (making the GI higher), the fiber binds the sugar, making it less available—lowering the GL. However, if you convert the carrot into carrot juice, much of the beneficial effect of the fiber is removed, releasing the sugar. This dramatically increases both the GI and GL. In other words, it is better to eat a carrot than drink carrot juice. Similarly, it is better to eat fruit than drink fruit juice. Then again, even carrot juice has a lower GI and GL than a sweetened bread roll.

The ideal food is highly nutritious with a low GI and a low GL. We therefore recommend a low-glycemic load (LGL) diet.

LGL foods are mostly whole grains, fruits, vegetables, beans, and nuts. These foods not only have less impact on your blood sugar, they generally are also powerful antioxidants and promote healthy detoxification in the liver. Many have anticancer and anti-inflammatory proper-

> Keeping your body healthy is an expression of gratitude to the whole cosmos— the trees, the clouds, everything.
>
> – Thich Nhat Hanh

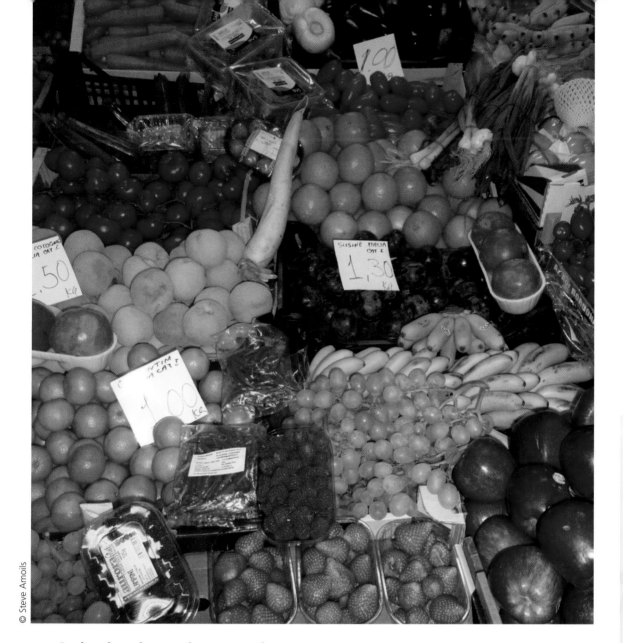

ties. Studies show that people on a LGL diet can eat as much as they want and still lose weight. No calorie counting is needed. This is because foods with a low glycemic load are high in fiber and will make you feel full quickly, and help avoid spikes in blood sugar.

Anti-inflammatory Foods

Foods high in omega-6 fatty acids (soy bean oil, corn oil) tend to be pro-inflammatory, while omega-3 (fish and flaxseed oils) and omega-9 fatty acids (olive oil and nut oils) are anti-inflammatory. The typical Western diet is filled with highly refined foods, high in omega-6 fatty acids. The agricultural shift from grass-fed to grain-fed meats is a factor in the dramatic increase of omega-6 fatty acids in the American diet. So is the shift to fried foods, prepared foods, and junk food.

You can ensure that you're getting the essential healthy or "good fats" you need by eating foods rich in omega-3s, such as fatty fish (e.g., wild salmon, sardines, and herring), flax seeds and flax seed oil, and omega-9 monounsaturates found in olive oil, avocados and nuts.

Probiotic Foods

A healthy balance of good bacteria in our gut play a major role in our health. Foods that promote the growth of these good bacteria include yogurt, kefir, sauerkraut, aged cheeses, cottage cheese, miso, tempeh, kombucha, and kimchi.

Healthy Herbs and Spices

Many spices have healthful, antioxidant, anti-inflammatory, and anticancer effects. Turmeric (and the curcumin it contains) is well known for all of these effects. Cinnamon helps to lower blood sugar. Garlic has antibiotic, anti-inflammatory, anti-nausea, and pro-detoxification properties. Rosemary, thyme, oregano, and hundreds of other herbs and spices used in foods abound with beneficial effects.

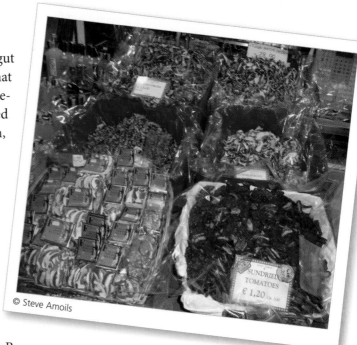

© Steve Amoils

What Is the **Best Diet** for You?

Because we each have a unique genetic makeup, we all have slightly different needs in terms of food and nutrients. Much of this is based on our genes, but also on our lifestyle and the nutrient content of our diet.

Match Your Food to Your Genes

In Ring 1, we talked about the Pima Indians, who have a strong genetic tendency to develop insulin resistance and diabetes. By adopting a diet similar to their ancestors, they can avoid this fate. You may be able to improve your own health by following a similar approach. We often refer patients to an excellent website called Oldways (www.oldwayspt.org) to help them understand the merits of a traditional diet. Following a diet similar to your ancestors may be helpful. They were genetically adapted to eat certain foods, which probably means you have

the same genetic tendencies. If your family is European, that probably means a cereal-based diet. If your family comes from the Mediterranean, that healthy diet may be best for you. If your family is Asian, that suggests a rice-based diet, with all the advantages conferred by this alkaline grain. If your ancestry is not northern European, you probably have lactose intolerance and should avoid milk. In short, you will want to pattern your nutrition after the genetic instructions encoded in your genes, established over the millennia in your ancestors.

Genetic Glitches

Why is it that a basically good diet may not be good enough for a particular person? Genetic variations may result in nutrient needs that vary dramatically between one person and another. An example of this would be someone who has the genetic variation or SNP called MTHFR, or methylene tetrahydrofolate reductase. If you have this variant, which can be detected by a blood test, you can't completely metabolize folic acid, a B vitamin, to its active form, called tetrahydrofolate or folinic acid. Even with a diet full of green leafy vegetables, the main source of folic acid, or even if you take a conventional folic acid supplement, this genetic SNP can block complete metabolism, or activation, of the vitamin. Fortunately, taking an activated folic acid supplement such as 5-methyltetrahydrofolate, 5-formyltetrahydrofolate or folinic acid lets you overcome this genetic problem by bypassing the glitch.

Traditional Diets and Health

Let's look at some common threads of traditional diets: generous use of vegetables and fruits, unrefined grains where possible, healthy fats in the form of vegetable oils, nuts, and seeds, herbs and spices, a lower intake of animal protein. Perhaps often overlooked is the relaxed social manner in which this food is eaten, and the sanctity which is afforded to it.

The traditional Mediterranean diet is a cuisine that emphasizes daily seasonal fruits and vegetables. The diet includes legumes and beans, a variety of daily grains (especially whole grains) in the form of breads, pastas, rice, and cereals. Olive oil is consumed liberally. Nuts and seeds are used as snacks or part of main dishes. Herbs such as garlic, oregano, basil, and rosemary are used to flavor foods (and happen to also be potent antioxidants). Dairy products are eaten in moderation, mainly as yogurt and cheese; milk is rarely drunk. Protein comes mostly from cold-water fatty fish (e.g., salmon), shellfish, eggs, and poultry. Red meat is used in small quantities. A glass or two of wine (usually red) complements main meals.

When we look at other traditional cuisines

> *Food should nourish life–this is the best medicine.*
> — Japanese proverb

from around the world, we see something similar: an emphasis on whole grains, beans, and fresh vegetables, with plenty of antioxidant spices. Dairy foods are eaten in moderation. Fats come from vegetable oils. Protein comes from soy, nuts, and meat, poultry, fish, and eggs in moderation. Many traditional cuisines are lacto-ovo vegetarian, using no animal foods except milk and eggs. In all traditional cuisines, alcohol is used in moderation or not at all.

Longevity and Diet

On the island of Okinawa in Japan, residents are known for their longevity and vitality. The traditional Okinawan diet (as described in *The Blue Zones* by Dan Buettner) is 20 to 25 percent lower in calories and grains than the average Japanese diet, but contains three times as many green and yellow vegetables. The Okinawan diet is low in fat and sugar and high in soy and other legumes. It includes a small amount of fish, and with the exception of pork, almost no meat. No eggs or dairy products are consumed.

In *The China Study*, Dr. T. Colin Campbell looked at dietary, lifestyle, and disease mortality characteristics in sixty-five rural Chinese counties over the course of twenty years. The study observed a genetically similar population that tended to live in the same way in the same place and eat the same foods for their entire lives.

In terms of meat consumption, Campbell concluded that "people who ate the most animal-based foods got the most chronic disease. People who ate the most plant-based foods were the healthiest and tended to avoid chronic disease. These results could not be ignored." He discusses how consumption of animal products can lead to illnesses such as autoimmune disease; cancers of the breast, prostate, and large bowel; coronary heart disease; degenerative brain disease; diabetes; macular degeneration; obesity; and osteoporosis.

Your **Personalized Nutrition Program**

To create your personalized nutrition program, start with the basics. In terms of pure simplicity, we like to quote author Michael Pollan, who states that we should eat:

1. **Real food**
2. **Mostly vegetables**
3. **Not too much**

Real food. The main point here is to remember that nature-made food is better for you than is man-made food. It is far better to shop around the side aisles of a supermarket, where the fresh fruit and vegetables are, than in the center aisles, where the boxes of ready-made, refined foods are kept. Even better than shopping in the supermarket is to get fresh produce from your local farmers' market. Eat seasonal, local, fresh, organic food whenever possible.

Mostly vegetables. Enough said.

Not too much. Learn to eat mindfully. Stop eating before you are full—the satiety center in your brain is about twenty minutes behind what you put into your mouth. Use a smaller plate, and definitely choose smaller servings. Meals that include large salads and generous servings of fresh vegetables will make this much easier than it sounds.

 What to Avoid

Processed and refined foods are low in nutrients but high in calories. They are also often high in added sugars, salt, and fat. In particular, decrease your intake of refined carbohydrates such as enriched white flour and sweeteners such as sugar and high-fructose corn syrup.

Avoid charred meat and other foods. The charred part can contain cancer-causing substances.

Avoid trans fats. These fats are associated with an increased risk of oxidative stress and diabetes. Read food labels carefully: food manufacturers are allowed to list any food with less than half a gram of trans fats per serving as having zero trans fats.

Avoid genetically modified (GM or GMO) foods where possible. In the U.S., this is very difficult, as the FDA doesn't require notification that a food is GM. We are concerned about the effects of GM foods and where possible believe it is better to avoid them until better studies are available.

Avoid artificial food colorings and additives. Many common food additives have been shown to interfere with normal vitamin and enzyme function. For example, yellow dye #5 can interfere with the action of vitamin B6.

Avoid irradiated fruits and vegetables. Like genetically modified foods, we have little information on the long-term effects of these exposures.

Avoid artificial sweeteners. Try stevia or agave nectar as natural alternatives.

Avoid fruit juices, even all-natural ones with no added sugar. Fruit juice is nothing but a glorified sugar drink. You wouldn't eat four oranges at a sitting, which is essentially what happens when you drink a cup of orange juice.

Creating a Nutrient-Rich Diet

Eat more vegetables and fruits. Aim to eat at least five servings of vegetables and fruits a day, but preferably seven to eight. Eat at least twice as many vegetables as fruit. Our "Supernutrition smoothie" (see page 126) can help you achieve this in a delicious way.

Eat seasonal, local, and organic produce, wherever possible. Especially aim to eat organic where the "dirty dozen" (see page 122) are concerned.

Ensure that you have good fiber intake. Benefits include lowering cholesterol, reducing risk of type 2 diabetes and colon cancer. Fiber comes in two forms: *soluble,* which dissolves in water; and *insoluble,* which doesn't. Don't worry about the difference. Aim for 35 grams of fiber daily through whole grains, fruits, and vegetables.

Eat meat sparingly, preferably grass-fed and finished (rather than corn-fed or finished) varieties free of antibiotics and hormones.

Rotate your foods. You are more likely to get food sensitivities if you eat the same food every day. Your body needs a variety of nutrients. Broadening your diet will help you get those nutrients.

Eat a variety of whole grains. Try some new ones, such as amaranth, barley, buckwheat, millet, oats, quinoa, and rye.

Eat less dairy. Although they often don't know it, many people are lactose intolerant and can't digest dairy foods well. If you can drink milk, choose organic, hormone-free milk.

Eat more good fats. Use first-pressed or cold-pressed extra virgin olive oil as your primary source of dietary fat. Avocados, as well as nuts and seeds, or oils and butters made from them, are excellent sources of good dietary fat.

Increase the omega-3s in your diet by eating fish, such as salmon, herring, mackerel, and tuna, two to three times a week, or consider a mercury-free fish oil supplement. If you don't eat fish or don't like it, consider alternative sources of good fats, such as chia seeds (*Salvia hispanica* or salba), flaxseed oil, hemp oil, or a small amount of evening primrose or blackcurrant oil. You can use these directly—a drizzle of nutty-tasting flaxseed oil on vegetables is a good alternative to butter—or take them as supplements.

Eat free-range eggs. Free-range organic eggs are higher in omega-3 fatty acids and are more humane.

Drink filtered water. Regrettably, it is almost impossible to measure the eighty thousand chemicals that abound in our environment and infiltrate into our water supply. An activated carbon charcoal filter on a tap or in a pitcher will remove most toxins. Reverse osmosis filtration and distillation are better ways of filtering your water but may also remove trace minerals that are healthy for you. Skip bottled water. Drink filtered water from your sink instead—it's free, it's environmentally friendly, and it doesn't use fossil fuel in the form of plastic bottles and truck fuel.

Spice up your diet. Many herbs and spices have proven anticancer and anti-inflammatory benefits. Dried herbs are as valuable as fresh ones. Examples include curcumin (turmeric), cinnamon, oregano and ginger.

Drink alcohol in moderation. Enjoy one (for women) to two (for men) glasses of red wine per day. Skip this if you are concerned about alcoholism or take drugs that interact with alcohol.

Add cultured and fermented foods. Fermented and cultured products, such as miso, tempeh, plain yogurt, and sauerkraut, can encourage the growth of the good bacteria in your gut.

The Dirty Dozen and the Clean Fifteen

The nonprofit organization Environmental Working Group (www.ewg.org) releases an annual list of fruits and vegetables that are highest and lowest in pesticides and other agricultural chemicals. The foods on the Dirty Dozen list are high in chemicals, so it is probably better to purchase these only if they have been organically grown. The Clean Fifteen list is lowest in chemical residue; these foods are safe to eat even if they are not organically grown. Below are foods that typically appear on the list, although it may change:

The Dirty Dozen Apples, cherries, and berries (strawberries, raspberries, and domestic blueberries), celery, spinach, lettuce, kale and collard greens, peaches, and imported nectarines, imported grapes, potatoes, sweet bell peppers. (Carrots, cucumber, green beans, squash and pears are also usually considered to have more pesticides.)

The Clean Fifteen Onions, avocados, sweet corn, pineapple, mangos, asparagus, sweet peas, kiwis, cabbage, eggplant, cantaloupe, watermelon, grapefruit, mushrooms, and sweet potato. (Broccoli, tomatoes, winter squash, cranberries, papaya, and bananas are often also considered as foods with fewer pesticides.)

Tips on Decoding Food Labels

Making better food choices requires that we pay attention to what we are eating. A crucial first step is learning to read the ingredient list on the food label.

1. Look at the list of ingredients:

Ingredients are listed by weight, so the most abundant ingredients are listed first. *If any of the first three ingredients are sugar, salt, or fat, avoid the product.* High-fructose corn syrup is just another way of saying sugar. So are pure cane syrup, beet sugar, brown rice syrup, dextrose, fruit juice concentrate, malt, and maltose.

Avoid products that contain more than five to seven ingredients. Make sure you recognize and can pronounce the names of the ingredients. If you can't pronounce them, you probably shouldn't eat them.

Avoid products with *artificial and hydrogenated ingredients*.

Avoid products that are *enriched or fortified*. These are indications that the food is chemically manipulated, rather than derived from nature. Also avoid products that claim to be low-fat, light, low-sodium, diet, or any other marketing term meant to fool you into thinking the product is somehow more healthful.

2. Look at the breakdown of servings, calories, fiber, fat, carbs and protein:

Look carefully at the *number of servings per container.* The label gives the number of servings in the container and the *number of calories per serving.* Often a container includes several servings. If you eat the whole thing in one sitting, you could be getting a lot more calories than you realize.

The *higher the fiber content*, the better.

Look at the *fat content.* Avoid saturated and trans fats (partially hydrogenated fats are trans fats). Trans fat less than 0.5 g do not need to be listed. Add up all the different fats. They should equal total fat content. If not, hidden trans fats may be present.

Remember, the Daily Value amounts are approximate guidelines only.

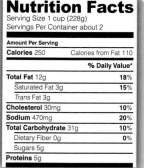

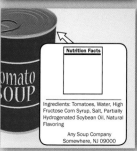

Fine Tuning Your Food Plan

A general rule of thumb for people who go on "a diet" is that about a third seem to do well, a third respond fairly well, and a third don't respond at all. Why is this? It's probably because people who go on a programmed diet end up on one that's wrong for their genetic type. Understanding nutrigenomics can help you find the right food plan for you.

In general, we summarize food plans into three types: Balanced, Low-Carb, and Low-Fat.

In March 2010, researchers at Interleukin Genetics, Inc. (Inherent Health) and Stanford University announced results from a diet study previously reported in the *Journal of the American Medical Association*. The conclusion: Subjects on a genetically appropriate diet lost two and a half times more than those on a genetically inappropriate diet over a one year period.

Here is how the study was conducted:

Patients were randomly assigned to follow a Balanced, Low-Carb, or Low-Fat diet. Typical examples of these are:

- **The Balanced Food Plan:** Modified Mediterranean diet, Volumetrics, Weight Watchers
- **The Low-Carb Food Plan:** South Beach Diet, Zone Diet
- **The Low-Fat Food Plan:** Dean Ornish's Eat More, Weigh Less; the DASH diet; New Pritikin Program; vegetarian; and many diets approved by the American Heart Association

When the genetic makeup of the people in the study was analyzed through nutrigenomics, those who were in the diet type that was also best for their genes lost the most weight.

Which Food Plan Is Best for You?

One way to decide what type of food plan will work best for you is to do nutrigenomic testing to see what food plan is most appropriate for your genes, or how to alter your food plan to affect your genes. Companies such as Inherent Health (www.inherenthealth.com/) offer this sort of genetic testing.

If you don't want do these tests, here are a few generalizations to help you decide which food plan to try:

1. **The Balanced or Modified Mediterranean food plan is appropriate for most people.** It is easy to modify a Standard American Diet into a modified Mediterranean food plan. Calories on this food plan are 50 percent carbohydrates, 20 percent protein, and 30 percent fat. Good candidates for a modified Mediterranean food plan have a family history of diabetes or heart disease. They may have a Mediterranean or European heritage. If you have difficulty deciding which food plan to choose, use this one.

2. **The Low-Carb Food Plan.** This approach was originally popularized by Dr. Robert Atkins in the 1970s. The Atkins diet is high in red meat and allows processed meats such as bacon, so for our patients, we prefer The South Beach Diet and the Zone Diet, which recommend more vegetables. The low-carb food plan works well for insulin-resistant people, especially "apples" with a waist larger than 35 inches. It is also appropriate for people with high triglycerides and type 2 diabetes. The low-carb calories are 30 percent carbohydrates, 40 percent fat, and 40 percent protein.

3. **The Low-Fat Food Plan.** Dr. Dean Ornish popularized this approach. He has shown that it can reverse both coronary artery disease and prostate cancer, while simultaneously reversing signs of aging. The calories from this food plan are 70 percent carbohydrates, 15 percent protein, and 5 percent fat. People who go on this food plan need to be prepared to eat a predominantly veg-

etarian diet. This food plan seems suitable for patients with high LDL cholesterol (including those with an Apo E4 SNP), heart disease and prostate cancer.

Eat More Often

Once you know what type of food plan you are going to eat, we would like you to think about eating five to six times per day. Here's how:

- A healthful breakfast.
- A midmorning snack
- A healthful lunch
- A midafternoon snack
- A healthful dinner
- Possibly a small evening snack before bedtime

Appropriate Portions

What you eat matters, but so does how much you eat. To give you an easy way to choose your foods and control your portions, we like to use the fist method.

For a bigger meal, one plate equals about four fist sizes.

As a snack, you don't need much. Consider ½ fist or two thumb sizes.

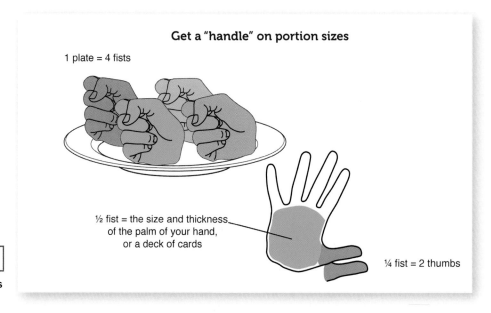

Get a "handle" on portion sizes

1 plate = 4 fists

½ fist = the size and thickness of the palm of your hand, or a deck of cards

¼ fist = 2 thumbs

Figure S3.1

Portion Sizes

Food Choice Guidelines

We want you to learn to choose your foods wisely in order to *Get Well and Stay Well*. Rather than just counting calories, count food groups. We recommend using these categories:

1. **Vegetables and fruit**

2. **Protein**

3. **Whole grain carbohydrates** (starches) and **legumes** (beans, lentils etc.)

4. **Good (monounsaturated) fats**

Note: Remember these are just guiding principles to help you decide which foods to eat. It is important to understand that foods may fall into two or three different categories. For instance, we place lentils and hummus into the starch group, but they are also good sources of protein. Avocados could be placed in the fruit or vegetable sections. We place them in the good fats section.

We list common foods below. It is important to note that all lists, including the food plates are not complete lists. We want you to use these as guidelines only.

You can eat unlimited amounts of the following Low Glycemic Load (LGL) foods:

Vegetables: artichokes, asparagus, bamboo shoots, bean sprouts, bell or other peppers, brocco sprouts, brocco flower, broccoli, brussels sprouts, cabbage (all types), cauliflower, celery, chives, cucumber/dill pickles, eggplant, garlic, green beans, mushrooms, okra, onion, pumpkin, radishes, salsa (sugar-free), sea vegetables (kelp, etc.), spaghetti or summer squash, sprouts, tomato or mixed vegetable juice, tomatoes, water chestnuts, zucchini.

Greens: beet greens, bok choy, collards, dandelion, escarole, kale, leeks, mustard greens, spinach, swiss chard, watercress.

Lettuce/mixed greens: arugula, butter lettuce, chicory, endive, herb mix, radicchio, red and green leaf lettuce, romaine, spinach and baby spinach, watercress.

These are good for you but should be limited to serving sizes below:

Vegetables (1/2 fist per day): beets, carrots, parsnips, rutabaga, sweet potatoes (yams), winter squash (acorn or butternut), potatoes.

Fruit (fresh, not dried or canned, about 1–2 fists per day): apples, apricots, berries (blackberries, blueberries, boysenberries, cranberries, goji berries, raspberries, and strawberries), cherries, fresh figs, grapefruit, grapes, kiwis, kumquats, lemons, limes, mango, melons (cantaloupe, honeydew, and watermelon), nectarines, oranges, peaches, pears, plums, tangerines.

Nuts (1/2 fistful or 1 tablespoon of nut butter per day): almonds, cashews, hazelnuts, macadamia, peanuts, pecans, pistachios, walnuts, seeds (poppy, pumpkin, sesame, and sunflower seeds).

Grains (1/2–1 fist per day) : amaranth, barley, buckwheat groats, bulgur (cracked wheat), kamut, millet, oats, quinoa, rice (basmati, brown, and wild), rye, spelt, triticale, wheat germ, and whole wheat, whole grain rye crackers, 1/2 whole wheat tortilla or pita, mixed, whole grain or 100 percent whole rye bread (1 slice).

Legumes (1/2 fist): Beans–black, cannellini, edamame (green soy beans), fat-free refried, garbanzo, kidney, lima, mung, navy, and pinto; hummus, lentils, snow peas, split peas, sugar snap, and sweet green peas.

Typical Meals and Snack Choices

Nutrition is complicated. To make your food choices a bit simpler, we give you some ideas for meals and snacks based on a low-fat, modified Mediterranean, and low-carb approach.

Breakfast

If you are following a low-fat or modified Mediterranean food plan, here are some good breakfast choices:

Cold whole grain, low-sugar cereal with rice, almond, soy, low-fat or skim milk

Oatmeal or multigrain porridge

Nonfat plain regular yogurt or nonfat plain Greek yogurt

Nonfat cottage cheese

Thin slice of low-fat cheese, e.g., mozzarella

Fresh fruit

Vegetable omelets (for low-fat diet, use egg whites only)

Tofu with scrambled eggs (for low-fat diet, use egg whites only)

Whole wheat toast

A Supernutrition Smoothie

Medical food shakes, as suggested by your doctor for your health conditions

If you are following a low-carb food plan, avoid carbohydrates/sugar in the morning (even fruit) where possible, as this tends to increase insulin levels. Instead, *try these choices for breakfast*:

Vegetable omelet

Tofu with scrambled eggs and tomato

Low-fat cottage cheese

Plain nonfat Greek yogurt and a handful of nuts

Medical food shake, e.g., UltraMeal Plus 360 or UltraglycemX (Metagenics)

Consider a nontraditional breakfast—use the previous night's protein leftovers!

A Supernutrition Smoothie with no or minimal fruit

Snacks

Consider 1-2 thumb sizes of nuts or nut butters, fruit, vegetable sticks or low fat cheeses.

Supernutrition Smoothie

Most of us struggle to get the necessary nutrients without a lot of extra calories. One easy way to achieve this is with what we call a Supernutrition Smoothie. This makes a great breakfast. Here is the basic recipe:

One glass of filtered water.

Add protein. Options are 2 tablespoons of organic tofu or a powdered protein such as a whey protein or spirulina-based powder.

Add vegetables. You can do this by blending 2 cups of leafy green vegetables. Use spinach, kale, parsley, and others to taste. Alternatively, use an organic, vegetable-based powder, available from your health-food store. Look for one that contains cruciferous vegetables, such as kale and brussels sprouts, as well as flax seeds. We recommend a product called SP Complete by Standard Process.

Add fruit. Use 1 cup of fresh or frozen fruit or 1 cup of 100 percent pomegranate juice. Berries are always a good choice; a banana will give the smoothie a creamier texture.

Add good fats. Try freshly ground flax seeds or 1/2 tablespoon of flax seed oil, or 1 tablespoon Salvia hispanica, better known a chia seeds. (If you don't like the taste of these, take 1000 to 2000 mg omega-3 mercury-free fish oil capsules as a separate supplement).

Add fiber. Add in 1 tablespoon of fiber. We suggest unflavored psyllium husk or inulin fiber.

Add flavorings to taste. Some ideas are 1/4-inch ginger root, peeled and grated; cinnamon or nutmeg; 1/4 to 1/2 teaspoon of powdered green tea; 1 to 2 teaspoons of a nut butter; yogurt or probiotic powder.

Blend together and enjoy!

© Shutterstock/ sutsaiy

Lunch and Dinner

The following illustrations are examples of the fist method showing what your meal would look like on a Mediterranean food plan, low-carb food plan, and low-fat food plan. These are maximum portion sizes for your main meal. No matter what size your plate, try to keep the proportions the same as those shown.

What your main meal looks like on a Modified Mediterranean Food Plan

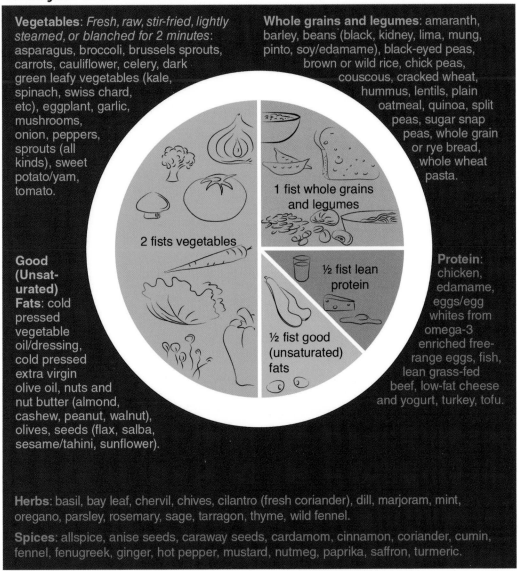

Vegetables: *Fresh, raw, stir-fried, lightly steamed, or blanched for 2 minutes*: asparagus, broccoli, brussels sprouts, carrots, cauliflower, celery, dark green leafy vegetables (kale, spinach, swiss chard, etc), eggplant, garlic, mushrooms, onion, peppers, sprouts (all kinds), sweet potato/yam, tomato.

Whole grains and legumes: amaranth, barley, beans (black, kidney, lima, mung, pinto, soy/edamame), black-eyed peas, brown or wild rice, chick peas, couscous, cracked wheat, hummus, lentils, plain oatmeal, quinoa, split peas, sugar snap peas, whole grain or rye bread, whole wheat pasta.

Good (Unsaturated) Fats: cold pressed vegetable oil/dressing, cold pressed extra virgin olive oil, nuts and nut butter (almond, cashew, peanut, walnut), olives, seeds (flax, salba, sesame/tahini, sunflower).

Protein: chicken, edamame, eggs/egg whites from omega-3 enriched free-range eggs, fish, lean grass-fed beef, low-fat cheese and yogurt, turkey, tofu.

Within the plate:
- 2 fists vegetables
- 1 fist whole grains and legumes
- ½ fist lean protein
- ½ fist good (unsaturated) fats

Herbs: basil, bay leaf, chervil, chives, cilantro (fresh coriander), dill, marjoram, mint, oregano, parsley, rosemary, sage, tarragon, thyme, wild fennel.

Spices: allspice, anise seeds, caraway seeds, cardamom, cinnamon, coriander, cumin, fennel, fenugreek, ginger, hot pepper, mustard, nutmeg, paprika, saffron, turmeric.

| Figure S3.2 | Modified Mediterranean Food Plan |

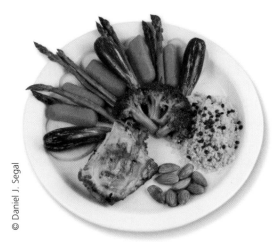

A Modified Mediterranean Food plate example:

½ fist lean protein (grilled chicken)
½ fist good fats (almonds plus olive oil dressing)
1 fist whole grains and legumes (brown rice and lentils)
2 fists LGL (Low Glycemic Load) vegetables

127

What your main meal looks like on a Low-Carb Food Plan

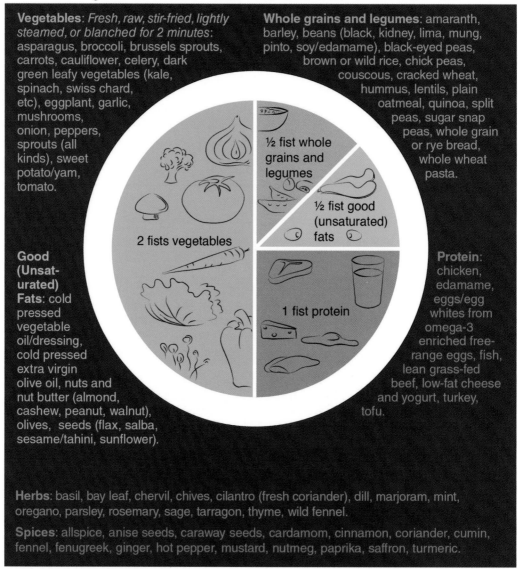

Vegetables: *Fresh, raw, stir-fried, lightly steamed, or blanched for 2 minutes*: asparagus, broccoli, brussels sprouts, carrots, cauliflower, celery, dark green leafy vegetables (kale, spinach, swiss chard, etc), eggplant, garlic, mushrooms, onion, peppers, sprouts (all kinds), sweet potato/yam, tomato.

Good (Unsaturated) Fats: cold pressed vegetable oil/dressing, cold pressed extra virgin olive oil, nuts and nut butter (almond, cashew, peanut, walnut), olives, seeds (flax, salba, sesame/tahini, sunflower).

Whole grains and legumes: amaranth, barley, beans (black, kidney, lima, mung, pinto, soy/edamame), black-eyed peas, brown or wild rice, chick peas, couscous, cracked wheat, hummus, lentils, plain oatmeal, quinoa, split peas, sugar snap peas, whole grain or rye bread, whole wheat pasta.

Protein: chicken, edamame, eggs/egg whites from omega-3 enriched free-range eggs, fish, lean grass-fed beef, low-fat cheese and yogurt, turkey, tofu.

½ fist whole grains and legumes

½ fist good (unsaturated) fats

2 fists vegetables

1 fist protein

Herbs: basil, bay leaf, chervil, chives, cilantro (fresh coriander), dill, marjoram, mint, oregano, parsley, rosemary, sage, tarragon, thyme, wild fennel.

Spices: allspice, anise seeds, caraway seeds, cardamom, cinnamon, coriander, cumin, fennel, fenugreek, ginger, hot pepper, mustard, nutmeg, paprika, saffron, turmeric.

| Figure S3.3 | Low-Carb Food Plan |

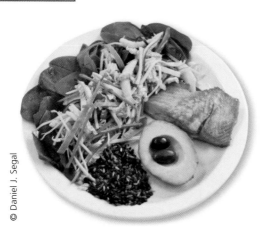

A Low-Carb Plate example:

1 fist lean protein (grilled salmon)
½ fist good fats (avocado and olives)
½ fist whole grains (wild rice)
LGL (Low Glycemic Load) vegetables
(2 fists)

What your main meal looks like on a Low-Fat Food Plan

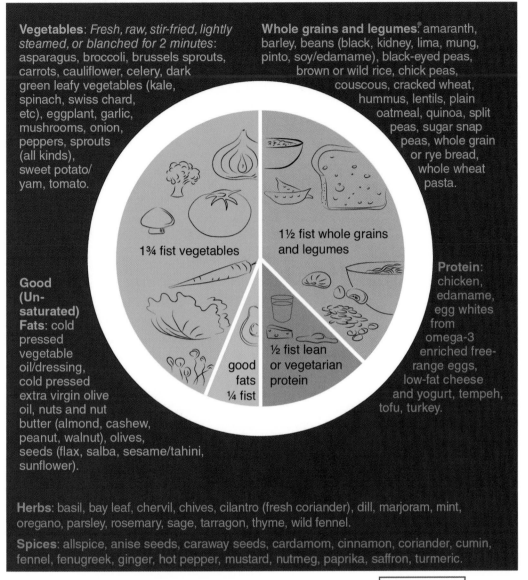

Vegetables: *Fresh, raw, stir-fried, lightly steamed, or blanched for 2 minutes*: asparagus, broccoli, brussels sprouts, carrots, cauliflower, celery, dark green leafy vegetables (kale, spinach, swiss chard, etc), eggplant, garlic, mushrooms, onion, peppers, sprouts (all kinds), sweet potato/yam, tomato.

Whole grains and legumes: amaranth, barley, beans (black, kidney, lima, mung, pinto, soy/edamame), black-eyed peas, brown or wild rice, chick peas, couscous, cracked wheat, hummus, lentils, plain oatmeal, quinoa, split peas, sugar snap peas, whole grain or rye bread, whole wheat pasta.

1¾ fist vegetables

1½ fist whole grains and legumes

Good (Un-saturated) Fats: cold pressed vegetable oil/dressing, cold pressed extra virgin olive oil, nuts and nut butter (almond, cashew, peanut, walnut), olives, seeds (flax, salba, sesame/tahini, sunflower).

good fats ¼ fist

½ fist lean or vegetarian protein

Protein: chicken, edamame, egg whites from omega-3 enriched free-range eggs, low-fat cheese and yogurt, tempeh, tofu, turkey.

Herbs: basil, bay leaf, chervil, chives, cilantro (fresh coriander), dill, marjoram, mint, oregano, parsley, rosemary, sage, tarragon, thyme, wild fennel.

Spices: allspice, anise seeds, caraway seeds, cardamom, cinnamon, coriander, cumin, fennel, fenugreek, ginger, hot pepper, mustard, nutmeg, paprika, saffron, turmeric.

Figure S3.4 | Low-Fat Food Plan

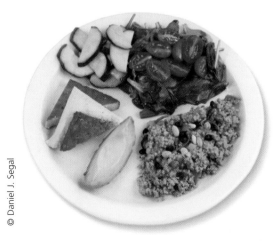

© Daniel J. Segal

A Low-Fat Plate example:

½ fist lean protein (tofu)
¼ fist good fat (avocado)
1 ½ fist whole grains and legumes (quinoa and lentils)
1 ½ fists LGL (Low Glycemic Load) vegetables

Nutritional Supplement Guidelines

Do we really need dietary supplements? You may have heard that all supplements do is make expensive urine, or that you just need a one-a-day multivitamin with minerals. These statements are both incorrect. Supplements can dramatically improve health. Yet, on the other hand, they may not always be good for you. They can fuel various diseases and interact with certain drugs.

Let's look at some factors to consider:

Supplements for Nutritional Deficiencies

As medical students in South Africa, we watched a young woman enter the hospital in heart failure. She struggled to breathe as her heart beat rapidly. Her swollen legs and altered mental status were a clue to the cause of her illness—a form of beriberi, or vitamin B1 (thiamine) deficiency. An intravenous infusion of thiamine resulted in an astounding recovery. She was better within hours, an example of how vitamins can make a difference. Does that mean we should give thiamine to everyone with heart failure? The answer is clearly no. Understanding nutritional deficiencies helps us use the correct nutrient for the correct problem.

Vitamin D is another good example. In general, excessive sun exposure can lead to an increased risk of skin cancer. In attempting to avoid this risk through the use of sunscreen and protective clothing, many people have become deficient in this important vitamin, which is derived from the sun on your skin. Checking your vitamin D level is a good idea. If it is low, supplementing with vitamin D3 (cholecalciferol) can help prevent or improve many conditions, including hypertension, depression, osteoporosis, and autoimmune diseases, as well as seasonal affective disorder. People with Seasonal Affective Disorder get cabin fever or depression in the winter months and crave warm, sunny climates. Vitamin D supplementation may be a much less expensive alternative!

Adriana's Story

We have found that a surprising number of people have amino acid imbalances. When the missing nutrients are added, the body can rebalance and symptoms resolve naturally. Consider the case of Adriana, a young woman who had suffered with chronic headaches for twenty years. During the five years before she came to us, her headaches occurred daily. She had seen several neurologists and headache specialists and been to a number of headache clinics. She came to us to try acupuncture for pain management.

We treated her with acupuncture, but it did not help. We prescribed medications, but they did not help. Finally, in desperation, we ordered a complete nutritional evaluation, which showed that all of her amino acids levels were abnormally low, including her essential amino acids.

We treated her with an amino acid powder that contained a full spectrum of these nutrients. The following day—after twenty years of chronic headaches—Adriana's headaches went away, and she has been almost free of symptoms for the last few years.

> Let food be thy medicine and let thy medicine be food.
>
> **– Hippocrates 460 BC–377 BC**

Breathe well. Stay well.
well. Love well. Relax w

Sophia's Story: Good Fats and the Brain

Sophia, a healthy-looking 24-year-old, came into our office complaining of a dull daily headache for the past five months. The headache started innocuously enough. She was helping her husband build a deck when she stood up suddenly and banged her head. She developed an immediate headache but didn't think much of it. A few days later, the headache was still there. Over-the-counter medications, ice packs, and rest didn't relieve the pain. Nothing seemed to help. Her physician thought she might have sustained a more serious trauma than she had reported. To make sure nothing was wrong, he ordered an MRI of her head. It was completely normal.

A trial of stronger narcotic medications helped the headache slightly, but made her feel sick. She tried an array of headache-prevention medications, but they did not help. A visit to a neurologist who specialized in headaches also offered no benefit. An EEG (electro-encephalogram) and MRA (magnetic resonance angiogram) were both normal. The neurologist thought Adriana might be suffering from a post-concussive headache, which would resolve over time. He told her to come back if the headache didn't improve. Unfortunately, it didn't. That was when she came to see us, frustrated about her progress.

A trial of acupuncture, nerve blocks into her scalp, and gentle manipulative neck treatments also didn't offer any relief. We began to think of other potential causes of the headache. Sophia had shared with us that she suffered from anorexia as a teenager. Although she was no longer anorexic, she still watched her diet very carefully. We thought she might have an amino acid deficiency, just as Adriana had. However, a nutritional evaluation revealed something entirely different: a severe deficiency of omega-3 fatty acids. This made sense. Sophia never ate fat—and that meant her bad saturated and her good unsaturated fat levels were both very low.

A trial of supplementation with mercury-free fish oil high in EPA and DHA was used. Sophia's headaches slowly subsided and disappeared over about eight weeks!

A Question of Quality

The quality of dietary supplements is extremely important, but the supplement industry isn't as carefully regulated as drugs are. Consumers are pretty much on their own when it comes to finding top-quality products. Look for products from reputable manufacturers that are made using pharmaceutical grade ingredients. The manufacturer should also guarantee the potency levels on the label and state that good manufacturing processes (GMP) were followed. A supplement should be safe and effective, as evident from safety and efficacy in clinical trials, case control reports, and other clinical documentation. The products you purchase should be batch-tested to ensure a scientific evaluation of ingredients.

They should be free of heavy metals, pesticides, and contamination by fungus, bacteria, or toxins. (Unregulated supplements from China notoriously are tainted with drugs and even toxins.) The products should meet the quality and purity standards set by the United States Pharmacopeia (USP, or USP-NF), NSF International and the Natural Products Association. The most effective products are manufactured by companies with scientific knowledge about the products they sell. Finally, look for companies that employ fair trade practices and are concerned about sustaining the environment and the area where they harvest the herbs.

Supplements for Better Metabolism

We can use nutritional supplements to take a functional approach to helping the body detoxify, lower oxidative stress, reduce inflammation, improve methylation at the correct time, improve digestive function, improve probiotic balance, and maintain equilibrium of the immune system. This only helps, however, if the correct, high-quality supplements are used.

Many supplement companies would have us believe that if we just take their trendy new antioxidant pill, powder, juice, or whatever, we will live forever and avoid illness. We are continually bombarded with ads for the latest supplement *du jour*.

What is important to realize here is that no one particular supplement will be the ultimate solution to preventing illness. The food plans we have outlined above will help promote normal function of all the systems we are concerned about. However, if clinical evaluation and functional lab testing still point to an imbalance, supplements can be added to promote normal functioning. The benefit here is that dietary supplements tend to have multiple benefits. For example, good antioxidants will usually help detoxification and lower inflammation. Used wisely, supplements offer us a way to help correct genetic predispositions to illness. In essence, they can act as a way for us to have an epigenetic tune-up! In the future, we will likely see the development of more functional foods or medical foods that will help us do this.

Supplements for Improving Detoxification

Numerous supplements can help improve your detoxification. N-acetyl cysteine (NAC) has been used in emergency rooms for decades to treat acetaminophen (Tylenol) overdoses, protecting the liver from damaging free radicals as it helps excrete the drug. Doses of 500 mg to 1000 mg twice daily can help the liver with its detoxification function. NAC also helps increase glutathione levels, a major antioxidant. It also appears to help an agitated mood. Supplements with watercress, ellagic acid, artichoke leaf extract, juniper berry powder (*Juniperus communis*), red clover powder (*Trifolium pratense*), collinsonia powder, fenugreek powder, and milk thistle (*Silybum marianum*) can also all help improve detoxification.

Antioxidant Supplements

The classic antioxidant supplements are vitamins A, C, and E, and the minerals zinc and selenium. These are often touted as the solution to macular degeneration and other degenerative diseases. However, studies on these supplements have not been positive. Smokers who took vitamin A had higher lung cancer rates. Vitamin C, when injected in extremely high doses, appears to help reverse early atherosclerotic disease. However, oral doses do not seem to do the same. Men with higher blood levels of vitamin E level tend to have lower levels of prostate cancer, but studies on supplementation with synthetic vitamin E showed that this could actually increase prostate cancer rates. Another confounding variable is that a substance that appears to be an antioxidant in the lab may turn into a pro-oxidant in the body.

Green tea (EGCG) is believed to be one hundred times more potent as an antioxidant than vitamin C and at least twenty-five times more potent than vitamin E. Even more impressive are resveratrol and pycnogenol, the antioxidants found in red wine, and enzogenol, an antioxidant derived from New Zealand pine bark. These products appear to mimic the benefits of a calorie-restricted diet, without the food restriction. Resveratrol appears to regulate the sirtuin family of our aging genes. Resveratrol is also thought to be a possible explanation for the so-called French Paradox—why the French can smoke, eat a high-fat diet, never go to the gym, and yet have a lower heart attack rate than Americans. It is possible the resveratrol they get from regularly drinking red wine with meals protects them. Products with resveratrol derivatives are being studied for their impact on aging and illness. Enzogenol fed to mice helped them live longer, healthier lives. It also appears to help regulate brain function, help prevent migraines, and regulate eye disease, heart disease, and even attention deficit hyperactivity disorder (ADHD). However, the correct doses of these supplements have yet to be determined. Antioxidants appear to work better when multiple supplements are used in combination with one another. So while they are promising, we suggest you review antioxidants with someone familiar with current research data on nutritional supplements before taking them.

Supplements for Lowering Inflammation

Curcumin, or turmeric, has great anti-inflammatory benefits when tested in the lab. However, in humans, study outcomes are variable. This may be because turmeric is 2,000 percent better absorbed if it is taken with pepper or a pepper extract (as it might be, for instance, in an East Indian diet). EPA, found in fish oil, has anti-inflammatory benefits, as do the botanicals boswellia (*Boswellia serrata*), devil's claw (*Hrapasgophytum procumbens*), cat's claw (*Uncaria* species), willow bark (*Salix* species), and ginger (*Zinziber officinale*).

Supplements for Maintaining Immune Balance

Supplements can be used to support immune function while simultaneously dealing with stress. Examples here are astragalus, Siberian ginseng, ashwagandha (Indian ginseng), and rehmannia. Mushroom extracts and echinacea can help prevent colds. Plant sterols and sterolins can help regulate T-cell or immune function, helping chronic fatigue, allergies, and boosting immunity.

We list only a few supplements to help you understand how to think about them. There is a broad array available. Find a health care practitioner who is knowledgeable in this area and can help you understand which is the best one to take.

The 4R Program to Improve Gut Health

The 4R model is a program promoted by the Institute for Functional Medicine. We find it to be an excellent approach to helping all diet-related disorders.

The four Rs are:

1. **Remove.** Use an elimination diet to discover and remove offending foods. Food sensitivity testing can be helpful here. Check the stool for bacteria and parasites and treat these, if necessary.

2. **Replace.** Enzymes, acids, or other digestive factors may be inadequate and may need replacement or supplementation.

3. **Reinoculate.** If the gut flora are imbalanced, reinoculate with the correct probiotics. Probiotics can neutralize pathogenic bacteria in the gut, reduce toxins in the gut, improve cell maturation, enhance metabolic turnover, and improve enzyme production.

4. **Repair.** Healing the gut wall remains the most important step. Common supplements that are used for this include L-glutamine, zinc, fish oils, arabinogalactans (from larch gum), cinnamon (*Cinnamomum cassia*), plantains (*Musa paradisiacal)*, apple pectin or apple fruit powder, aloe vera gel or juice, slippery elm bark, and marshmallow root.

Food as Medicine

In Ring 3 and Star 3, we discuss the myriad benefits of a proper diet. This will send the correct message to your genes, as well as help to optimize your metabolism. Beyond the benefits of a nutrient-dense diet, you can do even more for your health with food.

As discussed in Ring 3, when you get sick, you may develop altered intestinal permeability, or leaky gut syndrome. In this case, a food rotation diet may be useful when dealing with irritable bowel syndrome and inflammatory bowel disorders. It can also help with autoimmune disease in general and with nonspecific symptoms such as headaches, fatigue, bloating, urticaria (hives) and other skin conditions such as eczema and psoriasis, spontaneous bruising, memory problems, and a host of other health issues.

In Star 4 we will discuss how you can alter your diet to help balance insulin resistance and optimize your hormone function.

Food or Drug?

One of the big differences between food supplements and drugs is that drugs in general are new-to-nature molecules. In other words, we may not have detoxification pathways to adequately deal with the metabolic by-products of drugs. In addition, drugs tend to have side effects and interactions, especially when you start taking more than one. Sometimes we only find out years later what these interactions are.

Food supplements in general are much less likely to have side effects and interactions. In general, Mother Nature has helped us decide which foods humans have tolerated over thousands of years. In effect, the human race has functioned like a big experiment, showing us where an intervention has worked or not worked.

Food supplements are often, but not always, better tolerated than drugs. While a drug may have one or two benefits, it may also have multiple side effects. One food supplement, on the other hand, is likely to have multiple benefits. Vitamin D, for instance, may benefit osteoporosis and depression, may decrease pain, may reduce autoimmune disorders, and may even lower hypertension. Fish oil supplements may help heart disease, arthritis, osteoporosis, depression, and host of other problems. The body is used to foods in combination. This is not true with drugs.

Synergistic Nutritional Benefits

The more drugs we take, the more likely we are to suffer from drug interactions and side effects. Nutritional substances are different. In nature, foods have multiple elements all working together to benefit us. Supplement companies may tout the benefit of the latest antioxidant. New scientific studies may show the benefit of a supplement on a certain antioxidant response or inflammatory pathway. However, we need to remember that in nature, these nutritional substances work together with one another. By understanding the various systems of the body, we can learn to analyze this and design specific programs that affect multiple systems.

You may need some nutritional supplements to antidote a subclinical nutritional deficiency, others to speed up detoxification, and others to act as antioxidants or anti-inflammatories. We can still use others to balance or modulate the immune system. Finally, we can use these in addition to medications if necessary.

When we analyze and understand the body from a nutrigenomic and functional medicine standpoint, we learn that the treatment that reverses illness is often the same treatment that promotes health. What's more, the same process appears to help multiple disease processes at the same time. This is the essence of Transformational Medicine. We use one program to transform your illness process into a wellness process.

A Transformational Supplement Program

A transformational supplement program can include vitamins, minerals, amino acids, enzymes, herbs, and medications. It should ensure that hormones and mood are balanced. Your program should be selected in conjunction with a comprehensive lifestyle approach. We strongly recommend working with a doctor who has an understanding of nutrigenomics and functional medicine.

If you are taking any sort of dietary supplement, always tell your doctor. Supplement-medication interactions may create unexpected side effects.

You will know when your Transformational Nutrition Program is working when:

1. You feel better.

2. Your lab markers change.

3. Your illness begins to improve.

4. You develop a sense of resilience— the ability to bounce back.

5. You develop a new, positive sense of vitality.

A Transformational Nutrition Program =
A nutritionally dense, genetically appropriate diet + appropriate supplements

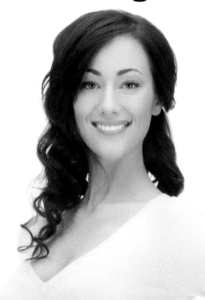

Alex Learns to Transform His Body Chemistry

When Alex discovered he had insulin resistance, he realized that the low-fat food plan he was following was incorrect for him. His new approach was to follow a low-carbohydrate food plan and stay away from white bread, white flour, pasta, and sugar. He began adding more and more green vegetables to his diet, often making a super smoothie for breakfast or having a nutritional food shake. He made sure to get vegetable oils in his diet every day, usually in the form of some avocado with a liberal amount of a cold-pressed, extra virgin olive oil mixed with balsamic vinegar. He also began experimenting with a rotation diet to see if that helped. He found that he felt much better when he removed dairy and wheat from his diet. He added some daily supplements, including a combination B vitamin, (Vitamin B6 50 mg, Vitamin B12 500 mcg and L-methyl tetrahydrofolate 800 mcg), vitamin D3 2000 IU, mercury-free fish oil 1500 mg oil, and a high dose of human strain probiotic. He also added a digestive enzyme supplement three times a day with meals.

Six months after seeing us, Alex returned to his primary care physician for a follow-up visit. He was pleased to report that his knees were better, although his back still ached at times. His bowel function seemed to have completely normalized. He no longer suffered from indigestion or flatulence. What he really wanted to find out, though, were his clinical results. His doctor congratulated him on his twenty-two-pound weight loss and then opened his chart to review the results. Alex's blood pressure was now normal at 124/78. His total cholesterol had dropped from 210 mg/dL to 168 and his LDL (bad cholesterol) from 135 mg/dL to 87. His triglycerides were 320 mg/dL but had fallen to 116, and his HDL (good cholesterol) had risen from 28 to 34 mg/dL. What's more, his fasting blood glucose had dropped from 106 mg/dL to 78, his homocysteine level from 14 to 7 and his hs-CRP level from 4.2 to 1.3.

"Whatever you're doing, Alex, keep it up," his doctor said. Alex smiled. He had transformed his body chemistry, all without medication. Even more important than his body chemistry, though, he felt great!

4

RING FOUR

Understanding Your Hormones

Hormone Imbalances Can Lead to Fatigue, Weight Gain, Hot Flashes, Low Libido, Impotence, and Depression—

but Hormone Testing Can Help Restore the Balance

Hormones are chemical messengers—tiny messenger molecules that serve as a means of communication between our cells, regulating body functions. Hormones are manufactured inside glands, such as the thyroid or pancreas, and are secreted into the body, usually directly into the bloodstream.

In Greek, "hormaein" means "to set in motion," and that is exactly what hormones do. They set in motion activity that ultimately affects every cell in our bodies. Our body chemistry is an invisible web of relationships—vast complex networks that ultimately make us who we are. Our hormones are always behind the scenes, calling the shots, defining everything that happens. They are everywhere at once, interacting with the microscopic receptors on every single cell. The entire system is called the endocrine system; it comprises both the hormones and the glands that make them.

Master Hormones

Many of our hormones, no matter where they are made or what they do, are controlled by a complex feedback mechanism that begins in the brain: the hypothalamic–pituitary–adrenal axis. The system begins in the hypothalamus, the part of the brain that links the nervous system to the endocrine hormone system through the pituitary gland. Among other crucial functions, the hypothalamus controls body temperature, sense of hunger and thirst, and sleep and circadian cycles. It also makes and secretes neurohormones known as hypothalamic-releasing hormones. These hormones travel to the pituitary gland where they may stimulate or inhibit the release of hormones.

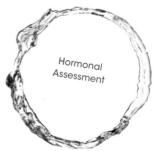

Hormonal Assessment

The pituitary gland is a pea-sized organ also located in your brain, close to the hypothalamus. In response to hormones released by the hypothalamus, the pituitary gland produces pituitary hormones. Sometimes called the master gland, the pituitary orchestrates the entire symphony of hormonal chemistry. As the conductor, it sends messages to the adrenal gland, thyroid, testicles, ovaries, breasts, uterus, kidneys, and other organs and tissues throughout the body.

Pituitary hormones send chemical messages to the adrenal glands, small organs that sit on top of each kidney. The adrenal glands respond by producing hormones which help us deal with stress (adrenaline, noradrenaline and cortisol), regulate our water and salt balance (aldosterone), and produce sex hormones (estrogen and testosterone). Because the stress hormones have such an impact on our health, we will discuss them in detail in this section.

Stress Hormones

We tend to view stress hormones as harmful and stress as a negative. In reality, stress is how we adapt to our lives—it's part of being alive. The issue of stress is really more a question of balance. How do we react to stress? Can we maintain a balanced response when stress intensifies?

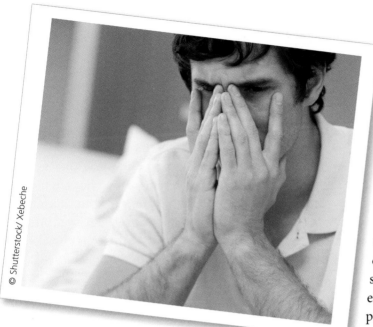

If the blood sugar/pancreas feedback loop is working properly, enough glucose enters the cells to keep them fully fueled; excess glucose gets carried off to be stored as fat. When this happens, the blood sugar or glucose level drops down to a baseline until you eat carbohydrates again.

The glucose/insulin loop can be disrupted. Some people don't produce enough insulin to carry the glucose into their cells. More commonly, some people develop resistance to the effect of insulin. In either case, these people have diabetes mellitus, a disease marked by high blood sugar levels.

In type 1 diabetes, an autoimmune disease, the insulin-producing cells of the pancreas are destroyed, usually in early adolescence, although the disease can sometimes develop earlier in childhood or in mature adults. In this case insulin levels are low.

In this section, we will focus primarily on type 2 diabetes, because it is so prevalent. Insulin resistance is the hallmark of type 2 diabetes. Insulin levels may be normal or even elevated, but it's not doing its job of carrying glucose into the cells. The causes of insulin resistance are complex and not fully understood, but the result is that while blood sugar levels are abnormally high, the cells are unable to accept the glucose because of insulin resistance. The high levels of blood sugar or glucose circulating in the bloodstream can cause extensive damage to blood vessels, particularly in the heart, eyes and kidneys.

Ultimately, we want to redefine stress as adaptation. Our stress hormones allow us to stay up all night to push through on a project that's due or study for an exam. This same response enables us to pull our child out of the path of danger in the blink of an eye. It is actually quite a marvelous survival mechanism.

Under acute (short-lasting) stress, the adrenal glands secrete the hormones adrenaline (also called epinephrine) and noradrenaline (also called norepinephrine.) Under chronic (long-lasting) stress, the adrenals secrete the hormone cortisol. Stress hormones are essential to our adaptation and to our survival. Stress is fine—until it becomes relentless and depletes us. Then it can be dangerous to our health. (See Ring 2, where we reviewed the changes that happen to cortisol under chronic stress.) In the end, it is always a question of balance.

Insulin

When you eat sugary or starchy foods (carbohydrates), they enter the bloodstream as glucose, also called blood sugar. A rise in blood sugar stimulates the pancreas to produce the hormone insulin, which then carries the glucose into cells, where it can be used for energy.

Sex Hormones

Procreation is one of the primary drives for human beings. Sex hormones help us carry out this function. All occur in both men and women, although in different ratios. The sex hormones are primarily produced in the ovaries in women and the testes in men.

139

As we get older, these organs begin to produce hormones at reduced levels. The sex hormones are also produced in smaller amounts by our adrenals. Since all the sex hormones use cholesterol, a chemical steroid, as their main building block, they are called the steroidogenic hormones.

Sex hormones fall into three major classes

Androgens include testosterone and anabolic steroids, the primary hormones of the male body. In men, testosterone is secreted by the testes; women secrete much smaller amounts of testosterone from the ovaries. Testosterone is needed to develop the male reproductive organs; it also gives men their male characteristics, including larger muscle mass, heavier bones, and body hair. Anabolic steroids build up the body's muscles and give us a sense of well-being. That's why so many athletes are tempted to take synthetic anabolic steroids to improve performance.

Estrogens are the primary sex hormones for women, although men also produce this hormone in much smaller amounts. The word estrogen comes from *estrus/oistros* (a period of fertility for female mammals) and *gen/gonos* (to generate). In other words, estrogen helps generate female fertility. It also produces fe-

Myth #5. Getting older means aging.

— **Mark Hyman, M.D.,** *Ultraprevention*

male secondary sexual characteristics—making women sexually attractive and curvy. Women actually produce three different estrogen hormones. Which form of estrogen hormone that is dominant depends on the stage of a woman's life. For women who are still menstruating but are not pregnant, estradiol is the primary form. During pregnancy, estriol is the primary estrogen. After menopause, the primary estrogen is estrone. (We will talk about those in a bit more detail later in this section.)

Progestagens include progesterone, which supports the health of the uterine lining. Low levels of progesterone can result in premenstrual syndrome (PMS) in younger women and can contribute to menopausal symptoms later in life. Progesterone appears to counterbalance some of the effects of estrogen.

Thyroid Hormones

The thyroid, a butterfly-shaped gland at the front of the neck, just below the voice box, produces the hormones that control the metabolic flame—turning the heat up or down. You could think of the thyroid as the thermostat of metabolism, because it affects energy level, mental focus and function, sleep cycles, heart rate, digestion, muscle tone, and even strength. The thyroid has an impact on every system in the body.

Hormones Out of Balance

The elegant chemistry of hormones is like a beautiful symphony, with messages constantly feeding back to controller glands in order to balance and regulate the system, affecting the entire body and every aspect of its function. When a part of the hormonal system becomes out of tune, however, the result can be cacophony.

Physicians, especially the hormone specialists known as endocrinologists, are well trained to look for abnormal hormonal pathways. These vary from mild thyroid imbalances and type 2 diabetes to more complex hormonal problems, such as adrenal hyperplasia (excessive or deficient production of sex steroids), pituitary tumors, and Cushing's disease.

Hormones 101: How Hormones Affect Tissues, at a Glance

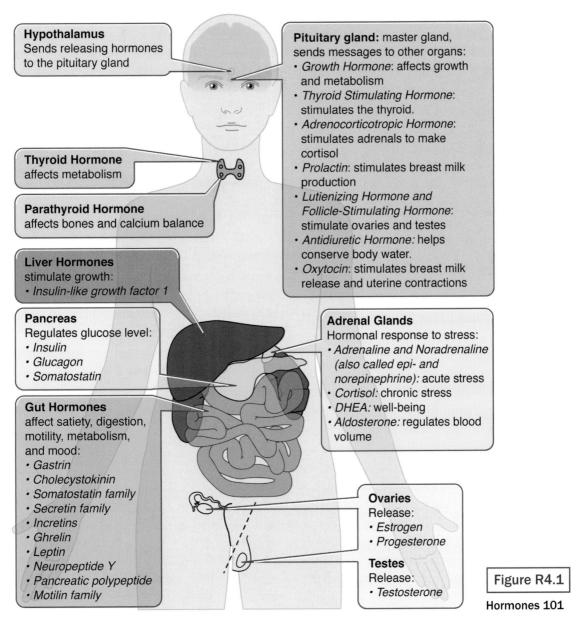

Hypothalamus
Sends releasing hormones to the pituitary gland

Pituitary gland: master gland, sends messages to other organs:
- *Growth Hormone*: affects growth and metabolism
- *Thyroid Stimulating Hormone*: stimulates the thyroid.
- *Adrenocorticotropic Hormone*: stimulates adrenals to make cortisol
- *Prolactin*: stimulates breast milk production
- *Lutienizing Hormone and Follicle-Stimulating Hormone*: stimulate ovaries and testes
- *Antidiuretic Hormone*: helps conserve body water.
- *Oxytocin*: stimulates breast milk release and uterine contractions

Thyroid Hormone
affects metabolism

Parathyroid Hormone
affects bones and calcium balance

Liver Hormones
stimulate growth:
- *Insulin-like growth factor 1*

Pancreas
Regulates glucose level:
- *Insulin*
- *Glucagon*
- *Somatostatin*

Adrenal Glands
Hormonal response to stress:
- *Adrenaline and Noradrenaline (also called epi- and norepinephrine)*: acute stress
- *Cortisol*: chronic stress
- *DHEA*: well-being
- *Aldosterone*: regulates blood volume

Gut Hormones
affect satiety, digestion, motility, metabolism, and mood:
- *Gastrin*
- *Cholecystokinin*
- *Somatostatin family*
- *Secretin family*
- *Incretins*
- *Ghrelin*
- *Leptin*
- *Neuropeptide Y*
- *Pancreatic polypeptide*
- *Motilin family*

Ovaries
Release:
- *Estrogen*
- *Progesterone*

Testes
Release:
- *Testosterone*

Figure R4.1

Hormones 101

W e often see patients who are convinced that they have hormonal problems, yet their physicians have told them that all the conventional tests are normal. This is due to one of two reasons. The patient may be attributing symptoms to a disease he or she doesn't actually have. We often see patients, for example, who attribute their weight gain to thyroid problems, but they don't have thyroid disease. Today, thyroid testing is very sensitive and accurate. In these cases, patient needs to look elsewhere, especially at lifestyle, for the cause of the problem. Alternatively, the patient may truly have a hormone imbalance, but conventional lab tests are not detecting the problem. Hormones fluctuate from day to day and over the course of the month, so doing a single test may not reveal a problem. Ultimately, the only way to diagnose a hormone problem is with a hormone test.

Insulin Resistance: When Sugar Becomes a Poison

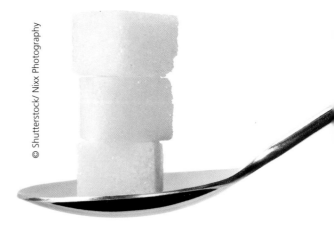

Why is it so easy to gain weight and so hard to take it off—and keep it off? It just doesn't seem fair. One reason weight gain can be so difficult to reverse is that it is often caused by insulin resistance or prediabetes, the preliminary stage that eventually leads to type 2 diabetes. If you have insulin resistance, you are also likely to have high cholesterol, high blood glucose, high blood pressure, and high inflammation markers. The group of signs and symptoms occurs together so often that it's called the metabolic syndrome and is the first leg of the journey on the road to diabetes.

The Snowball Effect of Weight Gain

If we look at the data on obesity and diabetes incidence, we see that they generally parallel each other. In other words, the fatter we get as a nation, the higher our incidence of type 2 diabetes. It's a vicious cycle. Obesity increases insulin resistance, which only makes us fatter. We used to call type 2 diabetes adult-onset diabetes. Unfortunately, these adult-onset conditions now affect children as well. And they are affecting them at younger ages. Children as young as 8 are being diagnosed with type 2 diabetes, a disease that will almost certainly cut their lives short.

Insulin resistance describes an aspect of our body chemistry that probably evolved as a way for our bodies to adapt to famine. Many thousands of years ago, people who had insulin resistance were more likely to survive periods of starvation. When food was plentiful, insulin resistance meant they could quickly add fat around their bellies; when food was scarce, the stored fat helped them survive. Some scientists also believe that insulin resistance prevented frostbite.

Fast forward to current times. No more starvation. We now live in the land of plenty—more than plenty, in fact. Almost all of our food contains added sugar. In 2003 in the United States, the average American consumed a whopping 142 pounds of sugar and 61 pounds of corn syrup—and downed 46 gallons of soft drinks. In 2010, the average American ate about 21 teaspoons of added sugars every day. A lot of that came from sugary sodas and juice drinks—an average can has 10 to 12 teaspoons of sugar, and half of all Americans drink at least one can of soda a day.

Our bodies are genetically adapted to a lifestyle of scarcity, not abundance. The bodies of people who are genetically inclined toward insulin resistance react to all that sugar as if the growing season that year had been especially good. Their insulin resistance kicks in, and their body stores the excess sugar as fat in anticipation of the scarce food supply that is sure to follow any period of abundance. But if the abundance never ends, insulin resistance stops being a survival mechanism and instead becomes a disease that leads to increasing complications, disability, and premature death. Not only that, but insulin may also be a tumor growth factor, making people with high insulin levels more likely to get cancer or making their cancer worse if they get it.

The Metabolic Syndrome

According to the American Heart Association and the National Heart, Lung, and Blood Institute, the metabolic syndrome exists if you have any three of the following five conditions:

- Waist measurement > 40 inches for men; >35 inches for women
- Triglyceride levels >150 milligrams per deciliter (mg/dL), or taking medication for elevated triglyceride levels
- HDL, or "good," cholesterol level < 40 mg/dL for men and < 50 mg/dL for women, or taking medication for low HDL levels
- Blood pressure levels >130/85, or taking medication for elevated blood pressure
- Fasting blood glucose levels >100 mg/dL, or taking medication for elevated blood glucose levels

Similar definitions have been developed by the World Health Organization and the American Association of Clinical Endocrinologists.

Individuals with the metabolic syndrome are at high risk for type 2 diabetes, heart disease, peripheral vascular disease, and stroke.

In addition, we use the following criteria to look for trends toward the metabolic syndrome and insulin resistance:

1. HbA1C levels > 5.6%
2. C-Peptide levels should be 0.6 - 4.7 ng/mL
3. Rising total proinsulin levels > 22 pmol/L
4. Leptin Levels > 20 ng/mL (females) or > 6.9 ng/mL (males)
5. Adiponectin levels < 1.4 mcg/mL (males) or < 2.7 mcg/mL (females)

Newer Biomarkers for Weight Control

Newer biomarkers for insulin resistance include adipocytokines (chemicals produced by fat tissue), which include adiponectin, ghrelin, leptin, and resistin. The hormones pancreatic polypeptide and glucagon-like peptide 1 (GLP-1) play a role in digestion and satiety. These factors can be used in the evaluation of obesity, the risk for metabolic syndrome, and the risk for type 2 diabetes.

- Leptin and resistin make tissues more resistant to insulin, thereby increasing the risk for diabetes.
- Adiponectin does the opposite, by sensitizing the tissues to insulin. Falling adiponectin levels mark the first stage of progression to diabetes.
- Ghrelin lets us know that we feel full.
- Pancreatic polypeptide (PP) is a hormone released after eating. It slows the movement of food through the gut and causes a release of hormones and enzymes that help digest the food. It also lets us know we are full. Reduced levels are associated with obesity.
- Glucagon-like peptide (GLP-1) is released proportionally to calories ingested. It also helps to decrease appetite.

As patients progress toward diabetes, other markers often rise. These include inflammatory markers such as:

- hs-CRP (high-sensitivity C-reactive protein)
- IL-6, IL-8 (interleukin-6 and -8)
- Tumor necrosis factor alpha (TNFα)
- Plasminogen activator inhibitor type 1 (PAI-1)

Other markers include elevated uric acid, ferritin, fibrinogen, and low red cell magnesium levels.

Oleg's Story

Oleg is a 57-year-old man with a gregarious personality. He came to us for acupuncture treatment for osteoarthritis of his right knee. Football injuries in his youth were taking their toll years later. His swollen knee was keeping him from exercising. Since his college days, he had gained forty pounds. His cholesterol levels had soared, his blood pressure had shot up, and he had been diagnosed with type 2 diabetes.

Soon he found himself on a statin drug for his cholesterol, an ACE inhibitor for his hypertension, and metformin for his diabetes. Clearly, Oleg needed to lose weight, but the standard low-fat diet his doctor recommended wasn't working. Oleg wanted acupuncture for his knee pain. A transformational approach suggested he needed to treat both his meta-bolic syndrome and his knee pain.

Because his blood tests showed excessive inflammation, we discussed a different approach with Oleg. Instead of a low-fat diet, we put him on a low-carbohydrate diet with lots of anti-inflammatory foods. To start off the day, Oleg had an UltraMeal Plus 360 Shake by Metagenics. We supplemented this with fish oil, an anti-inflammatory hops extract, and a specialized turmeric extract. Within weeks, his weight started to come off.

In seven months Oleg lost twenty-five pounds and found he was able to dramatically cut the dose of his medications. With acupuncture, he was better able to manage his knee pain. The benefit extended past his pain and metabolism. As he said, "I feel awesome and in control of my life and health."

Endocrine Disrupting Chemicals and Obesogens:
Substances that Can Make Us Sick and Fat

Hormones are chemical messengers that turn processes on and off in our bodies. Just as a key fits into a lock, a particular hormone fits into receptor sites on the cells in order to set the process in motion or turn it off. Some chemicals in our environment can do the same thing, because their molecular structure is very similar to the molecular structure of some natural hormones, such as estrogen. These chemicals are called endocrine disrupters, because they can mimic and disrupt the body's normal endocrine (hormone-producing) system. Unlike hormones, which break down when they're no longer needed, endocrine disrupting chemicals break down slowly and persist in the body for a long time. They turn the lock to the on position and leave it stuck there, possibly for years.

What are these chemicals and how are they gaining access to our bodies? Endocrine disrupters are in the hormones used to process our meat, fish, and milk, the pesticides on our fruits and vegetables, the additives in our processed food, the plastics in our bottles, and the solvents in the cleaning fluids we use. Examples of these chemicals include plastics such as BPA, PFOA (perfluorooctanoic acid or C8), and PVC. BPA is a synthetic estrogen found in some plastic bottles and in the lining used in some tin cans. C8 is found in nonstick pans, spatulas, and spoons, microwave popcorn containers, and pizza boxes. PVC contains chemicals called phthalates that lower testosterone and affect metabolism. PVC is found in the plastic wrap on commercial meat products, shower curtains, and air fresheners.

Atrazine, a common food additive, can affect thyroid hormones. Tributyl tin, which has been linked to obesity, is a fungicide used on the bottom of boats, which then enters the food chain in fish.

Endocrine disrupting chemicals have been linked to diabetes, heart disease, breast and prostate cancer, thyroid disease, and infertility. Some of these chemicals are obesogens: They seem to alter the metabolism and make us more insulin resistant and even recruit more fat cells, contributing to type 2 diabetes, obesity, and polycystic ovary syndrome (PCOS).

Endocrine disrupters also have an adverse affect on detoxification (check back to Star 3 for more on this). What happens when we place a bigger load of endocrine disruptors on the detoxification system than it can handle? In Cambodia and Vietnam, there has been a striking increase in the incidence of diabetes over the past decade, yet the population continues to eat a mostly traditional diet and isn't getting fatter. We think that an important yet unaddressed factor is endocrine disruption due to the increased use there of petrochemicals, creating an environment laden with heavy metal byproducts such as arsenic.

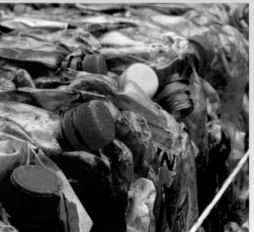
© Shutterstock/ Borys Khamitsevych

Our **Natural Steroids**

Can stress cause us to get fat and lose our sex drive? Yes. The hormones our bodies make from cholesterol are referred to as steroidogenic or steroid hormones. They are the natural steroids in our bodies—the same steroids that bodybuilders and athletes use to bulk up and enhance their performance. Our bodies actually make the very same hormones, but in much lower doses—and they are essential to our well-being.

Steroid Pathways

Steroid hormones flow down two main pathways: the stress hormone pathway to form cortisol and the well-being hormone pathway to form DHEA, testosterone, and estrogens. DHEA (dehydroepiandrosterone) is the most abundant steroid hormone in the body. It is produced mostly in the adrenal glands. DHEA is the basic hormone used by the body to manufacture testosterone and estrogens.

When we are living a balanced life, our hormones reflect this. We have just enough cortisol (our primary stress hormone) to keep inflammation in check, and just enough of our well-being hormone, DHEA. People with high DHEA levels experience a sense of well-being and comfort in their bodies and have been found to have the lowest incidence of cancer, arthritis, and chronic disease.

When we are dealing with intense stress—or relentless low-level chronic stress—the body will "steal" sex hormones so it can continue to produce stress hormones. As a result, our well-being hormone levels drop. Testosterone levels go down, causing a decrease in libido and a loss of muscle mass and strength. Estrogen drops too, which is why menopausal women notice more hot flashes when they have been stressed. You can see how the pathways flow and how stress affects them in the diagram on page 146.

How Our Bodies Wear Down— and How They Get Restored

Ideally, we have a balance between the two hormone systems—between the production of stress hormones and well-being hormones. Stress hormones, such as cortisol, tend to break our bodies down and are referred to as catabolic. In a famine or time of stress, the body needs to repair damage and find protein to make hormones and enzymes, so it breaks down muscle. It also needs to store fuel, so it builds fat. Is it any surprise that stress makes us weak and flabby?

Hormones that restore and heal us, such as DHEA, testosterone, and estrogen, are described as anabolic hormones. They make our muscles grow and give us a sense of well-being.

Chronic stress is very different from acute stress. Acute stress gives us a "fight or flight" response, which triggers the production of adrenaline and noradrenaline. These brief bursts of hormones are a survival mechanism that our bodies are designed to handle. However, when stress becomes chronic and long-term, our bodies eventually wear down. Cortisol initially climbs, but then bottoms out as our adrenal glands become overworked and depleted. The exhausted adrenals also result in low DHEA levels. Chronic stress is associated with higher inflammation and altered immunity. As the body shifts to produce more stress hormones, it also decreases the amount of well-being hormones—DHEA, testosterone, and estrogen—it produces.

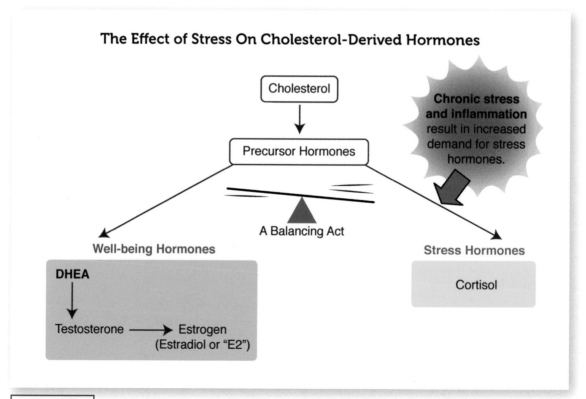

Figure R4.2 | The Effect of Stress on Cholesterol-Derived Hormones

Trevor is a 54-year-old man who came to us with recurrent episodes of back pain. During his examination, he mentioned that he was more tired than usual. Despite working out, he noticed that he needed to use lighter weights, and his muscles were getting smaller and his belly larger. Finally, he admitted that his libido was very low and that he suffered from erectile dysfunction. Another physician had prescribed sildenafil (Viagra®) for him. While it had helped his erectile dysfunction, it did little to change his libido.

A simple blood test confirmed a low testosterone level due to andropause, or male aging. After counseling on the risks and benefits, Trevor decided he wanted to try a testosterone gel. The results after a month were excellent. His libido and zest for life had returned, and his muscles were stronger.

Three months later we checked Trevor's urinary hormone metabolites. While his testosterone and anabolic/catabolic balance were normal, his test showed an abnormal ratio of estrogen metabolites, placing him at an increased risk for prostate cancer. To counteract this, we placed him on a supplement containing a derivative of broccoli (indole-3-carbinol). A repeat hormone test four months after his first visit showed that his ratio of estrogen metabolites had normalized, which indicated that his risk of cancer had been reduced.

Sex Hormones in Midlife

For our ancestors, the cycle of life was quite different than it is for us today. In 1850, the average life span for women in the United States was just 40 years; in 1900, it was 48 years. Consequently, only a minority of women lived to experience menopause. Today, things are different. The majority of women reach menopause and may live several decades beyond it. Once women reach menopause, it's time to decide how to live the second part of their lives.

Similarly, in the past, men didn't have options as to how they would age. Until fairly recently, we didn't hear much about erectile dysfunction and lower libido, because nothing could really be done. In 1998, the erectile dysfunction drug Viagra (sildenafil) was approved and changed everything. Today, however, even with Viagra and similar drugs, men want better and different approaches to improve their virility.

Menopause and Andropause

As the body ages, production of well-being hormones naturally begins dropping—we make less DHEA, testosterone, and estrogen. This results in a decreased sense of vitality and lowered libido. Men may notice more difficulty getting an erection or loss of muscle mass and strength.

In women, the typical symptoms of menopause—the complete stop of menstrual periods—include night sweats, hot flashes, mental fog, insomnia, vaginal dryness, and loss of libido. A woman's pituitary gland will begin producing excessive amounts of FSH (follicle stimulating hormone) as it tries in vain to get the ovaries to make more estrogen. In fact, a high FSH level is one of the normal signs of menopause. Once the ovaries start shutting down production, estrogen is produced primarily by the adrenal glands. The adrenals must also still produce cortisol in response to stress. Since they have only so much capacity, when a postmenopausal woman is under stress, her adrenals will gear up to produce more cortisol and stop making estrogen. As a result, she will become catabolic, lose muscle, and gain weight. Her testosterone will also drop, so her libido will decrease.

For men, hormone chemistry during andropause—the slowly decreasing levels of testosterone that happens as men age—can vary widely. Men have fewer complications due to waning levels of sex hormones compared with those experienced by women. Andropause symptoms are often subtle and slow to develop. A man may be less likely to notice the symptoms or to connect them with andropause.

As testosterone levels drop, libido goes down and erectile dysfunction develops. In addition, men in andropause develop more body fat and have a higher propensity to develop insulin resistance. Testosterone levels also affect mood, mental functioning, endurance, bone health, and muscle strength.

Of course, some men maintain high testosterone levels well into their later years. Others find that their hormones start dropping in their forties, earlier than average. The word andropause has become a popular term for the overall impact of lower testosterone. It is also sometimes called male menopause. This isn't really a good description, because men in andropause don't experience the more dramatic changes that affect a woman in menopause. Andropause develops gradually and less predictably than female menopause.

Tyrone's Story

Tyrone is a 56-year-old businessman who came to see us for recurring episodes of back pain. Tyrone explained that he had struggled with the effect of the recession on his business. He was working sixty- to seventy-hour weeks to keep his business afloat as he tried in vain to stop the financial bleeding. Ultimately, he was forced to dismiss more than a third of his employees. After a few acupuncture treatments, Tyrone reported that his back felt much better. However, he needed to share a troublesome problem that was affecting his marriage. He admitted tearfully that his libido was low and that he suffered from erectile dysfunction.

Tyrone initially attributed his weight gain and lack of sex drive to his poor eating habits, long work hours, and increased stress. Eventually he went to see his urologist, complaining that he couldn't get an erection. His doctor prescribed Viagra, which worked, but as he confided to us, he "still didn't have his mojo back."

Lab testing revealed low testosterone as well as a low DHEA level. Fortunately, low hormone levels from andropause can be treated effectively. In Star 4, we will explain how we helped Tyrone.

The Domino Effect of Stress in Men

Stress = need to cope = need for more cortisol

Testosterone "stolen" to make cortisol

Less testosterone = lower libido and erectile dysfunction

Less testosterone = less protection against inflammation

More Inflammation = more work-related injuries, sports injuries, and joint pain

The Domino Effect of Stress in Women

Stress = need to cope = need for more cortisol

Body makes cortisol at expense of DHEA, testosterone, and estrogen

More cortisol = more body fat

Less testosterone = lower libido

Less estrogen = more hot flashes and night sweats

Less estrogen = lower serotonin = more depression, more irritability, and hot flashes

Eleanor's Story

Eleanor kept complaining to her husband that she felt "frumpy and grumpy." She hadn't been sleeping well and was feeling tired all the time. Work was too busy, and she didn't have enough time for herself. She found her teenagers irritating.

She wasn't enjoying her husband's company that much any more. Normally, she felt very sexually attracted to him, but something had changed. She had gained weight, especially around her waist, so she wasn't feeling good about herself. Sex itself wasn't as enjoyable either. At times, it was somewhat painful, as she struggled with lubricants. Her orgasms were less intense. A few months earlier, her gynecologist had reassured her that at age 49, with her periods becoming more and more irregular, she was probably in perimenopause, the months or years of change that lead up to the final cessation of menstrual periods, or menopause.

Then hot flashes started overwhelming her. She found herself dripping sweat at all times of the day and night. She had no doubt menopause had arrived. But what should she do? Should she take hormones? A second cousin had died of breast cancer. She wasn't sure she could get through this without help. Someone had suggested antidepressants, but she didn't think that was the answer.

When Eleanor came to us, we suggested a hormone and metabolite test. Her stress hormones were understandably high. Her FSH (follicle stimulating hormone) level was high, and her estrogen (estrodiol or E2) levels were low, consistent with her menopausal state. Her testosterone and DHEA levels were also low, as reflected in her low libido and loss of vitality. In Star 4, you will see how we were able to help Eleanor restore her health and her sanity, safely.

Measuring Your Sex Hormones

Sex hormones can be measured using blood, urine, and saliva tests. Each type of testing has its pros and cons. Because hormone levels naturally fluctuate with normal day/night diurnal rhythms, the results can be different depending on what time of day the test is performed. In addition, estrogen and progesterone levels fluctuate with the menstrual cycle.

Blood tests. Measuring FSH and the main form of estrogen (estradiol or E2) in the blood can be helpful in diagnosing menopause. Measuring testosterone levels can be helpful in determining if that is the reason men are suffering from erectile dysfunction.

Urine tests. We have found that urine tests correlate very well with patients' symptoms, more so than blood tests. Urine tests help in determining how testosterone and estrogen are being broken down or metabolized in the body. We use this test to see whether unsafe estrogen metabolites are building up in the body or being safely cleared out.

Saliva testing. Saliva testing is an easy way

to check hormone levels at different points throughout the day. All you have to do is collect saliva at regular intervals. Salivary testing is helpful in testing cortisol levels, but it might not be reliable for evaluating sex hormones. We did an informal "study" in our own medical office. Some of our female physicians collected their saliva samples on the same day, and then sent them off for estrogen and progesterone testing at three different laboratories. The results from the three laboratories were completely different for each physician, even though the samples were all taken at the same time. One of the physicians also had blood hormone levels drawn at the same time and sent off samples to two different labs. The results on the blood samples were almost identical.

Estrogen By-products and Cancer

As estrogens are naturally broken down by enzymes in both the female and male body, they are converted into by-products, or metabolites, that can sometimes be harmful. The chances that the by-products will be harmful are increased if the body's detoxification pathways are not working well.

Breast Cancer

The incidence of breast cancer has tripled, from one in twenty in 1960 to one in eight today. Breast cancer is currently the sixth leading cause of death in women in the United States. Why has this happened?

Elevated estrogens and their metabolites can increase breast cancer risk (we will discuss this in more detail later in this section). Interestingly, after a slow but steady increase in the incidence of breast cancer through the last few decades, there was a statistically significant decrease in both incidence and death from breast cancer between 2001 and 2004. The most likely reason for this is the decrease in use of estrogen therapy, which was likely prompted by the findings of the Women's Health Initiative (www.whi.org), a study which looked at over sixteen thousand women and lasted for over ten years. This study showed that taking a synthetic (not bioidentical) estrogen, Premarin®, and a synthetic progestin, Provera®, caused an increased risk of blood clots, heart attack, strokes, and breast cancer.

For decades, women were urged to take estrogen hormones during menopause to relieve hot flashes and prevent osteoporosis. Some doctors even touted these as a way of remaining youthful. When the results of the Women's Health Initiative were published in the summer of 2001, millions of women panicked and stopped taking their hormone supplements. Suddenly, the elixir of youth had become a toxin to be avoided. Women began to realize that the decision whether to take hormones should not be taken lightly.

Other risk factors for breast cancer include a family history of breast cancer, increasing age, higher socioeconomic status, ionizing radiation, and excessive alcohol consumption. In addition, endocrine disruptors appear to have an influence.

We know that gene mutations such as BRCA 1and BRCA 2 predispose women to breast cancer. Yet women with these SNPs who were born before 1940 have a 24 percent lifetime risk of breast cancer, while those born after 1940 have a 67 percent risk. This seems to suggest that something in the environment is affecting the way breast cancer genes turn on. While medicine has focused on what causes women to develop breast cancer, no one seems to have looked at the flip side. We know that BRCA 1 and

BRCA 2 SNPs confer a greater risk on women for breast cancer. Today, women with BRCA 1 have a 50 to 80 percent greater risk, while those with BRCA 2 have a 40 to 70 percent greater risk of developing breast cancer. So the question we should ask is: why are some of these women *not* getting breast cancer? What are they doing differently, and what can we learn from them? Are they less exposed to estrogen-disrupting chemicals in the environment? Do they eat a diet higher in detoxifying fruits and vegetables? Do they get more vitamin D exposure? Do they detoxify estrogen metabolites better? We don't know for sure. But there is more to breast cancer than just genetic susceptibility.

Prostate Cancer

About one in six men will develop prostate cancer during his lifetime—aside from skin cancer, it is the most common cancer in American men. Only one man in thirty-six will die of prostate cancer, however. By age 85, 85 percent of all men will have prostate cancer, but very few will actually die of it or even have troublesome symptoms.

Prostate cancer is the fifth leading cause of death in men over age 45 in the United States. The largest long-term outcome study of intermediate grade prostate cancer confirmed that early treatment improves survival rates significantly. Prostate-specific antigen (PSA) levels are used for early detection, because PSA is a protein that is produced by prostate cancer cells. Unfortunately, normal prostate cells stimulated by inflammation or infection can also produce an elevated PSA, as can benign prostatic hyperplasia (BPH), a relatively common change in the prostate that occurs with age.

Early Detection Is Not the Same as **Prevention**

We have tended to rely on PSAs and mammograms for early detection of prostate and breast cancer. It is important to realize that while these tests have saved thousands of lives, they are not perfect. They only pick up cancer that has already developed. They also have false positives, which have resulted in unnecessary procedures on many men and women.

What about going one step further than early detection? Can we prevent these illnesses?

Detoxification and Cancer Prevention

The human body is more complex than any factory system ever developed. Every substance that passes through the body must be broken down and disposed of safely. That applies to toxins we breathe in, foods we eat (healthful and unhealthful), and medications we take—as well as our own hormones.

The body's ability to fully detoxify hormones depends on several factors:

- Genetic predisposition
- The level of toxic by-products produced within the body
- The toxic burden from the environment
- The body's ability to detoxify its own hormones
- A diet rich in nutrients that support detoxification

When the harmful byproducts of hormone metabolism are not broken down completely and quickly, they may contribute to conditions such as breast cancer and prostate cancer.

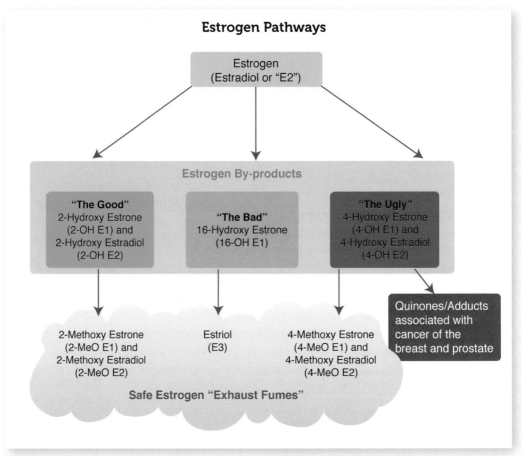

Estrogen By-products and Breast and Prostate Cancer Risk

The Good, the Bad, and the Ugly Estrogens

Both men and women produce estrogen, although women produce far more of it. In both sexes, the primary active form of estrogen is estradiol, or E2. When estradiol is metabolized, it is broken down into three different metabolites, which we term "The Good" (2-hydroxy estrone or 2-OHE1), "The Bad" (16-hydroxy estrone, or 16-OH E1), and "The Ugly" (4-hydroxy estrone, or 4-OH E1).

Good estrogen (2-hydroxy estrone) has a naturally protective effect on the breast and prostate. Bad estrogen (16-hydroxy estrone) has a damaging effect on breast and prostate tissue.

The ratio of good to bad estrogen is very important. The more good estrogen we have, the better.

When it is metabolized in your liver, Ugly estrogen (4-hydroxy estrone) can be converted to a toxic by-product called a quinone (or an adduct) that is found in high amounts in cancerous breast and prostate tissue. Some people are genetically prone to producing more of the Ugly estrogen by-products.

The Good, the Bad, and the Ugly estrogens can all be safely converted to what we call "safe exhaust fumes" or by-products that can be excreted from the body before doing any damage. When it is successfully detoxified, Bad estrogen is converted to estriol (E3), which appears to actually protect against benign breast disease, breast cancer, and endometrial cancer.

SNPs and Estrogen Detoxification

In Ring 3, we discussed the detoxification process in the liver. Estrogen is one of the hormones detoxified in the liver by Phase I and Phase II pathways. SNPs or genetic glitches in the detoxification pathways can result in more Bad and Ugly estrogens, as well as unsafe metabolites.

SNPs in Phase I:

- CYP1B1 results in more of the Ugly estrogens (4-hydroxy estrone, or 4-OH E1)
- CYP3A4 results in more of the Bad estrogens (16-hydroxy estrone, or 16-OH E1)

SNPs in Phase II:

- Catechol-o-methyl-transferase (COMT) decreases the ability to convert or methylate the Good estrogen (2-hydroxy estrone or 2-OHE1) to its safe by-product (2-methoxy estrone or 2-MeOHE1) as well as the Ugly estrogen to convert to its safe by-product (4-methoxy estrone or 4-MeOHE1)

- Glutathione-s-transferase (GST) helps neutralize the toxic quinones or adducts that are found in high amounts in cancerous breast and prostate tissue

- NAD(P)H:quinone oxidoreductase 1 (NQO1) decreases the ability of the liver to convert the unsafe quinones to safe by-products for excretion

More on Estrogen Disruptors: Toxins in the Environment

Earlier in this chapter we discussed endocrine disrupting chemicals. Estrogen disruptors are chemicals that we are exposed to in our environment, including chemicals from plastic bottles, automobile exhaust, pesticides, and herbicides. They all affect the body by mimicking estrogen, yet unlike estrogen they can hang around in the body for years. In young girls, estrogen disrupters can cause early puberty, with the development of breasts and menstruation at an early age. This prolonged estrogen stimulation should be taken seriously. In women, estrogen disruptors are associated with an increased risk of breast cancer and in men, with an increased risk of prostate cancer.

Estrogen Replacement or Hormone Therapy

Estrogen replacement therapy (ERT), now more commonly known as hormone therapy (HT), is sometimes recommended for women as a treatment for severe menopause symptoms, such as disruptive hot flashes, night sweats, and vaginal dryness. While HT can be helpful for relieving symptoms, it can also have serious side effects, including an increased risk of uterine cancer, breast cancer, heart attack, and stroke. (We will look at pros and cons of HT in Star 4.)

Just as there may be a time lag between [pollution] emissions and exposure, there may also be a time lag between exposure and [human or ecological] damages.

—U.S. Environmental Protection Agency, *Unfinished Business: A Comparative Assessment of Environmental Problems*

The Thyroid:
Revving Your Body's Engine

Faru's Story

Faru is 45 years old and of Indian descent. He was essentially healthy, but he had noticed over a six-month period that he was feeling progressively more fatigued. He was also mildly constipated and thought his skin felt much dryer than usual. Many people in his family, including his mother and sister, have hypothyroidism. Because this condition can have a genetic basis, we didn't have to think too hard about running thyroid tests when Faru came to us. His tests showed high TSH levels and low free T3 and free T4 levels, consistent with a diagnosis of hypothyroidism. In addition, further testing was positive for antibodies to thyroid tissue. The testing revealed that Faru had a genetic condition called Hashimoto's thyroiditis, in which his body was producing antibodies targeted at his own thyroid gland.

The thyroid gland works in concert with the hypothalamus and the pituitary gland. It is a complex process, so we'll outline the simple version. The hypothalamus tells the pituitary gland to secrete thyroid stimulating hormone (TSH). As the name suggests, TSH stimulates the thyroid to make the hormone thyroxine (T4).

TSH and T4 work in a feedback loop. Normally, when T4 is low, it will kick the "on switch" and TSH will rise, stimulating the thyroid to produce more T4. When T4 is high enough, it will kick the "off switch," and the pituitary gland will stop secreting TSH. This loop is how the body keeps thyroid levels within a normal range.

Common Thyroid Conditions

The most common thyroid condition is hypothyroidism, or low thyroid function. When the thyroid isn't producing enough T3 and T4, the body's metabolism slows, causing us to feel tired and weak. Hypothyroidism can also cause depression, weight gain, memory problems, dry skin and brittle nails, intolerance of cold, constipation, and menstrual irregularities.

Killing Itself Slowly: Hashimoto's Thyroiditis

Hashimoto's thyroiditis is an autoimmune disease in which the body attacks its own thyroid gland. Surprisingly, autoimmune diseases of the thyroid gland are the most common of all autoimmune conditions. This disease usually comes on very slowly, taking years to damage the thyroid enough to reduce hormone production. Patients might think that their forgetfulness and tiredness, for instance, are just from getting older, but it could be the result of Hashimoto's thyroiditis finally causing noticeable symptoms.

Catching on Fire, Then Fizzling Out: Graves' Disease

Graves' disease is another autoimmune condition of the thyroid. Graves' disease initially causes excessive thyroid production, or hyperthyroidism. In the early stages, patients usually have palpitations, insomnia, diarrhea, and unexplained weight loss. Their symptoms are triggered by high thyroid levels, which are amping up their metabolism. The patient may develop an enlarged thyroid gland (goiter) and may also develop a protrusion of one or both eyes. Like Hashimoto's disease, Graves' disease has a genetic component; several members of one family may have it.

A Final Note on Hormones

Our body's hormone system functions in tandem with the neurological and immune systems. Stress and depression can have a major effect on our hormones, as can detoxification, oxidation, and inflammation. Together, all of these processes affect our metabolism.

The important thing to understand is that altering hormonal balance is not just accomplished by using medications. By changing lifestyle, diet, and environment, using appropriate nutritional supplements, and dealing with stress, you can make a dramatic difference in how you look, feel, and age.

When the hormones are in balance, they orchestrate a beautiful symphony, maintaining the normal function of the body. If they are imbalanced, we want to know why. When we look for hormonal imbalances, we do so while looking at the patient's body and his life as a whole—and then we help the patient regain balance. In Star 4, we will discuss how we do this.

Alex Learns to Understand His Hormones

Alex's high ratio of triglycerides to HDL (> 10) and his slightly high blood glucose pointed to a problem with insulin resistance. No wonder he was gaining weight. Alex already knew his genetic risk for prostate cancer was increased (see Ring 1, page 38). Urinary hormone testing confirmed this. He had an altered 2:16 OH estrone ratio. In other words, he had too few good estrogen by-products and too many bad estrogen by-products. In addition, his ugly 4-OH estrone levels were abnormally high.

Rather than seeing these issues as problems, we discussed how Alex could deal with these challenges now, averting the real problems before they manifested later.

Alex continues to pursue Health and Wellness

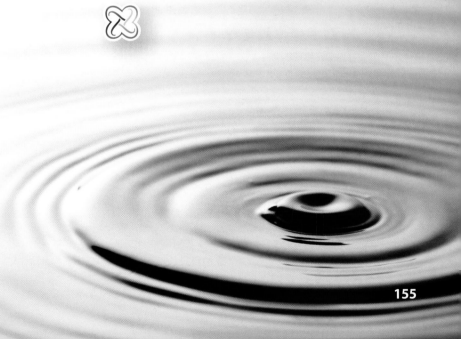

4

STAR FOUR

How to Optimize Your Hormonal Balance

What to Do

- **If You Are Overweight**

Or If You Have

- **High Blood Sugar**

- **Unexplained Fatigue**

- **Decreased Libido**

- **Hot Flashes or Menopausal Symptoms**

- **PMS or Irregular Periods**

- **Erectile Dysfunction**

Optimize Your Hormonal Balance

We have been primed to think that the only way we can help our hormone system is to take hormones. This isn't true! Taking hormones replaces hormones if they are deficient, as they might be if you have low thyroid hormones. There is a lot more you can do to improve your quality of life without taking hormones, especially in the early stages of midlife changes.

To rule out illness, however, we suggest that you have your hormones tested by a medical practitioner who understands how to diagnose and treat endocrine issues. Some fairly common diseases do need medical treatment with hormones. Diseases such as congenital adrenal hyperplasia, Cushing's disease, Conn's syndrome, Hashimoto's disease and Graves' disease are but a few.

However, you may simply be suffering from what we refer to as mild endocrine dysfunction. In that case, you don't have an endocrine disease per se—your hormones are simply out of balance.

Five Steps to Balancing Your Hormones

Once we've ruled out a disease as the cause of our patients' symptoms, we help them with a five-step approach to balancing their hormones.

Step 1. Balance your stress hormones (also see Star 2).

Step 2. Conquer insulin resistance.

Step 3. Balance your well-being and sex hormones, DHEA, testosterone, and estrogen.

Step 4. Protect against breast cancer or prostate cancer by reducing estrogen metabolites.

Step 5. Balance your thyroid hormones.

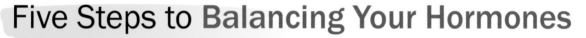

Step 1. Balancing Stress Hormones

We consider good stress management the essential first step in balancing your hormones. You want to manage stress effectively, because your body uses the same cholesterol to make both stress hormones such as cortisol and what we call the "well-being" or sex hormones such as DHEA, testosterone, and estrogen. Our bodies are designed to handle chronic stress by shunting hormone production toward cortisol. (Check back to Figure R4.2 on page 146 in Ring 4 to see how this works.) Think of it this way: In times of famine, our ancestors would have needed to survive, not make babies. Their bodies made more cortisol to store fat and survive the stress of their times. Although times have changed, our bodies have not. We still handle stress in the same way, by reducing our sex and well-being hormones and increasing our cortisol production. But now we complain that stress is making us fat and giving us hot flashes! We cannot change our hormonal responses, but we can learn how to modify them. In Stars 1 and 2, we discussed how to do this. Let's look at what else we can do to balance hormones.

Step 2. Conquering Insulin Resistance

To change the insulin resistance dynamic we discussed in Ring 4, we need to send our hormones a signal that there is an abundance of good, healthy food. The way to send this signal is by eating a diet rich in high-density nutrients, delivered regularly (six small meals are better than two or three large ones). This is different from sending the wrong message of an overabundance of high sugar, high fat, and inflammatory food filled with new-to-nature chemicals. This makes insulin resistance worse, leading to type 2 diabetes.

Just watching calories usually isn't enough to help insulin resistance. We need to do more to make our food and lifestyle work for us, not against us.

Improving Insulin Resistance

Diet will help improve insulin resistance quite a bit—it should be the first line of attack. After that, managing stress is the next step. Remember, the body is designed to store fat when it's stressed. If you're content and happy, your body is more likely to lose weight.

We suggest creating a healthy eating plan that includes small, frequent meals. If you have insulin resistance, you may also be likely to have episodes of hypoglycemia, when your blood sugar drops too low. Symptoms of hypoglycemia include irritability, feeling jittery, or feeling depressed. Low blood sugar can also make you feel lightheaded or confused and can even trigger an uncomfortable cold sweat. When you are having a hypoglycemic episode, you instinctively want to eat something sugary or starchy to raise your blood sugar. What happens then is that you eat a candy bar or some cookies, which does raise your blood sugar quickly. However, the sudden spike of blood sugar stimulates your pancreas to release a lot of insulin, which then drives your blood sugar down again, which can trigger another hypoglycemic episode. Switching your diet to a high-nutrient approach that is low in refined carbohydrates and processed foods will help you get off this endless roller coaster of blood sugar highs and blood sugar crashes.

> If I'd known I was going to live this long, I'd have taken better care of myself.
>
> —Eubie Blake, at age 100

In Star 3 we discussed a high-nutrient diet. The foods that are going to sustain us for the long haul are high in fiber and are nutrient-rich. Since fiber requires time to digest, the food is broken down slowly, resulting in steady energy from a gradual rise in blood sugar that your body can handle easily. Compare this with what happens if you drink a sugary soda or fruit juice or sugary or starchy snacks such as cookies or pretzels. Those foods give you a sudden rush of blood sugar, often followed by an energy crash.

A better diet means fewer highs and lows—no big shocks to the system that leave you feeling moody, flat, or depleted. With a nutrient-rich diet, you gain the following:

Stable energy. A steady release of glucose provides a constant supply of energy.

Less insulin needed. Foods low in carbohydrates such as salads, nonstarchy vegetables, and protein require little or no insulin and are referred to as insulin sparing. In contrast, foods high in sugars and starches break down quickly. They are definitely fast foods—with a fast energy spike—and a rapid crash. If this happens only now and then—the occasional treat of birthday cake or Sunday dessert—it's usually not a problem. But many of us live on these simple carbs daily.

Fewer spikes and crashes. When insulin spikes too often from a poor diet high in refined carbohydrates, the body becomes less able to cope with up-and-down blood sugar. Fluctuating glucose levels result in fatigue and high insulin levels. The high insulin results in high blood

Weight Loss and Stress

Have you ever tried to lose weight when you were also in a stressed state? Did you find it was difficult? If weight loss was as simple as lowering caloric intake, we wouldn't be facing the current epidemic of obesity. Despite calorie cutting, some people just seem to gain more weight. Clearly, evaluating insulin resistance and lowering calories are important aspects of weight loss. But there is more to weight loss than just calories.

Trying to lose weight by dieting during a stressed (and catabolic) state simply amplifies the message that starvation is imminent, piling another stress on an already stressed body. The body reacts by increasing cortisol levels, making it more difficult to lose weight. Emotional stress can affect your cortisol balance, causing you to go into storage mode in order to retain fat. In addition, emotional overeating is likely to cause you to binge on comfort foods, which are usually high in calories and low in nutrients. Being stressed and inflamed will make things even worse. The increased inflammation aggravates the insulin resistance, resulting in another vicious cycle! Losing weight is more than just reducing calories!

- It is also vital that your stress hormones are balanced and that your thyroid hormones are normal.

- Inflammation, oxidative stress, and detoxification problems can play a role in weight gain and weight loss.

- Normal gut flora seems to be an important component of a weight loss program.

- And you need to remove the obesogens from your life by limiting your chemical exposure wherever possible. (We discuss these later in the chapter.)

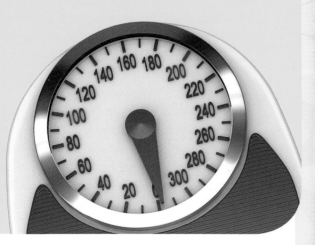

© Shutterstock/ ulegundo

pressure and obesity. Obesity causes more insulin resistance, which in turn causes more obesity and inflammation. The inflammation causes heart disease and even more weight gain. It is a vicious cycle. Fast foods are a fast way to poor health!

Some Food Advice for Insulin Resistance

- If you suffer from insulin resistance, fat, sugar, refined carbs, and salt are your nemesis. They are addictive. If you are feeling hungry, snack on vegetables, a small piece of cheese, a handful of nuts, a baked chicken leg—and not on sweet or starchy refined foods. Protein and healthy fats will give you a lasting sense of satisfaction and satiety

- Spread your meals evenly throughout the day by eating smaller main meals and supplementing with between-meal snacks. This way you signal abundance to your body, so it won't need to store fat.

- Eat breakfast and dinner early.

- Start your day with a high-protein, low-carb breakfast. We often recommend a medical food shake such as UltraMeal® Plus 360 (Metagenics) or a whey protein shake as a breakfast replacement.

- In Star 3, we discussed the low-carbohydrate diet, which we suggest for insulin resistance. Use this as a guideline, but remember that nutrition is a complex subject and everyone has individual needs, along with personal food preferences. A nutritionist can help you work out a meal plan that puts you on a better path while still letting you enjoy your favorite foods.

- If you fall off the wagon, don't be surprised. Everyone does, all the time. Don't waste emotional energy on guilt or self-blame. Instead, just get back on your healthy diet and try to stick to it for the next twenty-four hours. This will help reset your metabolism back to where it was before you slipped.

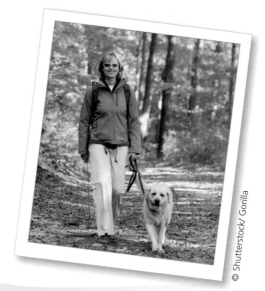

© Shutterstock/ Gorilla

- Daily aerobic exercise will help improve your insulin sensitivity. If you don't have much time, try taking a short, brisk walk after meals.
- Many natural supplements appear to improve insulin sensitivity. These include cinnamon, green tea, chromium picolinate, alphalipoic acid, L-carnosine, and gymnema.

Obesogens and Estrogen Disrupting Chemicals: Substances to Avoid

In Ring 4 (page 144), we discussed how certain foods and chemicals can make us fat by aggravating insulin resistance. These obesogens are another reason we should aim to eat natural, organic food.

At the top of the list is high-fructose corn syrup (HFCS). This very cheap sweetener is why fast food restaurants can offer to supersize your soda for just a few pennies more. HFCS came into widespread use in the 1980s, exactly when our current epidemic of obesity began, and may well be the primary cause. It has been implicated as a cause of insulin resistance.

Next on the list is the heavy consumption of corn-fed beef. Steers fed on corn instead of their natural diet of grass produce meat that is more marbled with fat. That fat is disproportionately high in omega-6 fatty acids compared to omega-3 fatty acids. Grass-fed beef has a much healthier ratio of fats. In addition, grass-fed steers are not usually given the hormones and antibiotics that are given to steers fed on feed lots.

Surprisingly, farm-raised salmon, which is now very popular, is no longer a source of good nutrition. While wild salmon is an excellent protein source that is high in omega-3 fatty acids, farmed salmon is now a different story. These fish are now low in omega-3s and are often contaminated with pesticides, antibiotics, and mercury. Farm-raised salmon has been associated with weight gain at the waistline (higher waist to hip ratios) and higher body mass index, two of the primary markers of insulin resistance.

Endocrine disrupting chemicals have been shown to cause obesity in a number of ways. This is another reason to be mindful of the use of pesticides, herbicides, plastics, cleaning agents, cosmetics and synthetic chemicals in your environment.

Step 3. Balancing Your Well-Being Hormones

As we discussed above in Step 1, sometimes just treating stress will normalize the production of well-being hormones. Hot flashes go away, erectile dysfunction resolves, and libido returns. However, in menopause or andropause, the levels of the hormones estrogen and testosterone begin dropping regardless of the level of stress. In this case, the use of supplemental hormones may be an option. We prefer to use these hormones for only brief periods of time.

We consider a number of issues before recommending hormones. We always do laboratory testing as the first step. If the lab tests results reveal that hormone levels are low, hormone therapy may be the most appropriate treatment. When we use hormone therapy, our goal is to bring levels back to normal, not to above normal, which may cause disease.

We prefer to use bioidentical hormones whenever possible. The structure of bioidentical hormones matches that of human hormones, right down to the shape of the molecule and the atomic weight.

Bioidentical hormones can be delivered to the body using pills, creams, gels, or patches. Bioidentical hormones are made by many pharmaceutical companies. They can also be made to order by compounding pharmacies in cream and gel preparations of various strengths. This is controversial, because the compounding pharmacy may not offer the same reliable dosing as a pharmaceutical company does. On the other hand, compounded hormones can be customized to include various hormones at differing doses to individualize your hormone therapy.

Both women and men taking supplemental sex hormones should be seen regularly by their doctors.

Hormone Delivery

We usually recommend using estrogen or testosterone patches, gels, or creams. This way, hormones are absorbed into the bloodstream transdermally, or through the skin, releasing the hormones directly into the blood. Transdermal absorption means that the hormones are not metabolized by the liver, as they would

> There is a fountain of youth: it is your mind, your talents, the creativity you bring to your life and the lives of people you love. When you learn to tap this source, you will truly have defeated age.
>
> –Sophia Loren

be in pill form. This avoids the risk of creating toxic metabolites, which have been associated with an increased risk of certain illnesses.

We recommend against hormone implants that are placed under the skin and left there for several months. Because these products release the hormone continuously, you can accumulate them at excessively high levels.

Is Hormone Therapy (HT) Safe?

In Ring 4 we discussed the Women's Health Initiative. This was the largest study ever undertaken to evaluate hormone replacement, and the results were unsettling. Hormonal replacement with Premarin and Provera, which are both synthetic hormones, resulted in an increased risk of blood clots, heart attack, strokes, and breast cancer. Women who stopped their hormones abruptly were often devastated by a resumption of hot flashes and menopausal symptoms.

Over the past decade, women have been increasingly using hormones which have a chemical structure identical to the hormones found in the human body. The general term for this is *bioidentical hormones*. However, it is important to note that there are two types—those manufactured by pharmaceutical companies, and those made by compounding pharmacists. Pharmaceutical companies believe that their drugs are better manufactured and standardized. Compounding pharmacists argue that they can uniquely tailor to your individual dosing needs.

Bioidentical hormones are now often touted as the new hormone solution. Proponents say that your hormones do not decrease because you age—rather, you age because your hormones drop. Advocates infer that since bioidentical hormones are the same as those your body makes, they must be safe. These are not just the sex hormones—estrogen and testosterone—but hormones such as growth hormone, or even β-HCG, the pregnancy hormone, which can be used for weight loss.

Factors to Consider with HT

As with most medical problems, the answer is a complex one relating to how our genes interact with medications, environmental toxins, life stress, and diet. Here are some things to consider, especially with estrogen and testosterone replacement.

Genes governing the way you detoxify hormones: Genetic glitches or SNPs on cytochrome P450 enzymes CYP1B1, CYP1A1, CYP3A4, COMT, NQO1, and GST are more likely to make procarcinogenic estrogen compounds and adducts (see Ring 4).

Genes governing clotting: Some SNPs will increase the risk of clotting. These include SNPs for Factor II, Factor V, and GP3A Pl(A). Women with these SNPs who take estrogen are more likely to suffer from clotting problems such as deep venous thrombosis (DVTs), pulmonary emboli (PE), heart attacks, and strokes. A SNP called PAI-1 (plasminogen activator inhibitor-1) also increases the risk of clotting. However, hormones such as estrogen or DHEA *turn down* this SNP, *decreasing* the risk for clotting. So, depending on which SNPs you have, estrogen may be bad or good. And if you have a mixed picture, the answer is even less clear.

Excessive exposure to estrogen or estrogen disrupting chemicals: Between 1940 and 1970, pregnant women were given a synthetic estrogen diethylstilbestrol (DES) in the mistaken belief that it would reduce pregnancy complications. It was also used to supplement cattle feed. Unfortunately, women who were exposed to DES had a higher risk of breast cancer. Their daughters were at higher risk for breast, vaginal, and cervical cancers. Their sons were at higher risk of transgender issues. Epigenetic changes persisted into the third generation. Although DES is no longer used, excessive use of synthetic estrogens through estrogen medications and excessive exposure to estrogen disrupting chemicals have been associated with illnesses such as reproductive disorders, endometriosis, breast abnormalities and cancer, polycystic ovarian syndrome (PCOS), and even breastfeeding problems.

Nutritional factors, lifestyle, and behavioral factors: Diets high in cruciferous vegetables, such as broccoli, and antioxidants, such as those found in colored fruits and vegetables, will help improve hormone detoxification through the liver and help prevent cancer. Smoking, stress, an inflammatory diet, and dehydration can aggravate the risk for clotting, while a diet high in fish oils will help prevent clotting.

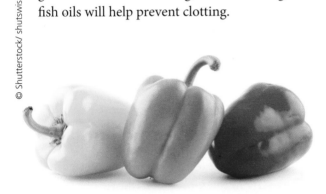

How Do You Know What to Do?

There is no way that the current gold standard of studies—the double-blind, placebo-controlled crossover study—can answer the question of whether hormone replacement is good or bad for you. There are simply too many variables. If you do decide to use any hormone replacement, you should thoroughly discuss the risks and side effects with your doctor. Ultimately, you must be the one to decide. The current opinion is to use hormone therapy only if needed and then for the shortest time possible. Women should take a break from estrogen after three to five years and reassess if they still need it. In men, we still don't really know if testosterone supplementation affects the risk of prostate cancer. That is why we generally adhere to using low doses for a shorter time, and then consider testing for estrogen metabolites.

Testing for both the SNPs involved in the breakdown of estrogen, as well as the estrogen metabolites themselves, can help you better understand your risks. A physician who understands these mechanisms can then advise you how to individually mitigate your risk factors by using appropriate hormone therapy, together with diet, nutritional supplements, stress reduction, and lifestyle techniques.

DHEA (Dehydroepiandrosterone)

Higher natural levels of DHEA are associated with lower levels of cancer, heart disease, metabolic syndrome, arthritis, and chronic disease. DHEA also helps sexual function, depression, immune function, and inflammation. However, it is not yet clear who best benefits from supplementation with DHEA.

Although DHEA is available over-the-counter from health food stores, it must be used cautiously. As a precursor hormone, it is metabolized into both testosterone and estrogen. In theory, supplemental DHEA may increase the risk of hormone-sensitive cancers affecting the prostate, breasts, uterus, or ovaries. On the other hand, higher levels of DHEA inhibit the action of enzymes that break sex hormones down into toxic by-products. In other words, higher levels of DHEA might help prevent breast and prostate cancer.

Unfortunately, there are no definitive studies at this time. Because DHEA is converted into testosterone, high doses of DHEA can be associated with typical symptoms of high testosterone such as alopecia (balding), as well as increased facial hair, prostate enlargement, and irritability.

DHEA dosage usually ranges from 25 to 200 mg a day. We prefer to use low doses, ranging from 25 to 50 mg. We also prefer sublingual sprays dissolved under the tongue rather than pills. The sublingual dose appears to be absorbed more quickly into the bloodstream.

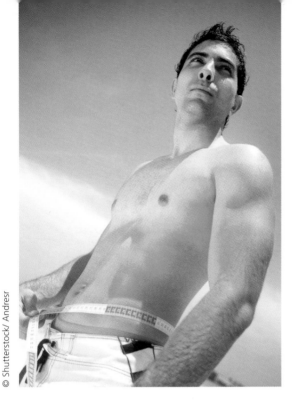

© Shutterstock/ Andresr

Testosterone

If your testosterone is low, you have a number of good treatment options.

Lifestyle changes that raise testosterone levels include reducing stress, losing weight, improving insulin sensitivity, increasing protein intake, quitting smoking, and minimizing alcohol consumption.

Testosterone Therapy

When needed, we recommend testosterone supplementation in the form of a gel, cream, or patch. We prefer transdermal forms to pills because that way, the hormone enters your bloodstream directly. In appropriately low doses, testosterone can sometimes be helpful for postmenopausal women. For men and women, we find testosterone is often helpful in correcting low libido, fatigue, and poor muscle tone.

Another way to raise testosterone is to stop it from being converted to estrogen. This strategy retains higher levels of testosterone in the body.

The enzyme that converts testosterone to estrogen is called aromatase, so aromatase-inhibiting drugs such as anastrozole (Arimidex®) letrozole (Femara®), and exemestane (Aromasin®) can be used to block the conversion of testosterone to estrogen. This approach is used as an anti-aging treatment by some physicians, but these drugs should be used with extreme caution in men and never in women except as a treatment to prevent breast cancer recurrence.

Many natural products can also slow conversion of testosterone. These include chrysin, stinging nettles, soy isoflavones, flaxseed, procyanidins, ECGC (from green tea), and vitamin C. DHEA supplementation can increase testosterone levels. If a zinc deficiency is affecting testosterone levels, zinc supplementation will help.

Baldness and Enlarged Prostate

In some men, testosterone is converted too rapidly to the form DHT (dihydrotestosterone). High DHT levels are associated with baldness. Drugs now used to treat both baldness and prostate enlargement (benign prostatic hyperplasia, or BPH) work by inhibiting an enzyme in this pathway. Medications that block this enzyme include finasteride (Proscar® and Propecia®), and dutasteride (Avodart®). Natural supplements such as saw palmetto, pygeum, and stinging nettles also appear to reduce this enzyme's activity.

> Aging is not lost youth but
> a new stage of opportunity
> and strength.
> —Betty Friedan

Are You Catabolic or Anabolic?

Anabolic steroids are the illegal substances that athletes and bodybuilders use to enhance their performance and make their bodies grow (super) big and strong. Anabolic refers to building up muscles as part of the normal growth and healing response. We need anabolic hormones to help us repair and rebuild, but too much is not good. Although bodybuilders may think they look great, they are putting themselves at risk for problems. Some men grow small breasts, and their testicles shrink. Likewise, women on steroids can develop clitoral enlargement and a variety of hormonal abnormalities. We need our bodies to make our own anabolic steroid hormones. If they do not, wounds will not heal and we feel tired and depressed.

The opposite of anabolic is catabolic, or breaking down. When you suffer excessive wear and tear or are seriously ill, you are catabolic—you are breaking down your body faster than it can repair itself. In general, we become somewhat catabolic as we get older and also when we are under prolonged or excessive stress. Our muscles become weaker and smaller, and we develop more fat around our bellies.

By measuring the ratio between your stress hormones and your well-being hormones, we can learn where you fall on the anabolic—catabolic continuum. Then we can balance these hormones through lifestyle changes and by using supplements and/or hormone replacements. These measures help to turn back the clock on the aging process.

Tyrone's Story (continued from page 148)

In Ring 4, we discussed Tyrone, a 56-year-old businessman who suffered from low libido and erectile dysfunction. While Viagra had helped his erectile dysfunction, it did little to change his libido. Tyrone wanted his mojo back.

We put Tyrone on testosterone gel and supplemental DHEA, with excellent results. Two months later, we checked Tyrone's urinary hormone metabolites. While his testosterone and anabolic/catabolic balance were normal, his test showed an abnormal ratio of 2:16 OH estrone (estrogen) metabolites, placing him at an increased risk for prostate cancer. (Remember, testosterone is converted to estrogen, even in men.) To counteract this, we suggested he increase his consumption of cruciferous vegetables, and placed him on a supplement containing a derivative of broccoli, called indole-3-carbinol. We kept him on the DHEA because of its beneficial effect on one of his genetic SNPs—it helped keep his ugly estrogen down. A repeat hormone test two months later showed that his ratios had normalized.

Happily, Tyrone can now continue testosterone replacement without worrying that he is at increased risk for prostate cancer.

Dance well. Get well. Be well. Stay well. Breathe well. Stay well. Sleep well. Think

Controlling Menopausal Symptoms

Women who reach menopause often come to us for help. "I feel desperate," they tell us. "My hot flashes wake me up at night. The bed is sopping wet. I feel moody and depressed. My libido has disappeared, and when I do have sex, it's painful."

Before you start any treatment for menopausal symptoms, check your follicle stimulating hormone (FSH), estradiol (E2), progesterone, and DHEA levels. FSH will go up as menopause develops, and estrogen levels naturally drop as women reach their 40s. If you are younger than that and have low estrogen, make sure your body mass index isn't too low. Women who are marathon runners, or those who exercise too strenuously, such as professional athletes and dancers, can deplete their estrogen levels.

Your progesterone level may also be low. In fact, often all that is needed for symptom relief in early menopause is progesterone replacement (without estrogen).

The next step is to check your DHEA levels. If you are not making much DHEA, you cannot convert it to estrogen and your levels drop. Remember that high stress can lead to low DHEA levels.

Nonhormone Options for Menopausal Symptoms

Women in perimenopause and menopause have a number of good options for treating symptoms such as hot flashes, vaginal dryness, and low libido without estrogen replacement or hormone therapy.

We recommend starting by checking your stress level. When you are stressed, your body makes less estrogen. (Check back to Star 2 for some helpful stress reduction techniques.) These, as well as acupuncture, can be very helpful in reducing hot flashes.

DHEA supplementation can be used, as discussed above. Women need to watch for increased facial hair as well as hair loss. If your progesterone is too low, consider herbal supplementation with chasteberry extract. Progesterone creams can be helpful, although the ability to absorb progesterone through the skin may vary considerably.

For older women with normal estrogen loss, we often suggest an herbal or nutritional supplement. Red clover, sage, black cohosh, and other herbs and supplements have mild estrogenic effects. Soy isoflavones also appear to be helpful, especially when they come from organic soy foods such as tofu. Heavily processed soy foods will not help, however. Some botanical supplements can raise estrogen. Rhapontic rhubarb (*Rheum rhaponticum L.*) root extract, sold as the nonprescription pill Estrovera (Metagenics), is a plant estrogen that has been clinically demonstrated to support a wide variety of benefits in menopausal women.

Hormone Therapy

We cannot overemphasize the importance of being under the care of a physician who is familiar with hormones and their metabolites—and with you and your health. This is not the time to experiment on your own with nonprescription products or work with a physician

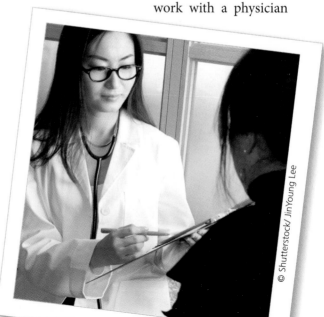

© Shutterstock/ JinYoung Lee

over the phone, by mail, or by e-mail. You need to have regular pelvic exams, Pap smears, mammograms and blood tests to assure that you are having a safe response to the hormones, even if they come from over-the-counter supplements.

For estrogen replacement, we usually recommend using a skin patch containing bioidentical estrogen. Examples include the estrodiol (Vivelle®) patch and gel (Divigel®). Another option here is compounded bioidentical hormones.

For progesterone supplementation, we usually recommend a progesterone pill called Prometrium® or a transdermal bioidentical form. For women with insulin resistance, we have found that glucose levels do better when we maintain the monthly menstrual periods by cycling estrogen and progesterone levels.

Testosterone can sometimes be helpful in aiding a sagging libido or stopping catabolism. Again, this is available as pharmaceutical gels and patches (Androgel®, Androderm®, Testoderm TTS®) and compounded creams and gels.

Healthy Menopause

Once a woman's hormone levels drop, she no longer has the protection provided by estrogen against heart disease and osteoporosis. If you are at that point, lifestyle becomes even more important as a way

Eleanor's Story (continued from page 149)

Eleanor is a 49-year-old woman who came to us with typical symptoms of menopause. Her lab tests confirmed that she was in menopause and that her estrogen levels had dropped. In addition, she suffered from decreased testosterone and DHEA levels. Her stress hormones were high.

Eleanor was a good candidate for HT (hormone therapy.) However, she needed more than just hormones. We started off by addressing her lifestyle, getting her to concentrate on stress reduction. Then, to address her low DHEA, we placed her on adaptogenic herbs, using a mix of rhodiola root, Asian ginseng, and a mushroom extract (cordyceps). We also started HT with a pharmaceutical estradiol gel and a daily low dose of progesterone (Prometrium).

Eleanor began feeling noticeably better within a few weeks. Her hot flashes disappeared, she began sleeping normally, and her mood stabilized. In fact, she was feeling herself again. After two months, she returned to see us. She still felt her libido was low. After discussing the pros and cons with us, Eleanor decided to try a testosterone cream. We began with a low dose, gradually increasing it until she noticed her libido return. We asked her to watch for signs of excess testosterone, such as the development of facial hair.

Eleanor came back to the clinic two months later, beaming. She had lost weight and was feeling wonderful. We did a urinary hormone test to check the balance of her hormones and to look for possible bad metabolites, to make sure she wasn't at risk for breast cancer. This test turned out to be well within the normal range. Not only were her estrogen metabolites normal, but all of her other hormone levels had normalized as well. Her DHEA level, stress hormones, and her testosterone were all within normal limits.

Eleanor's experience is a good example of what we feel a good hormone replacement program should look like. We asked her to see us every six months. She will continue to have regular Pap smears, mammograms, and gynecological checkups. In three to five years' time, we will talk about ending the hormone replacement therapy.

to protect your health. Address risk factors such as smoking, high blood pressure, high blood cholesterol, diabetes, physical inactivity, and being overweight or obese. If necessary, consider medications to control high blood pressure, high cholesterol, and high blood sugar levels.

The risk of osteoporosis increases with age. To help prevent osteoporosis, one key step is to follow an eating plan that is rich in calcium and vitamin D. Moderate exposure to sunlight also helps the body make vitamin D. Regular weight-bearing exercises help strengthen bones. Limit both alcohol and smoking, as these further aggravate bone loss. Other nutritional factors that can help prevent osteoporosis include vitamin K and strontium. Ostera®, a combination nutritional supplement by Metagenics, has been shown to beneficially support key factors in bone regeneration. Drugs that treat osteoporosis include bisphosphonates, such as alendronate (Fosamax®) or risedronate (Actonel®), and also selective estrogen-receptor modulators, such as raloxifene (Evista®). These drugs have potential side effects and should be used cautiously.

It is important to note that in the body, bones act as a bank for calcium. Bone is constantly being remodeled, a dynamic balance between bone being formed and resorbed. If not enough bone is being formed, osteoporosis can develop. That is why calcium supplements and vitamin D are usually recommended as a first line of prevention and treatment. What is just as important though is inflammation, which contributes to bone resorption. Stress, poor diet, and inflammatory diseases can all contribute to inflammation and the acceleration of bone loss. SNPs such as IL-6 and TNF-a (interleukin 6 and tumor necrosis factor-alpha) can increase your risk for inflammation.

Over and over we see the benefit of a Transformational Medicine approach. The same approach that helps one problem can also help many others. Here again we see how reducing stress (Star 2), reducing inflammation, and improving your diet (Star 3) helps yet another problem, counteracting bone loss and reducing inflammation.

Some Perimenopausal Success Stories

Joan is a physical therapist who had a hysterectomy five years ago after developing endometriosis. She began bioidentical hormones after leaving the hospital and never had a hot flash. Her estrogen metabolism is assessed yearly, and her nutritional status and stress management are continually reassessed.

Barbie is an administrative assistant who has experienced periodic hot flashes and sleep disruptions from menopause over the last three years. Her vaginal dryness occasionally caused pain with intercourse, and she found her libido had decreased recently. She chose to use nutritional supplements, estrogen vaginal cream, and monthly acupuncture treatments to keep her symptoms in check. She used a combination of Estrovera (a botanical from Metagenics) and the herb black cohosh to control her hot flashes and sleep disruptions.

Simone has menopausal hot flashes that leave her feeling mentally foggy. She has a clotting disorder, so she is not a candidate for hormone therapy because of the attendant risk of blood clots. She has found that guided imagery, paced breathing, and regular acupuncture appointments keep her symptoms in check. She says she always knows when it's time to come back in, saying, "It's time to pay attention again, Doc. The hot flashes are creeping back into my life!"

Conquering PMS and Irregular Periods Naturally

Symptoms of too much estrogen, known as estrogen dominance, include irregular periods, premenstrual syndrome (PMS), breast tenderness, bloating, irritability or anxiety, migraines, and weight gain. Chronic estrogen dominance can result in heavy periods, infertility, fibroids, and even uterine cancer.

Estrogen dominance may be caused by excess estrogen produced by the body, excess foreign estrogens from endocrine-disrupting chemicals, or inadequate estrogen detoxification in the liver. In some cases, estrogen dominance may be due to a relative deficiency of progesterone.

The conventional medical approach to these problems is to prescribe birth control pills, which increase the level of synthetic progestin in the body. If the woman wants to get pregnant, however, birth control pills are obviously not appropriate. Also, birth control pills can cause dangerous blood clots in women over age 40. Our approach is to first try to increase the level of progesterone by natural means.

We look carefully for clues of estrogen or progesterone excess or deficiency and then check hormone levels with standard lab tests. We also discuss lifestyle, stress, exercise, and diet.

If estrogen levels are too high, we use supplements that reduce aromatase activity. Aromatase is the enzyme that converts testosterone to estrogen; by reducing its activity, we reduce estrogen levels. We usually recommend green tea extract, flax seed, vitamin C, and chrysin.

We also use nutritional supplements that improve estrogen detoxification metabolism. These include isoflavones from natural soy products along with rosemary leaf extract, folic acid, vitamin B6 (pyridoxine), vitamin B12 (as methylcobalamin and cyanocobalamin), trimethylglycine (vitamin B15, also called betaine), and resveratrol. Evening primrose oil is often helpful for cramps. If p[...] low, we may suggest a herbal su[...] as chasteberry or a progesterone crea[...]

Acupuncture can also be useful in no[...] izing menstrual cycles, and the stress reductio[...] techniques outlined in Star 2 can be helpful in reducing mood swings.

Then, if none of these options work, consider using birth control pills.

Christine's Story

Christine is a 37-year-old woman who has premenstrual syndrome. Her symptoms include mood swings, from anger to sadness, as well as abdominal bloating in the two weeks prior to her menstrual period. She has a history of endometriosis and needed in vitro fertilization (IVF) to conceive her first child. She came to us because her PMS was making her miserable. We reviewed her health and lifestyle history. The birth of her child three years earlier had led to a drastic change in her exercise and nutrition—both were now very low on her list of priorities. She had gained weight, and her lack of exercise and poor diet were only making her PMS worse. Christine also felt pulled in several directions. Her husband travels frequently for work, and so she is left with the responsibility of her son, the household, and her job.

We started Christine on a medical food as a meal replacement (UltraMeal by Metagenics) to reduce her insulin resistance and help her trim down. We also recommended evening primrose oil, a regular exercise program, daily meditation, and acupuncture treatments the week before her period. She finds that this approach keeps her PMS symptoms at bay. In her words, "It's given me my life back!"

...rogesterone is too
...pplement is too
...pplement such
...m.
...mal-

...r conventional screen-
...ation, we recommend
...o protect yourself against
...rostate cancer.

The ... ...ncrease the risk for breast cancer in women ...e similar to those that cause prostate cancer in men. What has become clear in recent years is that we each have a unique genetic signature that controls how we detoxify and remove estrogen from our bodies. It is clear that some pathways of metabolism result in metabolites that are safer and less likely to cause DNA damage and cancer in our cells, while other pathways result in metabolites that are less safe. (Check back to Ring 4, page 153, where we discussed some of the SNPs that affect estrogen detoxification.)

Luckily, we can influence the pathways toward safer metabolism simply by providing plenty of the raw materials used by the body in estrogen metabolism. Specifically, this means eating more cruciferous foods such as broccoli or taking cruciferous extracts, such as indole-3-carbinol or DIM (di-indole methane), which helps improve the ratio of good to bad estrogen metabolites. A diet high in antioxidants, especially pomegranate juice and lycopene from tomatoes, appears to help by reducing production of the by-products.

In the illustration on page 171, you can see some of the factors that promote better or worse estrogen by-products.

> When estrogen (in men and women) isn't metabolized well by the body, the by-products can be harmful. Specifically, these hormones can be the triggers for breast cancer and prostate cancer.

Removing Endocrine Disrupting Chemicals from Your Environment

In Rings 3 and 4, we discussed the effect of environmental chemicals on metabolic pathways and detoxification. Unfortunately, many of these chemicals are widespread in our environment. Examples include herbicides, pesticides, solvents (cleaners) and cleaning agents, plastics, cosmetics, cooking utensils, flame retardants, synthetic fabrics, and food packaging materials. Because these chemicals don't break down in the environment or in your body, they're also known as persistent organic pollutants (POPs). In particular, POPs accumulate in the food chain, so they can be found in our food. It's impossible to completely eliminate our exposure to these chemicals in the environment. For example, studies show that BPA (bisphenol A), an estrogen disruptor, is detectable in most of us. So what should you do?

Here are some steps to reduce your exposure to endocrine disrupting chemicals in the environment:

- Use green products that are natural, non-toxic, biodegradable, and made without petrochemicals.
- Avoid heating food in plastic containers. Use glass or ceramic containers instead, especially when using a microwave oven. Heated plastics release more endocrine disrupting chemicals into your food.
- Air out dry-cleaned garments, mattresses, and fabrics that have been chemically cleaned or treated.
- Many cosmetics, shampoos, lotions, nail polish, sunscreens, perfumes, and chemical air-fresheners contain parabens and phthalates, which are known estrogen disruptors. Try natural or organic products free of these compounds.
- Non-stick cookware coatings contains PFOA (perfluorooctanoic acid or C8), a heat- and grease- resistant chemical that can affect thy-

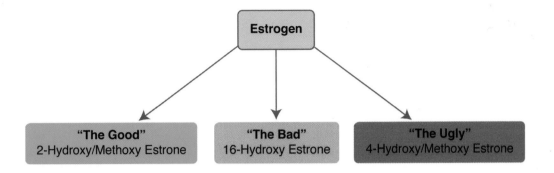

Protect Yourself from Breast and Prostate Cancer

Estrogen

| "The Good" 2-Hydroxy/Methoxy Estrone | "The Bad" 16-Hydroxy Estrone | "The Ugly" 4-Hydroxy/Methoxy Estrone |

Promotes "The Good" pathway and Safe By-products
- diet rich in antioxidants and cruciferous vegetables
- cruciferous vegetable extracts:
    Indole-3-Carbinol (I3C)
    Di-Indole Methane (DIM)
- DHEA
- exercise
- fish oil
- green tea
- hops
- magnesium
- resveratrol
- rosemary
- soy isoflavones
- vitamin E
- vitamins B2, B6, B12 and activated folic acid

Promotes "The Bad" and "The Ugly" pathways and Unsafe By-products
- certain synthetic estrogens
- excess alcohol
- excess sugar
- hypothyroidism
- overcooked meat
- obesity
- pesticides and endocrine disrupting chemicals
- smoking

Figure S4.1

Protect Yourself from Breast and Prostate Cancer

roid hormones and may increase obesity. In addition to cookware, this chemical is found in some microwave containers and pizza boxes. If you use non-stick cookware, discard it if it becomes scratched. Never scrape non-stick cookware with a metal spatula.

- Enhance your detoxification systems as discussed in Star 3.

Step 5. Balancing Thyroid Hormones

When we are experiencing chronic stress, the thyroid gland can be sluggish. In this case, the thyroid stimulating hormone (TSH) will rise slightly, free T3 and free T4 will be normal, and antithyroid antibodies will be negative. In our experience, supplements are helpful in returning the TSH level to normal. We often suggest iodine, selenium, tyrosine, bladderwrack, and rosemary leaf extract. If we need to treat using thyroid medications, we generally prescribe levothyroxine (Synthroid), which is bioidentical to T4. If necessary, we add cytomel, a synthetic form of T3. Many integrative medicine practitioners like to use Armour thyroid because it is natural in the sense of being derived from pig thyroid glands. We believe that while this product may be natural, it is not bioidentical to human thyroid hormones.

Achieving a More Balanced Life

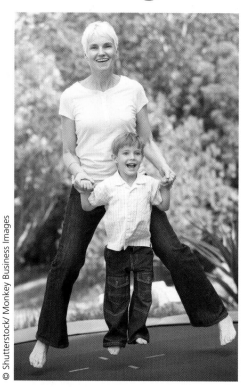

© Shutterstock/ Monkey Business Images

Balancing your hormones can help you achieve a more balanced life, and vice versa. You cannot do this alone, however. You need an accurate medical diagnosis based on a physical examination and laboratory testing. If prescription drugs are needed, you need regular follow-up visits to monitor your response.

We are often asked, "How do you know if balancing the hormones is working?" The answer is simple. When you are sick, your symptoms let you know. Then you need lab tests confirm what you feel. When you are better, you feel better, and the results on the lab tests will normalize.

The body is a complex matrix of systems. Even when replacing hormones, it is still a good idea to look at the body as a whole. This is a perfect example of how a systems approach provides a more complete understanding of the body. By supporting lifestyle, diet, oxidative stress, and detoxification processes, we support healing and balance.

Alex Learns to Balance His Hormones

Alex continues to pursue Health and Wellness

The changes that Alex made in his diet immediately helped his insulin resistance—he stopped feeling sluggish. His daily exercise and stress-reduction program made him feel twenty years younger. Earlier, he had questioned his attraction to his wife. As his vitality returned, so did his libido. His wife responded to all the new attention he seemed to shower upon her. Alex stopped worrying about his virility, but the risk for prostate problems still weighed heavily on him. To help prevent them, Alex continued on his daily supplements and added daily capsules of indole-3-carbinol, a broccoli extract. He made sure he regularly ate a large serving of organic broccoli, steamed for just ninety seconds.

When we repeated his urinary hormone testing a few months later, everything was normal! Even his ratio of 2:16 α-hydroxy estrone and his ugly 4-hydroxy estrone levels were now normal.

Alex had successfully balanced his hormones by changing his lifestyle, modifying his diet, handling his stress, and taking the appropriate supplements. Really, he had modified the way his genes were being expressed. As Alex told us, "I don't like science, but learning about epigenetics has been cool!"

All he needed now was to control his back pain.

5

RING FIVE

Understanding and Treating Pain

Your Body As Your Biography:
How Pain Can Give You a Different Perspective on Yourself and Your Life

Structural and Bioenergetic Assessment

Although acute pain can put us in agony in an instant, it is also a highly effective protective mechanism. If we accidentally put our hand too close to a fire, we abruptly feel pain. This normal physiological response is tied to saving our lives (or our hides). We respond quickly by pulling our hand away from the fire. Modern medicine is very good at using highly effective drugs to relieve acute pain.

The Reality of Chronic Pain

Chronic pain, defined as discomfort that persists for three months or longer, is different from acute pain.

Chronic pain may affect as many as 116 million Americans, but few receive effective treatment for it. Usually, there is a pain generator somewhere in the body, an underlying factor that is causing the problem. It may be the result of an injury or the secondary effect of some other condition present in the body, such as cancer, osteoarthritis, fibromyalgia, or endometriosis. It could be generated by a chronically inflamed disc or joint, or it might be coming from a knotted spasm in a muscle, referred to as a trigger point. In any case, the body often interprets that signal as a chronic problem.

Reverberating Pain Signals

Often, chronic pain is like a warning light stuck in the "on" position on your car's dashboard. You call the dealership, and they tell you not to worry. "It's just a mild malfunction—come in when you can and we'll fix it," they say. Despite this, the warning light continues to bother you. Eventually, you refuse to drive the car, convinced that something is going to happen.

Chronic pain is similar. The warning light is constantly on. Instead of saying, "OK, I know what's going on. You can switch off now," the body remains in a hyperalert state, constantly trying to figure out the source of the pain. This hypervigilant state becomes another source of stress, inflaming muscles and nerves and draining the body of energy.

Whatever the original source of the discomfort, the pain is sending a message up to the brain. The brain, once it senses pain, should send a "switch-off" message, an inhibitory signal that travels back down the spinal cord and turns off the pain. In other words, the body should recognize chronic pain and respond, "Oh, I know what that is, it's the site of my old injury, but I don't need to worry about it. It's not going to break, it's just hurting."

The "switch-off" or inhibitory signal is affected by your levels of serotonin and other neurotransmitters, such as norepinephrine. As discussed earlier, chronic stress depletes these neurotransmitters. When serotonin and norepinephrine levels get too low, the body cannot switch off the pain. This leads to vicious cycles of pain.

Vicious Cycle #1: Pain → Depression → More Pain

Here's how the cycle works. Stress leads to depression > which amplifies pain > which leads to more stress and depression. Get the picture?

If you have chronic pain, you're probably not sleeping well, which means you're not regenerating neurotransmitters such as serotonin very efficiently. You understandably become focused on the pain, which means you sleep less and suffer more. By definition, you quickly slip into the "inflamed and exhausted" mode of the stress curve (see Ring 2 to see the stress curve chart). As your inflammation levels rise, the inflammatory cascade is turned on, releasing cytokines and a whole array of other signaling chemicals that amp up the immune response and the pain.

Vicious Cycle #2: Pain → Spasm → More Pain

The body responds to chronic pain by causing muscle spasms in the affected area. Imagine you are a caveman and you break your forearm. Your muscles would go into spasm, forcing your bones together so they could bind. Once the fracture healed, the spasm would subside. In chronic pain, this natural healing mechanism persists, even though the original problem has healed. For some people, the pain of an injury leads to spasms that never really go away. The pain leads to spasms that further aggravate pain and spasms. In fact, this is described by doctors as the pain–spasm–pain cycle.

Conventional Medicine and Pain

Conventional medicine has succeeded in its approach to acute pain. Anesthesiologists are expert at relieving pain after surgery. Epidural steroids, nerve blocks, and medications have allowed physicians to master acute painful conditions. Unfortunately, chronic pain is different.

In our experience, when it comes to conventional medicine, chronic pain suffers the same fate as most chronic medical conditions. The longer the pain persists, the less likely conventional medicine is to cure it. If a patient has two or more areas of chronic pain, there is even less likelihood that there will be a cure. In addition, chronic pain is medically undertreated for fear of addicting patients to opioid medications.

This is where an integrative approach can be helpful. The Department of Defense has recently recognized this when it comes to caring for injured warriors and their families. In a report issued in May 2010, the Army's Pain Management Task Force developed 109 recommendations that led to a comprehensive pain management strategy that is holistic, multidisciplinary, and multimodal in its approach, utilizes state of the art science modalities and technologies, and provides optimal quality of life for patients with acute and chronic pain. Similarly, in June 2010, the Institute of Medicine of the National Academies, an independent organization that works outside of the government to provide advice on health and medicine, issued a report that calls for a cultural transformation in how the nation understands and approaches pain management and prevention.

A Shift in Perspective

If you're living with persistent pain or discomfort, it is useful to look at the body as a whole—as a structural marvel, and not just as a series of problematic parts. While patients and doctors alike focus on the painful part of the body, understanding the body as a whole will deepen your understanding of why you have pain and will help move you toward a solution.

Tensegrity: The Body's Elegant Balance

An idea common to both engineering and biology is *tensegrity*, the elegant balance between the continuous "pull" of muscles and connective tissue and the "push" of our bones. This balancing process is ongoing, synergistic, and dynamic. Like everything else in the body, tensegrity is a push toward the overall balance we call homeostasis.

Consider the miracle of how our bodies work. Basically, we are just a stack of bones held together by ropes we call muscles, ligaments, and tendons.

Our bones connect at our joints. Some joints, like our hips, fit together in a ball and socket, while others are much more complex. Our legs, for example, involve a thigh bone, or femur, elegantly poised above a multifaceted hinge joint (our knee) that connects it with two other bones, the tibia and the fibula. Our knees are an ingenious feat of engineering. They remain stable while still allowing us to perform all kinds of subtle, complex movements, like twisting, squatting, kneeling, and climbing. This is accomplished by the ligaments that hold the bony parts of the knees in place, while the muscles act as pulleys to enable us to move and bend. The cartilage, or meniscus, acts as a shock absorber, while guiding our femur and tibia to act as cantilevers that enable us to lean, stretch, reach, and balance.

Muscles surround the joints. They pull on the joints like levers, allowing us to move. The muscles are attached to the bones via the ropes called tendons, which sometimes get overworked and inflamed—a condition commonly described as tendonitis.

The muscles are surrounded by a white, sinewy connective material called fascia, which wraps around the muscles throughout the body. It also surrounds, supports, and penetrates all of our muscles, nerves, and organs. It binds us together, much as plastic wrap around a sandwich holds it together.

A clear example of the fascia can be seen in chicken meat—it is the white membrane that surrounds the muscles of drumsticks and envelops the breast. In fact, the fascia forms a structure that connects and envelops every major muscle and every organ in our bodies, extending uninterrupted from the tops of our heads to the tips of our toes! Fascia is made up largely of collagen fibers that can resist great forces pulling from different directions. It is important that the fascia remain free, flexible, and easy-moving. When it is bound or stuck, that can cause both pain and functional problems.

Another way to look at the fascia is as our body's Internet. It wraps around all muscles and nerves, acting as a massive unseen network of connectivity that can be compared to an Internet for the body. This is important because acupuncture and bodywork such as massage or Rolfing work in part by freeing the fascia or by sending messages through it.

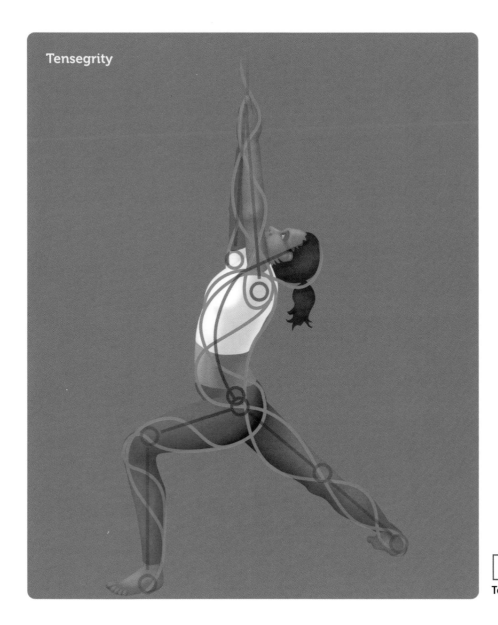

Figure R5.1

Tensegrity

The Domino Effect of Injury

Once you begin to think about the body in terms of tensegrity, a constant pull–push that interacts with the nervous system, it is easy to see that when the body goes out of balance after an injury or overexertion, that imbalance can ricochet throughout the system. The body compensates by attempting to balance the imbalance. A right ankle injury may throw the left hip out of balance. This can affect the right side of the chest, and ultimately the left shoulder.

While pain may be in one area of the body, it is always important to also understand pain as an expression of the body as a whole. Once again, we need to view the body from a systems perspective. Pain is a complex interaction between these systems. It is affected by tensegrity, stress and neurotransmitters, metabolic, inflammatory and immune problems, and even hormonal imbalances. To treat chronic pain, we need to view the whole person.

The Integrative Diagnosis of Pain

Pain is one of the top three complaints people bring to their doctor. It is possible you yourself have been in pain for a while and may not have found anything that relieves it. It is often difficult to identify the source of the pain. However, once you understand more about how pain is generated, your options for treatment will expand significantly. You may find someone who can do everything you need, or you may need to create your own health care team by working with several different integrative practitioners, such as a doctor and an acupuncturist, massage therapist, or a chiropractic physician.

A Stepwise Approach to Understanding Your Pain

Step 1. **A Medical Musculoskeletal Evaluation**

Step 2. **Understanding Body Mechanics, Structure, and Function**

Step 3. **Identifying Trigger Points and Myofascial Pain**

Step 4. **An Acupuncture Evaluation**

Step 5. **Understanding Your Biopsychotype: How Your Body Affects Your Mind**

Step 6. **How Your Mind Affects Your Body**

Step 7. **A Lifestyle Analysis: Finding the Causes and the Solutions**

Step 8. **An Integrative Diagnosis and a Transformational Treatment Plan**

Step 1.

A Medical Musculoskeletal Evaluation

A medical musculoskeletal evaluation is a typical examination done by physicians, such as a primary care doctor, orthopedist, physical medicine and rehabilitation physician, sports medicine physician, neurologist, or neurosurgeon. From a musculoskeletal point of view, in conventional medicine it is of primary importance to find the exact reason for the pain. This is what medical doctors are trained to do.

The standard examinations require a thorough knowledge of anatomy, neurology, and the musculoskeletal system. Testing typically employed in these conventional workups include x-rays, MRIs, CT scans, and EMGs (electromyograms, which show nerve conduction problems in the muscle and can be very helpful for finding the source of the pain).

An abnormal test result, however, does not necessarily mean that the test has revealed the source of the pain. Studies have shown that most people have one or two bulging discs in the spine that definitely do not cause pain. On the other hand, 50 percent of people with back pain have normal MRIs, with no apparent evidence of an abnormal disc. We always say, "We need to treat the patient, not the test!"

In some cases, by moving the body in a certain way or prodding the correct area, the doctor can reproduce the pain. This lets them know they are treating the right problem.

The diagnosis needs to correlate with the patients' symptoms. If not, the result may not be what you want. A good example is a patient who has back surgery when he should have had a hip replacement, or vice versa.

Dermatome Pain Patterns

As each nerve emerges from the spine, it supplies sensation to certain specific areas of the body, known as dermatomes. Damage to a nerve that comes from the thoracic (chest) part of the spine, for instance, can cause pain that wraps around the chest and goes into the abdomen, to the point where it can be confused with gallbladder pain.

The pain sensation is sometimes felt in an area that is far away from the actual source. Doctors call this referred or radicular pain. For example, a pinched nerve in the lower back may cause leg pain; a pinched nerve in the neck can result in arm pain. By identifying the distribution of your pain, tingling, or numbness, your physician can work backward to understand which disc is herniated and which nerve is being pinched. Similarly, the pain from angina, a heart problem, can be confused with neck pain, while leg pain from peripheral vascular disease (blocked blood vessels) in the leg can be confused with the pain from spinal stenosis. The diagram below shows the dermatomes—areas of the body that correspond to nerves as they emerge from the spine.

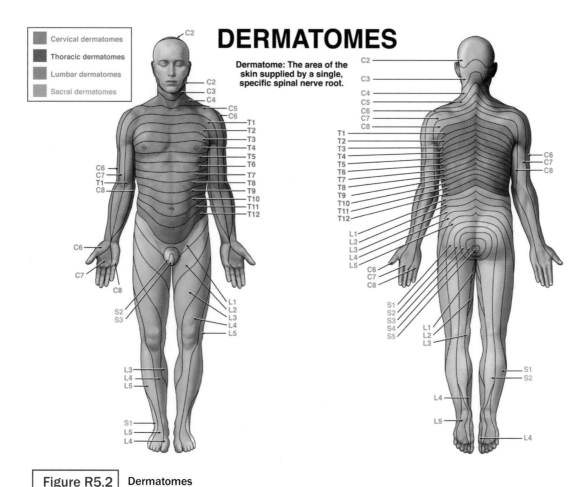

| Figure R5.2 | Dermatomes |

John's Herniated Disc in His Neck Causes Radiating Pain Down His Arm.

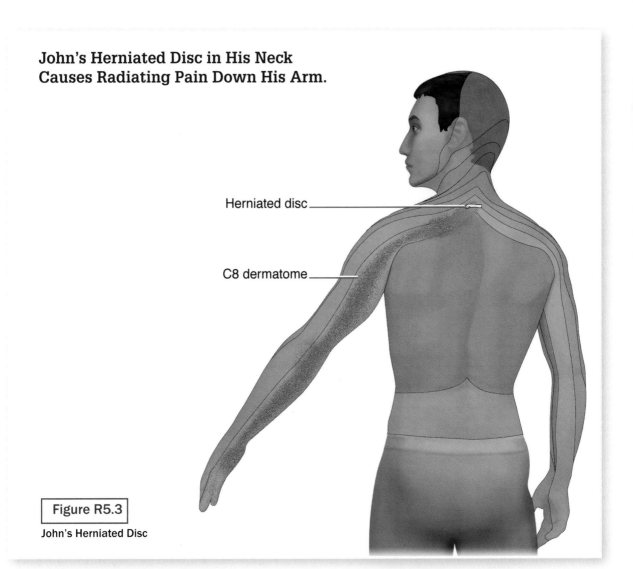

Herniated disc

C8 dermatome

Figure R5.3

John's Herniated Disc

Unraveling John's Story: A Pain in the Neck

John is a busy 47-year-old architect who went to see his orthopedic surgeon complaining of neck pain radiating down his left arm to his baby finger (his C8 dermatome). The physician quickly diagnosed a herniated disc in his neck between C7 and T1, prescribed some anti-inflammatories, and sent him for physical therapy. John returned three weeks later with no real improvement. At this point, his doctor ordered an MRI of the neck to confirm his diag-

nosis and referred him for a series of cortisone epidural injections. John knew the routine well. Only six months earlier, he had been through a similar problem with a herniated lumbar (low back) disc at L5/S1, causing radiating pain down his right leg. The cervical epidurals took his pain away for a few months, but then it returned. At that point he decided he wanted to try a different approach. That is when he came to see us....

Excluding Complex Regional Pain Syndrome (CRPS)

Complex regional pain syndrome (CRPS), also known as reflex sympathetic dystrophy or RSD, is one of the conditions a doctor will look for in a standard medical workup for chronic pain. Millions of people in the United States suffer from CRPS. The main symptoms are various degrees of severe pain, swelling, and hypersensitivity to touch, usually in an arm or leg. CRPS usually happens after a triggering event, such as an injury, surgery, stroke, or heart attack that causes nerve irritation and pain in the affected area. The pain continues past the time it should go away and is often out of proportion to the severity of the initial injury. A patient may feel burning, muscle or joint stiffness, rapid hair and nail growth, and constriction of blood vessels at the site. The pain then becomes more severe, often associated with weakening of the muscles, stiffening of the joints, and thinning of the bone (osteoporosis), until the joints can be fixed in a contracted position. Although CRPS usually follows an injury or surgery, sometimes no cause can be found. If you have unusual pain, discuss the possibility of CRPS with your doctor.

Step 2.

Understanding Body Mechanics, Structure, and Function

A biomechanical approach to diagnosing and treating chronic pain is based on the concepts of tensegrity—the pull and push that is always being exerted on the bones, muscles, ligaments, and tendons.

Chronic imbalance sets us up for injury. When one muscle group is always pulling harder than the opposing group, it creates tension in the system. If muscles are pulling too hard in a particular area around the spine, the excessive stress in that area puts us at risk for injury. The spine needs to move fluidly, with each vertebra moving just a little as we twist or bend. When there is spasm in a particular area, that segment of the spine will "lock up." A healthy disc in the adjacent segment must compensate, taking on some of the biomechanical stress of the spine and extending the range of motion beyond normal limitations.

Another tipping point. When an area of the body is in a state of chronic stress or weakness, it doesn't take much to tip it into crisis. If, for instance, there is a weakened disc in the lower back, falling or bending the wrong way may be enough to cause that disc to herniate.

Another vicious cycle. Chronic muscle spasms are the body's basic response to injury and pain. If a disc in the spine is injured, however, spasms only irritate it further. This triggers the vicious cycle of spasm–pain–spasm.

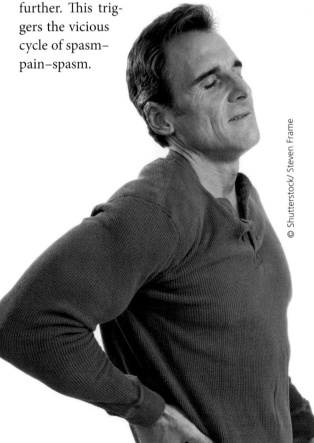

© Shutterstock/ Steven Frame

Evaluating Body Mechanics, Structure, and Function

When we work with a patient in pain, we do a complete exam to evaluate the person's body mechanics, structure, and function. We start by looking at the most painful part of the body. We want to know how well that area of the body moves. Is it stiff and sore, implying that it is in spasm, or is it red and hot, suggesting inflammation? Can we make the pain return by moving or palpating that area in a certain way? If we can reproduce the pain, we have a better idea of what's causing it. Is the area tender? If so, the pain is actually originating from that area. If not, it is being referred from somewhere else.

Next, we evaluate the spine. We apply gentle pressure to the spine to find areas of tenderness. We also look at how each vertebra moves to learn if there is any dysfunction in that area.

After that, we look at the whole structure of the person's body to see how it could be affecting or causing chronic pain. We check to see if the hips and shoulders are level and if they move well. Sometimes the problem is caused by a misaligned kneecap. Do the arches of the feet drop?

We view the patient's profile from the side, looking for posture problems. Is the head in a "head-forward" position? Are the shoulders directly above the ankles? If not, what kind of pressure is this placing on the system?

We look at the status of the person's muscles, ligaments, and tendons. How do all the parts move together? Does the person have chronic tension in the muscles? What does the person look like when sitting, standing, walking, or running?

And finally, we ask, what is the easiest, safest, most cost-effective way to get you better?

John's Story Continues

By the time John came to see us, the pain in his low back, leg, neck and arm had returned. While the cortisone in the epidural injections had reduced the swelling and inflammation, giving him symptomatic relief, his underlying problems hadn't changed. He had been working hard on a new architectural project, and the stress was getting to him. As we questioned him about his daily activities, it became clear that John spent much of his day multitasking, with his phone clamped between his ear and his shoulder. Sound familiar? Why was he having low back pain, though? As we worked with John, it became obvious that he stood in a way where one of his hips (or iliac crest) was continually elevated. The arch of his right foot tended to collapse, with resultant continual pressure on his low back. No wonder his disc was giving him trouble.

Treating John required us to treat both the problem as well as the underlying biomechanical cause. We needed to treat his whole body. We started him on acupuncture, chiropractic, and ACE Healing Treatment[SM] (a combination of acupuncture, chiropractic, and energy work). We helped solve his neck and shoulder problem by suggesting he wear an ergonomically designed headset for the phone. We helped treat his low back problem with hamstring stretches and abdominal strengthening exercises. He also needed corrective arch supports (orthotics) for his shoes.

John's story is a classic story of what we call "body unwinding." We systematically make our way through the issues and the logic of the body, like peeling away layers of an onion.

John's Pain

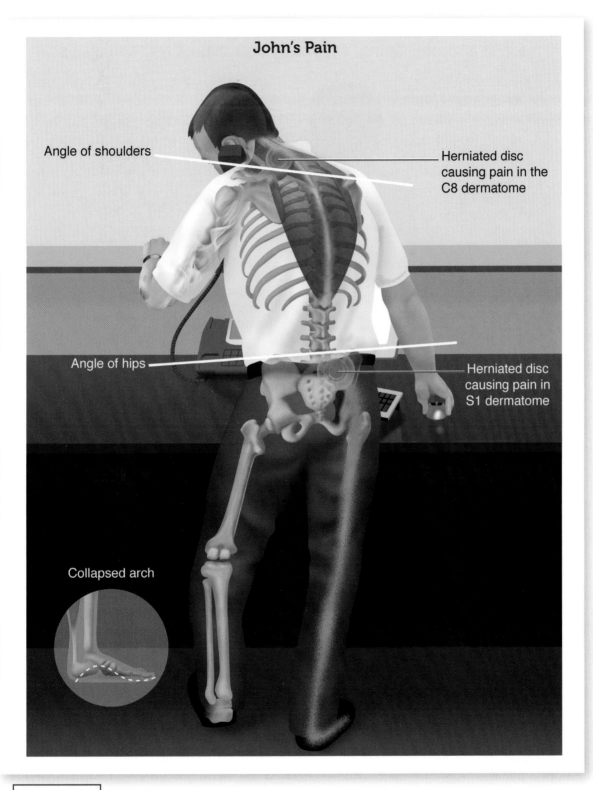

Angle of shoulders

Herniated disc causing pain in the C8 dermatome

Angle of hips

Herniated disc causing pain in S1 dermatome

Collapsed arch

Figure R5.4 John's Pain

John's Body Mechanics: The Forces That Caused His Herniated Disc

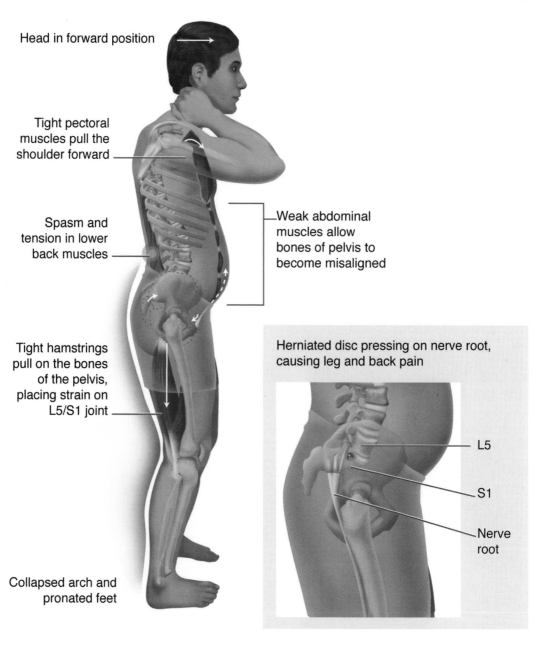

Head in forward position

Tight pectoral muscles pull the shoulder forward

Spasm and tension in lower back muscles

Weak abdominal muscles allow bones of pelvis to become misaligned

Tight hamstrings pull on the bones of the pelvis, placing strain on L5/S1 joint

Collapsed arch and pronated feet

Herniated disc pressing on nerve root, causing leg and back pain

L5

S1

Nerve root

Figure R5.5 | John's Body Mechanics

Identifying Trigger Points and Myofascial Pain

Trigger points are extrasensitive areas in skeletal muscle that often have palpable nodules (knots) or taut bands (tightness). Clearly, trigger points hurt. They also create referred pain patterns, meaning they can cause pain elsewhere in the body that doesn't seem directly linked to the painful point. We call this type of pain *myofascial pain*, meaning it comes from the muscles (*myo*) or the fascia. By injecting trigger points with local anesthetic, placing acupuncture needles into them, or even massaging them deeply, we can usually eliminate not only the pain in that area but also any referred pain. Deep massage can further help by freeing the blockages in the fascial planes, thus allowing the muscles to glide freely over each other.

> Pain is just another form of information.
>
> —Don Delillo, *Underworld*

Nerve Pain or Muscle Pain?

Nerve pain (sometimes called radicular pain) is caused by an irritated or pinched nerve, while muscle pain comes from an irritated trigger point. Sometimes differentiating between the two can be difficult. What makes this even more challenging is that both problems may occur simultaneously. To help diagnose this, we often recommend two tests: an EMG and an MRI.

EMG (electromyography) is a way of measuring the electrical activity in a nerve. The test is helpful for detecting altered nerve function. An MRI (magnetic resonance imaging) can show a bulging disc in the spine that is pinching a nerve. We have no good tests to detect trigger points, however. Instead, we check for them the old-fashioned way, with a physical examination.

Instinctively, we all know about trigger points, because most of us develop an inflamed trigger point at some time in our lives. Our instinctive response to the pain from a trigger point is to rub it hard, which can give an "ooh" sensation of relief.

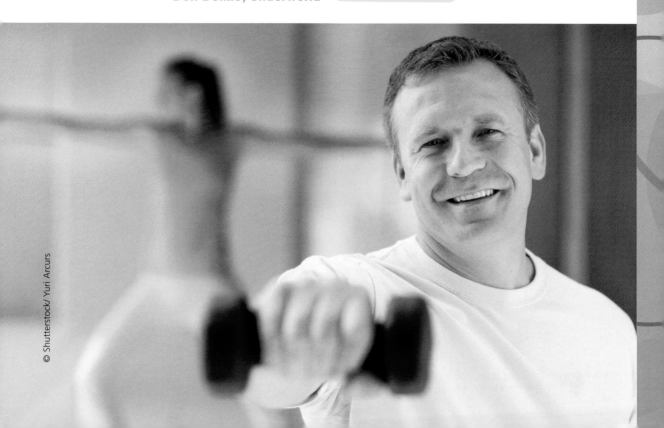

Is It a Pinched Nerve, Or an Irritable Trigger Point?

Referred myofascial pain and radicular pain (from a pinched nerve) can look and feel similar, but the treatment is different.

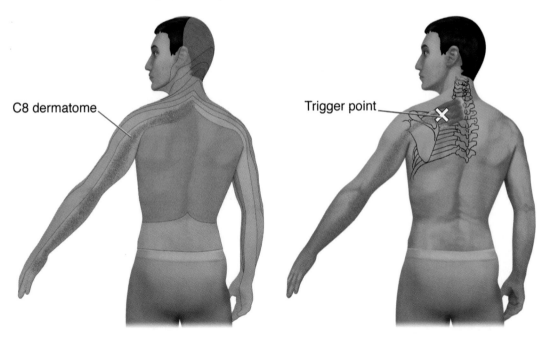

Dermatomal pain caused by a pinched nerve.   Myofascial pain caused by a trigger point.

Figure R5.6	Referred Myofascial Pain

President Kennedy's Back Pain

In 1955, Senator John F. Kennedy had major back surgery related to injuries he had suffered in World War II. Unfortunately, the surgery did not help the constant pain, and Kennedy and his family were concerned that this pain could result in his political career coming to a premature end. His orthopedic surgeon then consulted another physician, Dr. Janet Travell, for assistance. Dr. Travell was able to locate the source of Kennedy's pain in his lower back muscles. She described these painful areas as trigger points. By injecting low-dose local anesthetic directly into these muscles, she was able to alleviate his pain. Years later, President Kennedy appointed Dr. Travell to the post of Personal Physician to the President, making her the first woman to hold this position. Dr. Travell would go on to serve President Lyndon Johnson after the death of President Kennedy and remained in that post until 1965. Dr. Travell pioneered the understanding of trigger points and myofascial pain.

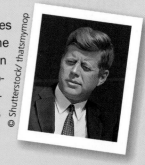

© Shutterstock/ thatsmymop

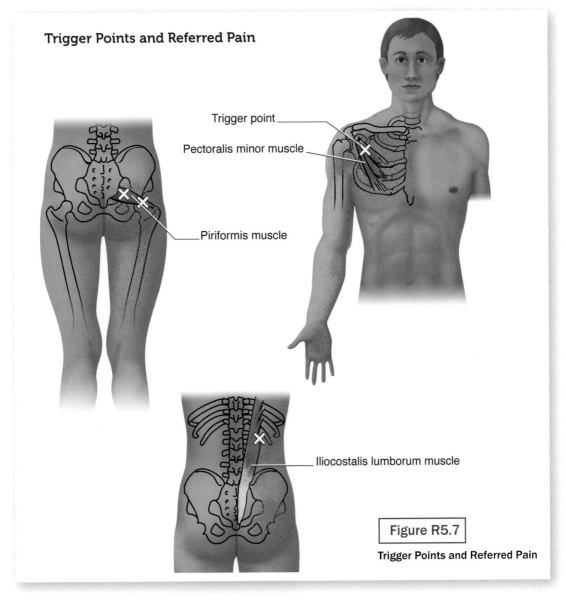

Trigger Points and Referred Pain

Trigger point

Pectoralis minor muscle

Piriformis muscle

Iliocostalis lumborum muscle

Figure R5.7

Trigger Points and Referred Pain

When Pain Becomes Self-Perpetuating

Pain can breed pain. A good example is pain that develops after a motor vehicle accident. Right after a car accident that causes a whiplash-type injury to the neck, the person usually has only mild pain. At that point, x-rays and neurological exams are usually normal. Hours later, however, the injured muscles often go into spasm, causing pain. Typically, the muscles in spasm then recruit adjacent muscles, which also go into spasm as the body attempts to immobilize and stabilize the area. Within a few weeks, the injured person may be experiencing pain throughout the entire body. Pain can interfere with sleep and neurotransmitter regeneration, especially if the person was already stressed. This pain can continue for months or even years if not properly treated.

Integrative Therapies for Myofascial Conditions

Integrative therapies can be very effective for myofascial conditions. Acupuncture, for instance, directly treats the myofascial network. Rolfing™ and other touch therapies can also be very helpful. Other alternative, complementary therapies that affect the fascia include osteopathy, massage, the Feldenkrais Method, the Alexander Technique, and energy healing.

Fibromyalgia

Fibromyalgia is a common condition characterized by long-term, body-wide pain and fatigue, often accompanied by problems with sleep, memory, and mood. It is officially diagnosed when there is widespread pain lasting at least three months and at least eleven specific tender points out of a possible total of eighteen. A tender point is a small spot on the body that is painful when pressed on firmly. Tender point locations are found all over the body, from the back of the head to the inner knees. Tender points are similar to trigger points, but they are not identical. The tender points of fibromyalgia are associated with body-wide pain, while trigger points usually cause pain that is focused in just one area of the body.

Understanding Pain from Autoimmune Disorders

Collectively, autoimmune diseases are a group of diseases affecting the collagenous connective tissue of several organs and systems. In autoimmune conditions, the body makes antibodies that attack our own tissues instead of attacking a foreign substance. Autoimmune disorders involving the musculoskeletal tissue include conditions such as rheumatic fever, scleroderma, rheumatoid arthritis, systemic lupus erythematosus, periarteritis, and serum sickness.

Autoimmune disorders almost always affect multiple systems of the body. The pain they cause may be due to multiple reasons. For example, they may cause arthritis, which is its own type of pain, as well as a separate pain caused by myofascial pain and fibromyalgia. They may be associated with stress and depression (Ring 2), nutritional problems, inflammation, oxidative stress, gut disorders (Ring 3), and hormonal problems (Ring 4). By understanding the Five Rings of Diagnosis, we can learn how each Ring influences the development of an illness. Then by using the Five Stars of Treatment, we can enhance the healing process by addressing each contributing system.

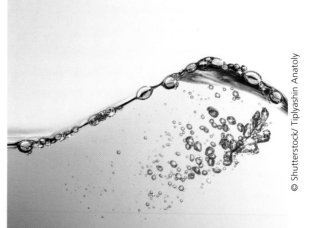

© Shutterstock/ Tiplyashin Anatoly

An Acupuncture Evaluation

Acupuncture—treating health problems by inserting and manipulating very fine needles into selected points on the skin—has been around for about three thousand years. Today the National Library of Medicine database contains more than eight thousand articles on acupuncture, including over eight hundred research studies on acupuncture and pain therapy. The World Health Organization has cited acupuncture as a legitimate therapy for more than forty conditions related to chronic pain.

Even as the debate still rages on about the effectiveness of acupuncture, millions of patients worldwide strongly attest to its many and very dramatic benefits. Acupuncture is not just a treatment, though—it is also a valuable diagnostic tool in dealing with chronic pain

Acupuncture to Diagnose Pain and Discomfort

Traditional acupuncturists were not taught to diagnose pain from a conventional medical point of view. Rather, they saw pain as an expression of blocked *chi*. In traditional Chinese medicine, *chi*, also called *qi*, refers to an invisible electrical-type energy that flows around the body through meridians (channels). Inserting acupuncture needles into the meridians at the right points unblocks areas of stagnant *chi* and restores the proper flow of energy, and unblocking *chi* is often helpful for relieving chronic pain.

Medical acupuncture builds on traditional acupuncture but takes a more scientific view of how acupuncture can achieve pain reduction. Acupuncture relieves spasm by deactivating trigger points, influences nerve and nervous system function, and seems to communicate with the whole body through the fascia.

Acupuncture is a wonderful tool to use for diagnosing chronic pain. There is a striking similarity between the location of acupuncture points and common trigger points. In fact, over 90 percent of these points overlap. Placing an acupuncture needle into a trigger point has a similar effect to injecting it with local anesthetic, although the pain relief is not immediate. In acupuncture, these points are referred to as "*ashi*" (pronounced *ah-shee*) points, meaning "ow," which implies a sensitive spot.

Acupuncture meridians also correlate with the fascial planes of the body. In fact, injecting acupuncture points with a radioactive substance shows the injected substance travelling down the fascial plane/meridian pathway. If the fascia is the body's Internet, the meridians are like software that helps the body make sense of information.

One important series of points along the acupuncture meridians are the command points, located on the arms between the elbows and the fingers, and on the legs from the knees to the toes. Most of these points overlie large nerves. Inserting a needle at these points

Professional Acupuncturists

Professionals trained to provide acupuncture include medical acupuncturists (M.D.s or DOs with additional training), Licensed Acupuncturists (LAcs), and, in some states, physical therapists and chiropractic physicians who have had additional acupuncture training. Having basic training in acupuncture does not mean the practitioner has a good grasp of neuro-anatomical and structural diagnosis. When choosing a practitioner, it is important to inquire about training and find out if the practitioner has had good results in treating the kind of problem you have.

is a way of manually promoting changes in the nervous system—it can be compared to reprogramming the body's software.

Overlapping Systems

Acupuncture meridians, trigger points, fascia, and dermatome (nerve) pathways all have a significant degree of overlap. As the diagram below shows, a pinched nerve at one of the vertebrae in the neck (C8), a trigger point in the shoulder, and an affected acupuncture (Small Intestine) meridian all involve the same area. After decades of experience of working with patients, we have come to see these systems as complementary. They are simply different dimensions of the body that provide a greater understanding of pain conditions.

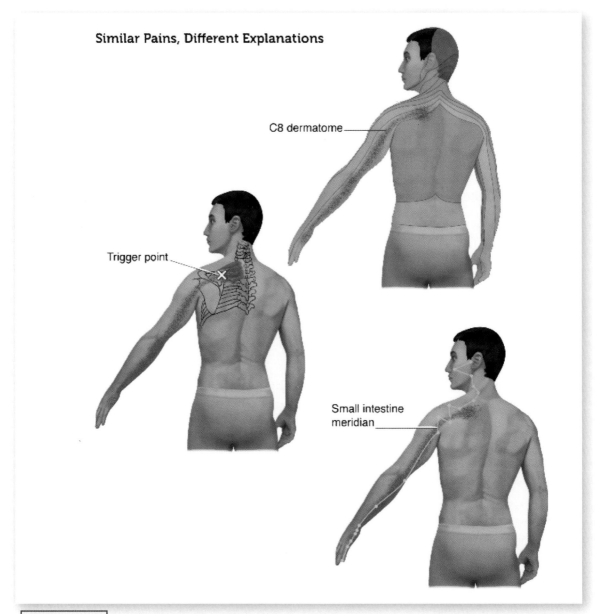

Similar Pains, Different Explanations

C8 dermatome

Trigger point

Small intestine meridian

Figure R5.8 | Similar Pains Different Explanations

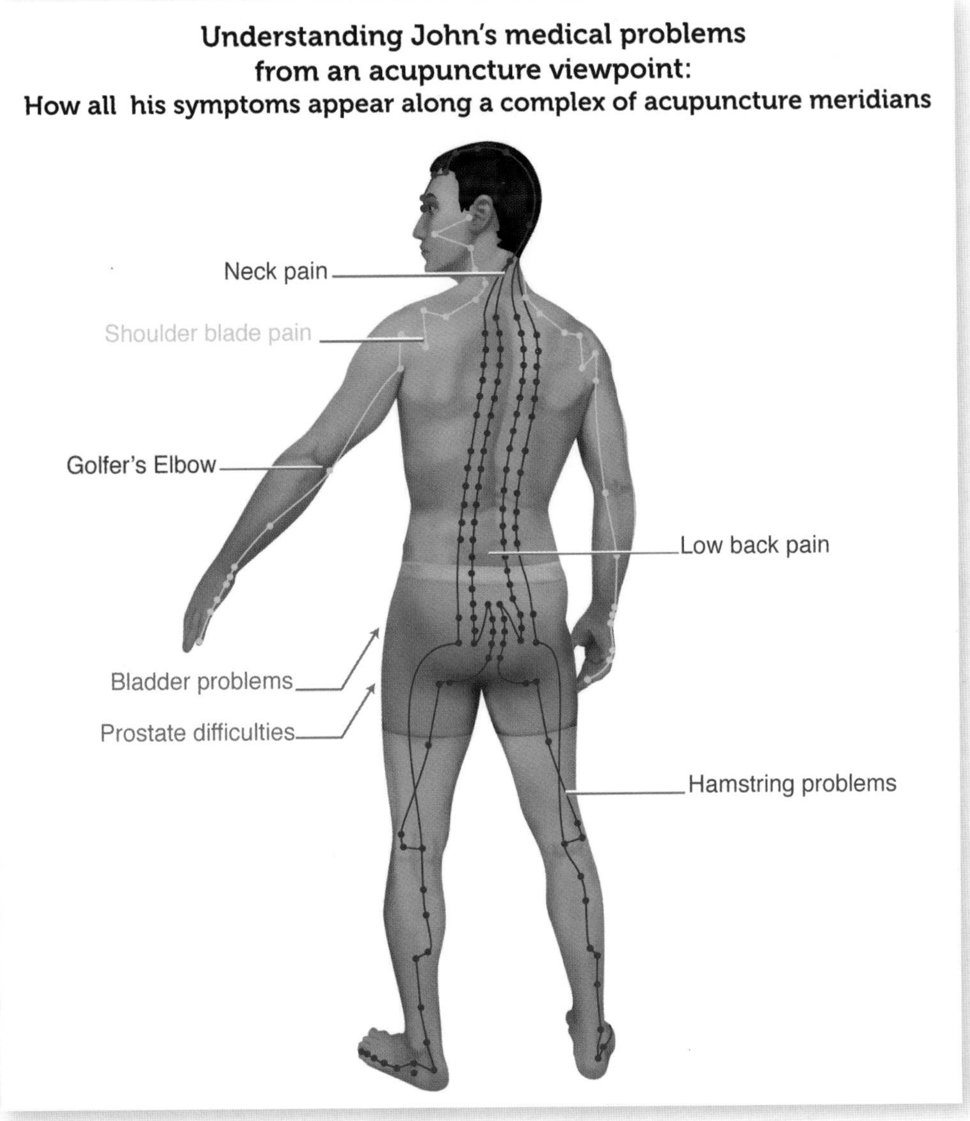

Understanding John's medical problems
from an acupuncture viewpoint:
How all his symptoms appear along a complex of acupuncture meridians

Neck pain

Shoulder blade pain

Golfer's Elbow

Low back pain

Bladder problems

Prostate difficulties

Hamstring problems

Figure R5.9

Understanding John's Medical Problems

John's Story Continues

John's initial problems were in his low back, neck, and shoulder. As we worked with him over several months, a number of other problems emerged. We treated John for golfer's elbow (medial epicondylitis), insomnia, and prostate and bladder problems. We even addressed a significant sense of fear and foreboding he suffered from in relationship to his work. As we diagnosed him from an acupuncture perspective, we showed him how all of his problems were on a single framework of interconnecting meridians.

Looking at the diagram above, you will see the same diagram we showed John. His golfer's elbow and insomnia related to the Heart meridian. His shoulder and neck problems related to the Small Intestine meridian. His lower back, prostate, and bladder symptoms related to the Bladder meridian. Finally, his fear and stress related to his Kidney meridian, which in turn affected his adrenal glands, as well as his lower back. These four meridians make up a single complex in acupuncture known as the Shao-Yin/Tai-Yang complex.

In other words, according to ancient Chinese medical theory, John did not have many problems, he had only one. It was as if the software program governing all the problems he was suffering from was malfunctioning, causing multiple problems at once. Acupuncture theory had predicted a person such as John would develop problems such as his thousands of years ago. This predictive ability to understand where someone will develop problems is called their biopsychotype. John has the problems common to his Will/Spirit biopsychotype.

Treating John with acupuncture meant we could treat all of his problems at the same time. Not only can we treat his physical problems, but we can also treat his emotional issues such as fear. In addition, the same treatment can address his old injuries as well as preventing him from developing new ones. In essence, we are able to use a Transformational Approach.

Understanding Your Biopsychotype: How Your Body Affects Your Mind

The propensity to develop certain illnesses—or to be healthy—is called a biopsychotype. Each biopsychotype is predisposed to certain physical and psychological problems. Understanding a person's biopsychotype is like understanding a computer's software program—it teaches us a person's strengths and weaknesses, attributes, qualities, and tendencies to dysfunction or disease. When we learn how to correct this software program, we can correct multiple problems at the same time.

Understanding Biopsychotypes

The term biopsychotype was coined by Joseph Helms, M.D., a wonderful teacher of ours. Dr. Helms has distilled his knowledge of acupuncture from Chinese, Japanese, Vietnamese, and French techniques. (The French missionaries were some of the early Western practitioners of acupuncture.) Dr. Helms goes into great detail in explaining these concepts in his excellent book, *Getting to Know You*.

Dr. Helms teaches how in each individual, four acupuncture meridians group together to form an archetype that is a predilection for both health and disease in that person. There are three main archetypes:

- The Vision/Action Biopsychotype
- The Nurture/Duty Biopsychotype
- The Will/Spirit Biopsychotype

Each biopsychotype is made up of four of the twelve traditional acupuncture meridians. When something goes wrong along any one of the four meridians, it is likely that there will be problems related to the other three as well. So when patients learn they have problems occurring along their meridians, they can begin to see themselves in a different way. Instead of seeing multiple problems, they see that they have one global dysfunction, and they feel an immediate sense of empowerment just by knowing this.

The real benefit, though, is that when we start using acupuncture to treat problems along the meridian complexes, other problems go away—simultaneously and effortlessly. In acupuncture, the body and mind are seen as interconnected. Because the meridians deal with both psychological and physical problems, acupuncture treatment does not differentiate between mind and body dysfunction. Treating a meridian complex or biopsychotype helps both.

Understanding Your Biopsychotype

Most of our patients readily recognize important aspects of themselves in one of the three fundamental biopsychotypes. Not every characteristic of the biopsychotype will match each of your characteristics. In fact, some may even appear to contradict each other. They do. They represent the yin and yang values of each biopsychotype. In real life, we usually fall mainly in one category but have smatterings of other qualities and disturbances. A good acupuncturist will treat your current symptoms while balancing the rest of the energetic system, with the goal of preventing future problems.

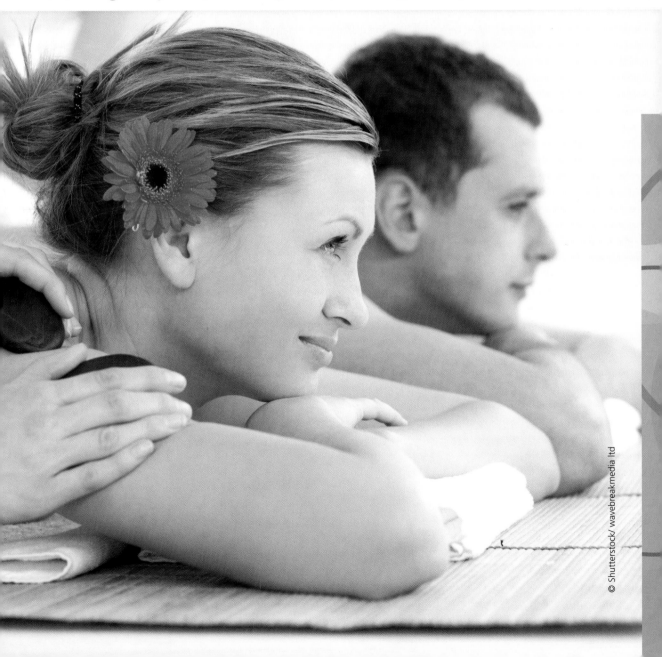

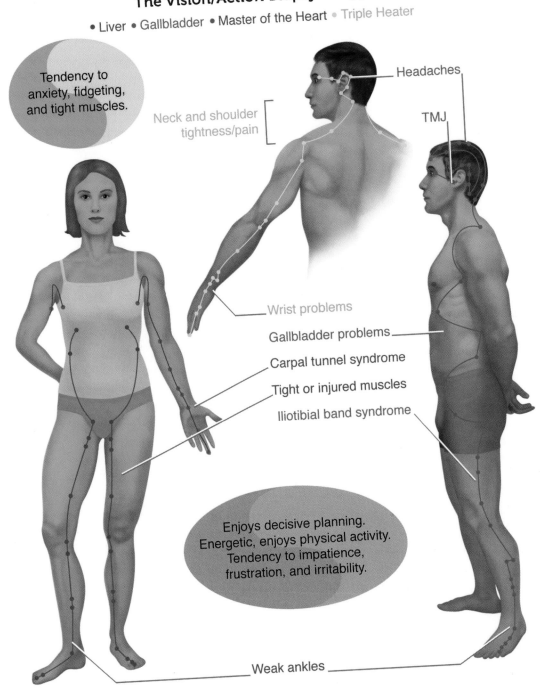

The Vision/Action Biopsychotype

• Liver • Gallbladder • Master of the Heart • Triple Heater

Tendency to anxiety, fidgeting, and tight muscles.

Neck and shoulder tightness/pain

Headaches

TMJ

Wrist problems

Gallbladder problems

Carpal tunnel syndrome

Tight or injured muscles

Iliotibial band syndrome

Enjoys decisive planning. Energetic, enjoys physical activity. Tendency to impatience, frustration, and irritability.

Weak ankles

Figure R5.10 | The Vision/Action Biopsychotype

The **Vision/Action** Biopsychotype

Ask yourself if any of these characteristics of the vision/action biopsychotype apply to you:

- Are you ambitious and driven?
- Do you have a tendency to impatience and irritability?
- Do you find that you really need to exercise?
- If you get stressed, do you find you tend to get very anxious, fidgety, and even hypochondriacal?
- Do you crave caffeinated beverages, coffee, or dark chocolate?
- Do you use alcohol to calm you when you get anxious?
- Do you experience problems along the Liver, Gallbladder, Master of the Heart, or Triple Warmer meridians?

Common problems are:

- headaches
- neck and shoulder pain or tightness
- carpal tunnel syndrome
- wrist problems
- tight or injured muscles
- dry eyes or vision problems
- gallbladder problems
- iliotibial band (ITB) syndrome
- weak ankles.

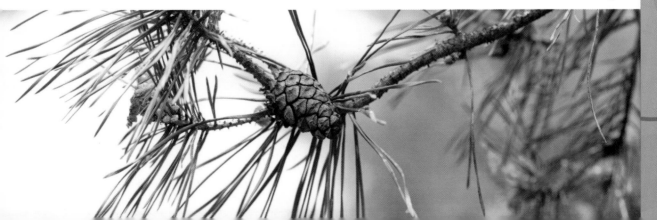

The **Nurture/Duty** Biopsychotype

Ask yourself if any of these characteristics of the nurture/duty biopsychotype apply to you:

- Are you organized and neat?
- Are you disciplined and responsible?
- Are you overnurturing? Do you sometimes feel the need to take care of everybody you know?
- Do you put on weight easily?
- Are you calm and easygoing?
- Do you tend to get colds easily?
- Do you have a melodic or soothing voice?
- Are you a perfectionist? Do you tend to be self-critical?
- Do you sometimes go overboard with the good things in life, like overeating or overdrinking?
- Do you have a build that is quite thin?
- Did you gray early?
- Do you tend to have problems with belching, heartburn, cramping, or diarrhea?
- Do you have painful or irregular periods?
- Do you tend to worry or easily become melancholic?
- Do you have any of the following physical problems found along the Spleen, Lung, Large Intestine, and Stomach meridians?

Common problems include:

- chronic respiratory problems
- difficulty getting pregnant
- fibroids
- a feeling of heaviness in your legs
- hemorrhoids
- varicose veins, diabetes, anemia
- De Quervain's tenosynovitis.

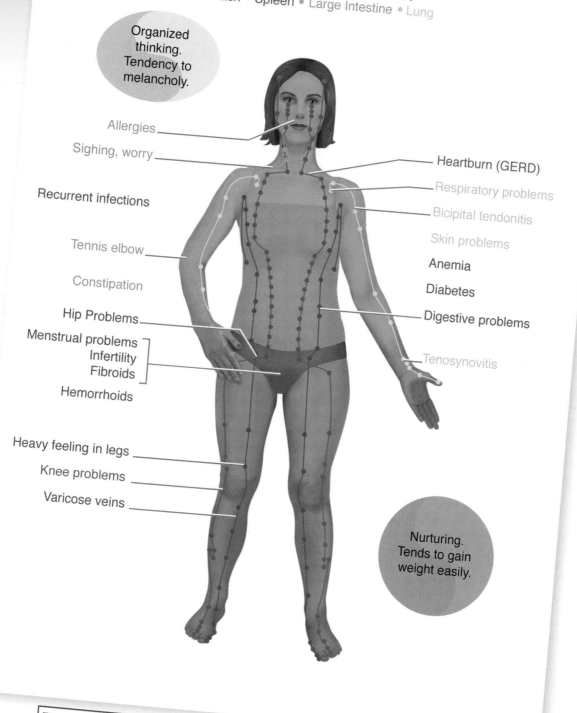

The Nurture/Duty Biopsychotype
• Stomach • Spleen • Large Intestine • Lung

Organized thinking. Tendency to melancholy.

Allergies

Sighing, worry

Recurrent infections

Tennis elbow

Constipation

Hip Problems

Menstrual problems
Infertility
Fibroids

Hemorrhoids

Heavy feeling in legs

Knee problems

Varicose veins

Heartburn (GERD)

Respiratory problems

Bicipital tendonitis

Skin problems

Anemia

Diabetes

Digestive problems

Tenosynovitis

Nurturing. Tends to gain weight easily.

Figure R5.11   The Nurture/Duty Biopsychotype

The Will/Spirit Biopsychotype

• Bladder • Kidney • Small Intestine • Heart

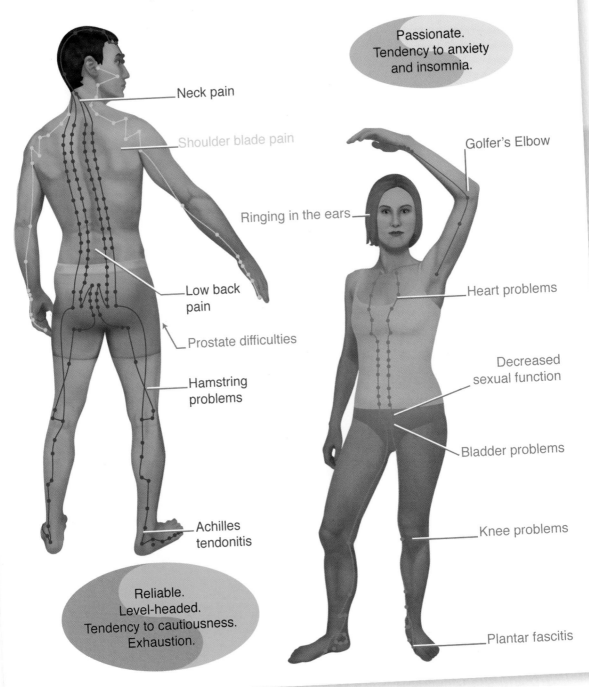

Passionate.
Tendency to anxiety
and insomnia.

Neck pain

Shoulder blade pain

Golfer's Elbow

Ringing in the ears

Heart problems

Low back
pain

Prostate difficulties

Decreased
sexual function

Hamstring
problems

Bladder problems

Achilles
tendonitis

Reliable.
Level-headed.
Tendency to cautiousness.
Exhaustion.

Knee problems

Plantar fascitis

Figure R5.12 | The Will/Spirit Biopsychotype

The **Will/Spirit** Biopsychotype

Ask yourself if any of these characteristics of the will/spirit biopsychotype apply to you:

- Are you reliable and level-headed?
- Are you a good leader or an ardent follower?
- Are you usually in good health and hard-working?
- Are you full of doubt or lacking confidence at times?
- Are you passionate, sexual, and creative?
- Did you start balding early?
- Do you suffer from back problems or joint stiffness?
- Do you have chronic sleep difficulties?
- Do you have physical problems along the Kidney, Heart, Small Intestine, or Bladder meridians?

Common problems include:

- plantar fasciitis
- Achilles tendonitis
- prostate difficulties
- bladder problems
- low back pain

- neck pain
- ringing in the ears
- golfer's elbow (medial epicondylitis)
- pain in your shoulder blades
- hamstring problems.

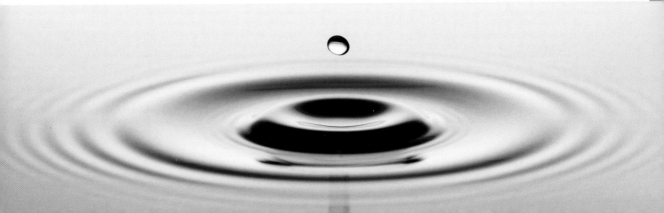

Bodywork and Suppressed Emotions

The biopsychotype is a helpful concept for understanding the mind-body connection. Physical problems are often associated with emotional issues, and vice versa. A legitimate but uncommon concern for massage therapists, yoga instructors, and other therapists who touch their clients is that a patient may sometimes become very uncomfortable or upset during the session. An example is a woman who starts suddenly sobbing uncontrollably when her thighs are massaged. The action of the massage therapist has possibly triggered a forgotten or suppressed memory of being sexually molested as a child. Similarly, physical pain may be related to traumatic events, such as a car accident or seeing a pet run over by a truck. Some bodywork therapies allow the patient to release hidden emotional issues and then process them in a safe way. Therapies combining touch and talk include Rubenfeld Synergy, the Rosen Method, and the Trager Approach.

Biochemical and Hormone Analysis

Biochemical factors and unbalanced hormones can affect pain, fatigue, and depression.

Hormonal problems in general can result in pain. Hyperparathyroidism can cause severe muscle pain. Hypothyroidism may also result in fatigue.

Vitamin D deficiency can lead to diffuse pain. Thiamine (vitamin B1) and vitamin B12 deficiencies can both cause nervous system problems such as tingling. Generalized inflammation can aggravate chronic pain. This list is extensive. That is where our Ring 2, 3, and 4 diagnoses are invaluable.

Energy Healing

Energy healing refers to a group of therapies such as healing touch, therapeutic touch, and Reiki. Energy healers train to increase their perception of the aura, or subtle physical energy of the body. They are taught to sense imbalances in the body and then correct them on a bioenergetic level. In our experience, the ability to do this can vary greatly. However, in a study we did at our center, we found that trained energy healers were able to perceive patients' areas of pain without even asking them where the pain was. One such person is Rosalyn Bruyere, who is well known for her abilities in this area. In our study, we recruited patients who had reported back pain and had recently had an MRI. We asked the patients to draw their pain on an anatomical chart. Rosalyn and another observer drew their perceptions of the patients' pain on a similar anatomical chart, without any input from the patient. We compared both of these charts to the results of a third chart, an MRI-generated image which showed a typical nerve-generated pain pathway. The observers' drawings resembled the subjects' drawings more closely than the MRI-generated images. In other words, they were able to perceive where the patient felt pain much as the patient did.

How the Mind Affects the Body

We often come across patients who give us some metaphorical clue to what is going on in their minds and in their lives. Their thoughts are a window to the subconscious. A patient with heartburn may confide that he "can't stomach" a certain situation. People with neck pain may tell us about the "pain in the neck" in their life. Patients with back pain may fear their support system is crumbling and may talk about feeling forced to "back down." Very subtly, they are giving us insight into the interrelationship between their mind and their body.

This idea was long dismissed by scientists. However, a very real syndrome that mirrors this is called the broken heart syndrome or Takotsubo cardiomyopathy, originally described by Japanese cardiologists in 1991. In this syndrome the heart enlarges shortly after a stressful situation, such as the death of a loved one. Patients feel sudden chest pain, often thinking they are suffering a heart attack. Fortunately—though frightening—the syndrome only rarely does any permanent heart damage or causes death.

There are many links between mind and body. One of the major connections is the interaction between neurotransmitters, stress hormones, and the pain generators that exist in our bodies.

Every time we have a thought or an emotion, our nervous system is flooded with neurotransmitters. Some, like serotonin and GABA, produce a sense of calm and well-being. Others can cause anxiety, fear, or anger. When we have the same repetitive negative thoughts or feelings, we bathe our bodies in stress hormones, depleting neurotransmitters such as serotonin. Since one of serotonin's jobs is to switch off pain, a patient depleted of serotonin will end up in the pain–depression–pain cycle.

Sometimes adding an antidepressant medication is all that is needed to break the cycle. For other patients, the addition of an antiseizure medication such as gabapentin (Neurontin®), pregabalin (Lyrica®), valproic acid (Depakote®), carbemazepine (Tegretol®), or topiramate (Topamax®) will help to calm down the nervous system and relieve pain. The pain fibers of people with chronic pain are switched on all the time. These medications help to soothe them and relieve the pain. Yet there are other times when even the best medication does not seem to help.

In these cases, we need to do more. This is where we find that looking at other systems can help. For example, rebalancing the adrenals or reducing inflammation might be what is needed to help improve a patient's mood and pain.

Previous Trauma and Pain

Imagine someone who has lived through a highly traumatic situation such as a rape, an accident, a disaster, or a war experience. Often, these people suffer from post-traumatic stress disorder (PTSD), an anxiety disorder that is triggered by experiencing an event that causes intense fear, helplessness, or horror. Every time something happens that reminds the victim of the original experience, the body is triggered into a highly reactive state—a flashback—that recreates the neurochemicals and the emotions associated with the original event. Emotionally, the person feels as if the traumatic event were occurring all over again. For example, someone who was traumatized by war may find that any loud noise can set in motion a biochemical and emotional cascade—a stress response in which the nightmare of the original war trauma will be replayed. Although not everyone who has

Energy in the Eastern Traditions

In every traditional healing system, working on the bioenergetic system of the body is integral to treatment. In China, the energy is referred to as qi or chi, in Japan it is called ki, and in India it is referred to as prana. In fact, almost every traditional culture has a word for the body's bioenergetic system. It denotes a physical vitality—a force that underlies and supports health. Each system differs slightly in how it achieves this. Acupuncture masters insert acupuncture needles to improve the level and flow of this energy in the body, while others suggest tai chi, chi gong (qigong), or acupressure. The Ayurvedic physicians of India suggest yoga. Practitioners of martial art cultivate their chi in order to become stronger, move better, and remain healthier.

Does this concept have a place in contemporary medicine?

We have a great deal of electrical activity in our bodies, much of which can be measured. An electrocardiogram (EKG) captures the electrical activity as it moves through the heart. An electroencephalogram (EEG) reads electrical brain wave activity, while an electromyogram (EMG) measures electrical impulses as they move along nerves. Magnetic resonance imaging (MRI) uses a magnet that creates a spin in our electrons, which is then translated into beautiful images of the inside of the body. On the other hand, the electrical activity in a cell wall or that occurs each time a nerve fires still cannot be measured. Measureable or not, any electrical impulse in the body creates an electromagnetic field—and every living object is surrounded by an electromagnetic field.

Today, no one would refuse to turn on the radio just because they cannot observe radio waves, and no one would stop using the microwave oven because they cannot perceive microwaves. After a century of breakthroughs in modern physics, we take these principles of electromagnetism for granted, even though we cannot see them and do not even really understand how they work. Is it possible that we just haven't yet developed a technology sophisticated enough to properly assess the bioenergetic systems described in Ayurvedic and traditional Chinese medicine?

Bioenergetic distortions in traditional healing systems reflect physical, emotional, and spiritual imbalances. In other words, the electromagnetic field seems to be an interface between physiology, psychology, and spirituality. In India, yogic theory suggests that this power is concentrated or stored at nerve nodules along the spine, described as chakras. The chakras serve as power grids, sending energy out to the extremities where smaller transducers around the joints, called nadis, then help transfer bioenergy to the tissues. If traditional Indian philosophy refers to the power grids of bioenergy or chakras, traditional Oriental medicine has been more concerned with the flow of energy between them. These are the meridian systems, which act as power lines, or the network on which the software of the body runs. The sum total of the bioenergetic field that exists in and around the body is thus called prana or chi (qi).This subtle physical energy is also referred to as the aura of the body.

experienced a horrific event suffers from PTSD, most of us have suffered events involving emotional trauma or even abuse. High-intensity pain or emotion, sexual abuse, or a change in consciousness due to trauma or even anesthetic, can be indelibly engraved into our minds.

Previous stress can trigger a state of chronic hypervigilance, with resultant anxiety, mood swings, and depression. This state of stress can lead to the domino effect of emotional trauma: inflammation, exhaustion, and depression. For someone who has lived through trauma or intense stress, sometimes even a minor event can easily topple them into a chronic pain condition.

A skilled mind-body therapist can play an important role in helping patients who are struggling to cope with their pain and also grapple with post-traumatic stress. Diagnosing mind-body problems is not always easy. Some disorders are obvious, such as mental suffering that clearly begins after an emotional trauma, while others are not. Emotional trauma should always be considered for unexplained cases of pain. Meditative practices can be extremely beneficial in making us less reactive to old traumas.

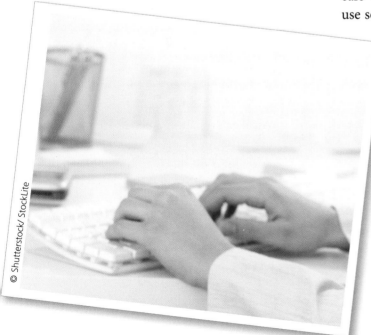

© Shutterstock/ StockLite

Lifestyle Analysis: Finding the Causes and the Solutions

To treat pain disorders properly, we need to know if the patient has counterproductive lifestyle habits that can reactivate the pain. Sometimes the causes are obvious, but in other cases, they are elusive. The solution is for the patient to have a good observer and coach, and also to become more self-aware. We look carefully at habits and activities that can affect body mechanics.

Habits that Affect Body Mechanics

Repetitive motion. The same movement repeated over and over again can cause an injury. Knitting, typing, hammering, digging, or even texting on a phone can be culprits here.

Posture. Are you slumping forward, slouching, or hunching your shoulders? Do you hold the telephone between your neck and your shoulder? What is your posture like when you sit at a desk? Are your shoulders close to your ears when you're on the computer? Do you use some kind of ergonomic rest pad for your wrists? All of these are factors can affect the physical stress you place on your body.

Clothing or accessories that affect the body. Are you sitting on a fat wallet that's in your back pocket? This can irritate your sciatic nerve. Knee-high socks can pinch the peroneal nerve, causing leg pain. Heavy purses, bags, and backpacks can cause neck, shoulder, and back pain. Pay attention to your areas of discomfort and see if any of these factors are irritating your discomfort.

Under- or over-exercising. Both of these lifestyles can cause problems. Too little exercise leads to under-conditioning. Too much exercise leads to overuse and repetitive stress injuries.

Lack of stretching or lack of strengthening. Both can affect the balance and tensegrity of the body, leading to a tendency to easy injury.

Sleep position and sleep deficiency. People who sleep lying on their stomachs with their neck twisted to the side place a significant amount of stress on the neck. In addition, sleep deficiency can lead to poor recovery from pain.

Habits that Affect Recovery

Smoking. Decades of research have shown that smoking leads to constriction of arteries and blood flow and, as a result, to poor healing. Smokers who have back surgery do much worse than nonsmokers. Similarly, smokers take longer to recover from injuries in general.

Alcohol or substance abuse. While one to two drinks a day seems to be beneficial to most people, alcohol abuse results in problems throughout the body. In addition to causing bodily damage, alcohol abuse can cause depression, leading to more pain. Street drugs can aggravate pain conditions in myriad ways.

Excess caffeine or overuse of other stimulants. Stimulant use can be associated with poor sleep and an adrenalized "wired and tired" state, leading to the need for more stimulants.

Stress excess and stress addiction. Ever notice how some people are drawn to drama? We all have a tendency to be sucked into drama, whether we are watching it in the movies or on the evening news—or feel as if we are involved in our own personal reality show. In our 24/7 world, we need to learn to switch off at times. The drama will always continue. We do not need to remain attached to it!

Negative self-talk. Every time you find yourself doing this, make a live well, and stay well conscious decision to get well, be well, live well and stay well!

Nutritional deficiency. Poor diet can lead to a lack of the nutrients necessary to repair our ligaments, tendons, muscles, and organs. For ideas on how to nourish your body, see Ring 3.

And lots more . . . . There are many other habits that can influence your recovery. Pay attention to what is going on in your life and see how it is affecting you!

Step 8.

An Integrative Diagnosis and a Transformational Treatment Plan

> Getting sick is a process.
> Getting well is a process too.

In a stepwise fashion, we just took a brief look at how chronic pain develops. The next step is to apply a systems approach to help the patient get better.

Here are some of the most important elements to focus on as you consider this:

- Your body is your biography—it can give you and us insight into many of the conditions you are suffering from.

- A physical examination and palpation of the body can give us an idea of your genetic makeup, your lifestyle, your hormonal balance, and your previous injuries. It can show us structural changes, as well as clues to underlying emotional states. We can then use this information to figure out impending problems. From there, you can take steps to avoid future illness.

- Draw on the knowledge of several disciplines. Learn to access information from different diagnostic and healing modalities. They need to make sense to you. They need to be safe and effective.

- Access new tools for diagnosis. As you explore this stepwise approach to diagnosis, you will gain access to the tools you need to resolve your health issues. This multidimensional understanding will give you the insight and tools to enable you to play a greater role in your own healing.

- Tap the resources of a health care team. In addition to medical diagnostics, an integrative team typically includes resources for evaluating biomechanical issues, nutritional problems, psychological concerns, and more. Working with more than one provider expands your treatment options and can have a synergistic effect on healing.

- Remain open to a range of reasonable solutions. There is no one way to achieve health and healing. You will need to assess safety, cost, and benefit before you decide what to do.

- Envision yourself as already well. The body is a homeostatic organism—that is, it tends toward balance. In order to allow it to heal, we need to tip the balance to favor factors that promote healing. As you read on, you will learn how to create a plan that will enable you to do this.

- Remember, we don't just want your problem to go away. We want you to use the problem to help you make your health and your life better. This for us is Transformational Medicine—the same treatment that treats a problem also prevents future problems before they happen!

Alex Learns to Understand His Pain (and His Body) as He Pursues His Quest for Wellness

Alex continues to pursue Health and Wellness

Alex had an aching back and knee pain. We investigated this with an MRI of his back, which revealed a mild disc bulge at L5/S1. His knees were normal. As we evaluated Alex, it became more clear to him and to us that he really had two separate issues. His back pain was being aggravated by a badly designed high-intensity exercise program: one night, unable to sleep, Alex had watched an infomercial showing young men and women marveling how they had shed pounds of fat and gained inches of muscle by following this program. Alas, Alex was soon to learn that his body did not respond the same way. The abdominal exercises he was doing were aggravating the pain from the bulging disc in his back. His aching knees, however, corresponded to his level of stress.

His IL-6 SNPs were causing a release of inflammatory chemicals that were making his pain worse.

As we worked with Alex from an acupuncture diagnosis perspective, he came to realize he was a nurture-duty biopsychotype—as shown by his knee pain, insulin resistance, irritable bowel problems, and allergies. As a classic nurturer, he was deeply offended by his boss's bullying antics. Alex tended to suppress his anger when he was stressed, often aggravating his pain. He began to see how his body was a barometer for both the physical and emotional stresses he was undergoing. What he wanted though was a way to control the pain and discomfort.

5

Healing Your Body

When, Where, and How to Use Conventional Medicine and Integrative Therapies to Both Optimize Health and Reduce Pain or Discomfort

Pain is that initial awareness that we need to choose another path. Chronic pain is often the impetus to help us make changes. The big question is: which changes? What will it take to make the pain go away? Obviously, if you already knew what you should be doing, you would have been doing it. Pain is the impetus to seek help.

That is why patients with chronic pain come to us. Patients want a quick fix. But, as we always say, getting better is a process. As health care providers, we want to partner with you. We want to find out what the best options are for you. We want to find out what we (or others) can do for you and what you can do for yourself.

The good thing about today's information age is that all of us can quickly learn about the various treatments that are available. On the other hand, claims sometimes abound with little validating evidence. That is why you need to be a key player on your own health care team. You will want to consider outcomes, safety and cost, and then decide what you want to do.

Heal Your Body

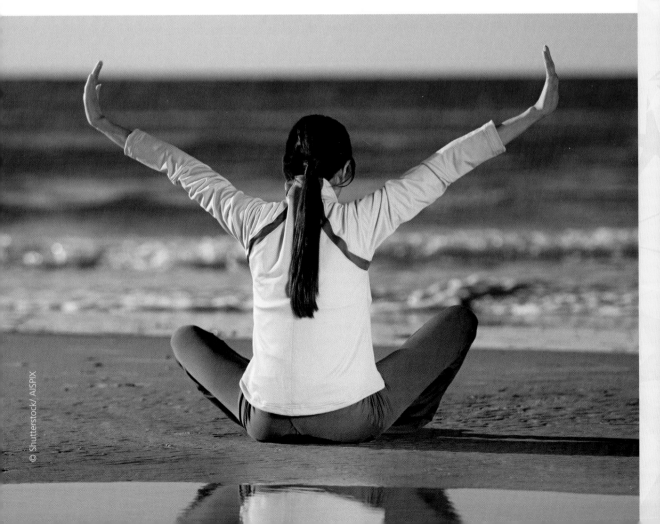

Your Transformational Treatment Plan

As you embark on your transformational treatment plan, remember that chronic pain doesn't just suddenly disappear. Typically, you will pass through several healing stages on the way to recovery.

Stage 1: Relief and Repair

In stage 1, people with chronic pain usually need consistent, relatively frequent care. At this point, if you are in enough pain, you may need rest to let your body heal. Your treatments will be starting to give you relief, but the process takes time, and you still need to take it easy. Depending on the type, cost, and availability of the treatment modalities you have chosen, you may need to be seen by one or more practitioners one or more times each week.

In general, we like our patients to have about 40 to 50 percent pain relief within four to five treatments. Range of motion should begin improving, and inflammation should start to subside. We create what we call a trajectory of improvement. Rapid improvement is usually an encouraging sign, while slower improvement signifies that your condition may be more involved than anticipated.

Most patients take longer to get better than they expect. Occasionally, someone needs up to ten treatments before we see any improvement. It's important to be open. If one type of therapy isn't helping, a different one may.

Stage 2: Restoration and Regeneration

In this second stage, your body has started to heal, and you can start to restore normal function and resume your usual daily activities. We want to return you to your previous, pain-free status. The aim here is to restore balance to the body's mechanics, with the emphasis on bringing you as close to a normal anatomical model as possible. By this second stage, you should be feeling better. Both you and your provider should get a sense that your body is healing. When you get to this point, your soft tissue begins to feel more compliant and responsive. Muscles become stronger, and ligaments feel more elasticized. Similarly, the joints and extremities regain smooth movement and function. Your body's tensegrity is starting to return to normal, without extra strains and stresses throwing it out of balance.

Stage 3. Realignment and Revitalization

In this stage, you're feeling good again. For you to keep feeling that way, it's important to remember that optimum health is a dynamic process. Ongoing maintenance is required to keep the body functioning well.

We have learned this through years of experience with our patients. When patients recovered from an injury and were pain-free, we would simply say, "Come and see us when you need us." When they did come back, they would be in severe pain again, and we would have to start over in stage 1 of treatment. We realized that if patients saw us regularly, we would notice little cues that indicated a problem was developing. In some cases, a segment of the spine would be a little stiff. In others, the person might not be able to rotate the neck as well. Many patients would have niggling aches and pains that meant they were likely to have an injury soon.

Now we take a proactive approach to prevention. By working with manipulative therapies, acupuncture, energy healing, massage and bodywork therapies, we are able to support health in several areas simultaneously: relieving current symptoms, preventing future problems, and working on healing past problems.

How Do You Know a Therapy Is Working?

With hands-on therapies such as massage or acupuncture, the benefit is often a direct reflection of the skill of the practitioner. A treatment with a good practitioner can be profoundly different than the same treatment provided by someone who is not as skilled. How do you know? The simple answer is, you should feel better. However, keep in mind that it is not uncommon for aches and pains to get a little worse after a treatment. This should be temporary (just a day or so) and should never be severe.

When you have a profoundly relaxing treatment that places you in a state of deep rest, your body will be able to do what it needs to do in order to heal. After a treatment, you may find yourself needing to sleep. This effect usually carries over—you will probably find that you sleep deeply that night and possibly for days afterward. Your body needs that deep rest to heal. We always tell our patients not to fight the effect with caffeine or other stimulants.

Finding a Good Health Care Provider

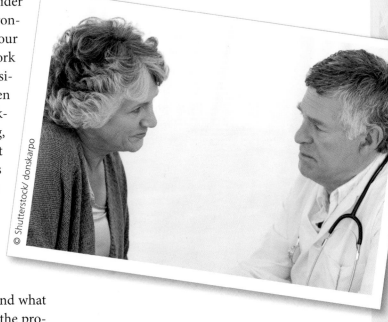

© Shutterstock/ donskarpo

To find a good health care provider with experience in treating chronic pain, start by looking in your area. You will need to do a little homework here. Ask for referrals from your physicians and from friends who have been seen by the type of provider you are seeking. Look initially for training, licensing, and certification. The U.S. Department of Health and Human Services provides a directory of health organizations that can be a great resource for finding a helpful professional organization (www.dirline.nlm.nih.gov). The next step is to look for skill. You need to find out how many people the provider sees with your kind of problem and what others' results have been. Finally, does the provider listen and respond to your concerns, adjusting treatment as necessary?

Effective Pain Therapies

Chronic pain can almost always be helped—it is usually just a matter of finding the right therapy or combination of therapies that is best for you. We always suggest starting with conventional medicine. Your primary care doctor or a specialist such as an orthopedist, physical medicine and rehabilitation physician, sports medicine doctor, neurologist, or neurosurgeon will usually have several good options for treating you.

If you have a severely arthritic hip joint, integrative therapies may help to relieve the pain for a time, but there will come a point when hip replacement surgery is the best option. If you have a large herniated disc causing pain or weakness in your arms or legs, then surgery is a good option. However, if you have spinal stenosis or several small herniated discs with chronic pain, surgery may not be the most effective treatment. Sometimes getting a second opinion can be extremely helpful.

Using a team approach to these issues from the perspective of several disciplines, we are able to provide earlier resolution of pain and deeper, more effective, and more permanent healing. Ultimately, we are looking for a synergy of treatments to put the patient back in balance so healing can happen. The core idea is to restore function to the body's structure as much as possible so the patient can then return to a dynamic physical balance.

Therapies for Well-being

It is important to realize that the therapies we offer are not just to treat pain. Our ultimate goal is to ensure that the patient feels comfortable in his or her own body. We like to see dynamic balance in the body, so whenever possible, we try to recreate the kind of fluid movement that one might see in a world-class athlete. This is a sense of equipoise—a balance between contraction and relaxation—that transcends the purely physical.

Manipulative Therapies

Manipulative therapy can be performed by chiropractors, osteopaths, and physical therapists. Manipulative therapies are effective for acute and chronic low back pain, neck pain, spinal stenosis, headaches, shoulder pain, hip and knee osteoarthritis, and vertigo. They work well with sports injuries, ankle sprains, and have even been shown to work with certain non-musculoskeletal disorders.

Adjusting the Spine

In chiropractic thinking, spine problems radiate throughout the body by affecting the entire nervous system; adjusting the spine can help relieve pain and other symptoms. The value and safety of chiroprac-

© Shutterstock/ Rainer Plendl

© Shutterstock/JKO

tic is documented in more than five thousand peer-reviewed articles in the National Library of Medicine database. This therapy has been evaluated in at least 350 clinical trials to date, showing both efficacy and cost-effectiveness in the majority of studies, particularly for treating low back pain.

A spinal adjustment can be performed in several different ways, but it is usually done by a quick, deft thrust or high-velocity manipulation. During a high-velocity spinal adjustment, you may hear a cracking or popping noise. This is normal and safe. Research has shown that small pockets of air or bubbles are found in the fluid surrounding a joint capsule. When the joint tissues are stretched during an adjustment, the pockets "pop," creating this cracking sound. The adjustment appears to increase the amount of joint fluid, which improves range of motion and the ease of movement of surrounding tissue and decreases pain. People who are concerned this technique may cause further injury may prefer a low-velocity adjustment, such as the counterstrain technique. In this technique, the patient is simply held in a specific position for one to two minutes. A physical therapist may achieve results similar to manipulation using a technique called mobilization, where parts of the spine are gently moved up and down to help improve range of motion and function.

The most common side effect of manipulative therapy is temporary soreness of the surrounding muscles. Occasionally, a patient may have a flare-up following a treatment. In this case, symptoms appear to be worse for a few days. In our experience, this can actually be a good sign and often heralds a movement toward healing. Manipulative therapy can have side effects, although they are rare. It is possible, though very unlikely, that manipulative therapy could cause stroke, disc herniation, or fractures of vertebrae and ribs.

Massage, Trigger Point Therapy, and Bodywork

There are literally hundreds of forms of massage and bodywork, including deep tissue massage, medical massage, myofascial release, postural integration, Rolfing, shiatsu, Swedish massage, Thai massage, Trager Approach, trigger point therapy, and watsu.

Massage and bodywork can be very helpful for relieving chronic pain. In the peer-reviewed medical literature, there are close to ten thousand journal articles on massage, including over nine hundred clinical trials.

Touch is a basic aspect of human experience that can have a profound impact on health. Studies done by Dr. Tiffany Field on premature babies showed that those who received massage gained weight much more quickly than those who were not massaged. Studies of massage for patients with back pain show they have less pain, depression, and anxiety, as well as im-

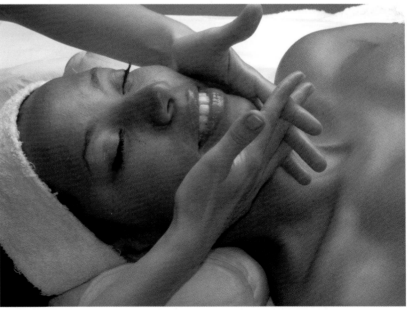

Treating Atypical Chest Pain

We often see patients with unexplained chest pain. Many of them have been worked up for cardiac conditions and treated with antacid medications for presumed gastric reflux with no benefit.

Many times we find that one of their ribs is slightly misaligned. Unfortunately, this misalignment is so slight that it will not show up on an x-ray. The resulting pain can occur where the rib attaches at the back to the spine, or in front where the rib attaches to the sternum or breast bone, or it can radiate around the entire chest wall. Frequently this condition is called costochondral pain, but may be misdiagnosed as everything from pleurisy to heart disease. (This type of pain may also be caused by a herniated disc in the tho-racic spine or even an irritated nerve in this area, commonly caused by shingles).

Fortunately, if these symptoms are due to rib misalignment, they respond quickly to a combination of manipulative therapies and acupuncture. Following the initial "pop" of the chiropractic adjustment, the patient will often take a deep breath and remark how the pain has disappeared. Acupuncture helps allay the associated muscle spasm and allows the rib head to remain in place, ensuring prolonged healing. In our experience most patients with this condition are better within two to three weeks. The rate of relapse is extremely low once the problem is actually resolved.

proved serotonin and dopamine levels. Other studies have reported that massage helps normalize cortisol levels in patients with fibromyalgia, depression, and post-traumatic stress disorder. Patients with cerebral palsy and Down syndrome receiving massage have shown enhanced flexibility and muscle tone. Massage research has also documented reduced pain in cases of carpal tunnel syndrome and juvenile rheumatoid arthritis and improved range of motion and strength in patients with spinal cord injuries. The healing benefits of touch have also been shown to boost general immune function and promote sleep. Massage has also been shown to improve our general sense of well-being.

Massage therapy is one of the safest and oldest forms of all the healing therapies. In hiring bodyworkers for our practice, we look for therapists who have both an innate sense of the body and a natural, intuitive gift of touch, as well as excellent clinical results.

Acupuncture

Acupuncture involves inserting very fine needles, only a little thicker than a human hair, at specific points, or *acupoints,* on the skin surface, following traditional acupuncture meridians. Typically, the patient feels nothing or feels only a slight pinch as the needles are inserted. During the session, patients usually feel very relaxed, and it is not uncommon for them to fall into a deep, comfortable sleep. They typically awaken feeling refreshed and rested, with a greater sense of well-being.

We strongly recommend working with a well-trained and experienced acupuncturist with good credentials. Results can vary among practitioners. There are many different styles, techniques, and backgrounds. If you find that acupuncture isn't helping, it is possible that treatment by a different practitioner could be more beneficial.

Both acute and chronic pain, ranging from acute injuries and sprains to chronic neck and

Live well. Eat well. Run well. Love well. Dance well. Get wel low back pain, often respond well to acupuncture. Arthritis, bursitis, fibromyalgia, frozen shoulder, and tennis elbow are just some of the pain conditions that can benefit from acupuncture. Post-surgical pain can be alleviated.

Acupuncture is sometimes thought of as a technique to treat only pain and musculoskeletal problems. This is not true. It is effective for a variety of problems, some of which include:

- Neurological disorders: strokes, migraine headaches, tension headaches, chronic daily headaches, Meniere's disease, neuralgias and neuropathies including trigeminal neuralgia, carpal tunnel syndrome, post-herpetic neuralgia (shingles), and Bell's palsy.

- Infections, allergies, and respiratory problems.

- Immune support. Studies show that acupuncture can improve the function of T cells in the immune system, which helps fight infection and inflammation.

- Stress, anxiety, depression, and insomnia.

- Adjunct treatment for drug addiction and smoking cessation.

- Chronic fatigue.

- Sexual health and prostate problems.

- Infertility.

- Menopausal symptoms, menstrual problems, and PMS.

- Nausea due to morning sickness, chemotherapy, and anesthesia.

- Interstitial cystitis.

- GI disorders such as GERD, irritable bowel syndrome and constipation.

Done well, acupuncture should treat current issues, help heal previous problems, while simultaneously preventing new ones. It will often leave a patient with a profound sense of well being. This is why we use it as a tool for Transformational Medicine.

Acupuncture in Our Practice

Over the past decade and more, our physicians have averaged over ten thousand acupuncture treatments per year. In doing so, we have amassed significant experience with regard to acupuncture. We have also met with, worked with, and observed acupuncture masters all over the world. As members of the American Academy of Medical Acupuncture, we have remained open to different professional perspectives on this approach to illness. We have seen seemingly miraculous turnarounds in situations ranging from asthma and allergies to strokes and pain.

However, in general, acupuncture really shines when used early on in an illness, or with what we call functional illness. Good examples include myofascial pain, migraine, and irritable bowel syndrome. What's more, acupuncture has almost no side effects.

Acupuncture excels in its ability to predict how certain people are predisposed to certain problems based on their biopsychotypes (check back to Ring 5 for the different biopsychotypes). Using this approach, we are able to individualize treatments to address several current problems simultaneously, while also addressing

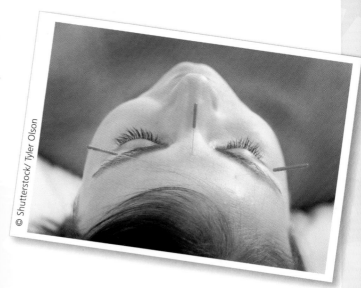

© Shutterstock/ Tyler Olson

older issues and preventing future problems. In this way, we can treat, for example, allergies, heartburn, and knee pain simultaneously. The same treatment will also boost the immune system and make the patient feel better and be more resistant to illness.

How Does Acupuncture Work?

We are often asked by skeptical patients, "How does acupuncture work?" The ancient Chinese theory of energy *(qi* or *chi)* flowing through meridians is one way to explain it, but we believe there is a more scientific answer based on modern medical knowledge.

Here is a glimpse of what we now know, based on more than 450 research studies.

- Acupuncture has been found to reduce pain signals as they travel to and from the brain and to modulate the signals in the brain.

- Functional MRI (fMRI) studies of blood flow in the brain show that when major acupuncture points such as those on the hand are stimulated, blood flow is improved in the brain. The influence of acupuncture on cerebral circulation helps explain why acupuncture relieves chronic pain.

- Acupuncture promotes the release of endorphins (pain-relieving chemicals) in both the brain and the spine.

- Acupuncture calms the sympathetic nervous system and improves activity in the parasympathetic nervous system. By balancing the autonomic nervous system, acupuncture helps switch the body out of the stress response into the relaxation response, a mode of healing.

- Placing a needle in a muscle in chronic spasm causes the muscle to relax and stops the pain almost at once.

- Research by Dr. Helene Longevin has shown that the fascial network, or as we call it, "the Internet of the body," is one of the ways in which different areas of the body

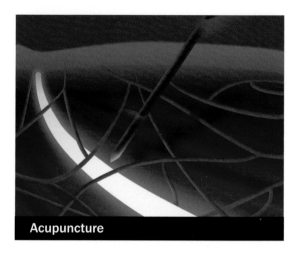

Acupuncture

communicate. Most major acupuncture meridians are now believed to run along planes of the fascia, the white sinewy material that surrounds and separates muscle groups and organs. Acupuncture seems to enhance this communication network, reprogramming the body's software.

- Many important acupuncture points turn out to overlie major nerves. Stimulating these points sends a message into the nervous system, telling it to behave differently.

- Acupuncture has been shown to alter gene expression. In other words, acupuncture can regulate the activity of your genes.

- Acupuncture creates a tiny injury at the site of the needle insertion. The body responds by sending healing chemicals to that area. Local release of chemicals (such as adenosine, bradykinin, histamine, and others) at the site of needle insertion appear to be involved in the healing process. Often the skin will turn red at this site, indicating that a healing process is occurring.

- Studies using functional MRIs (fMRIs) show that the same acupuncture point can have different effects on the same patient at different times. This helps to explain why an acupuncturist's ability to find the correct acupoint is so important, and also why acupuncture is difficult to research.

Risks of Acupuncture

In general, the risks of acupuncture are minimal. Infection from needles is very rare because disposable, single-use sterilized needles are the standard in treatment. The most common problem is occasional bruising or redness at the needle insertion points. As with other manual therapies, a flare-up of pain may occasionally occur after treatment. Very rarely, patients experience lightheadedness and sweatiness, especially during the first treatment. This is usually not a problem and goes away as soon as the needles are removed. An extremely rare complication is a puncture of an underlying organ such as the lung. However, extensive reviews conducted in the United Kingdom, Sweden, and Japan of records on more than 140,000 treatments found not one major adverse event.

Supplemental Therapies

Additional therapies for pain include mechanical and electrical units that can be used on their own or as a supplement to other therapies. These include TENS units (transcutaneous electrical nerve stimulation), interferential and horizontal microcurrent, low-level laser acupuncture, ultrasound, and frequency specific microcurrent (FSM).

In general, these therapies are nontoxic, noninvasive, and safe. They have minimal side effects, but their effectiveness varies. Depending on the type of therapy, they can improve blood flow and speed localized healing, reduce muscle spasms, prevent blood clots, train muscles to increase strength, prevent tissue and muscle degeneration, and stimulate peripheral nerves to help reduce pain or improve function.

Once again, work with a practitioner who is properly trained in the particular modality you are receiving. While these modalities are generally safe, be sure you are getting the results you have been promised.

Frequency specific microcurrent (FSM) utilizes a subsensory microcurrent (meaning you can't feel it) that is applied via graphite gloves or even directly through acupuncture needles. Dr. Carolyn McMakin, a well-known chiropractor and sports therapist, popularized this treatment modality when working with football players Bill Romanowski and Terrell Owens. The treatment can help reduce inflammation and heal injuries faster.

Serving a Healing Ace

Several years ago, we received a call from the distraught coach of a top professional tennis player, John Isner, who was playing in a tournament in Cincinnati. John had fallen and injured his ankle. An MRI showed three torn ligaments and a bruised ankle bone. Typical recovery for this type of injury is three to six months. We saw him immediately and treated him with acupuncture, gentle manipulation of his ankle, energy healing, and hours of FSM. Because John responded so well, he decided to purchase an FSM home unit, which he used diligently every day. A week later, his excited coach e-mailed us to say that his follow-up MRI was almost completely normal. Twelve days later, he played in the U.S. Open in New York!

Energy Healing Techniques

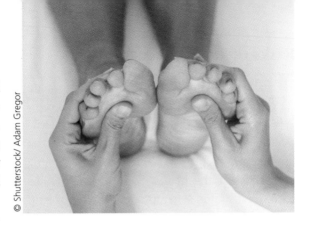

When provided by an experienced practitioner, energy healing induces a state of deep relaxation. These techniques, include craniosacral therapy, energy Healing Touch and Reiki. They appear to enhance and complement the body's natural healing mechanisms.

Therapists trained in these skills include osteopaths, who frequently receive instruction in craniosacral therapy, and nurses who have been trained in healing touch. There is currently no regulation or licensing of these therapies. Practitioners have a wide range of skill levels and natural talent.

Patients receiving energy healing often find that they melt into a state of well-being in which pain and anxiety are quickly relieved. These therapies also seem to boost the immune system and have myriad other benefits. More than three hundred studies have been conducted on Healing Touch and three hundred on Reiki. However, good studies are lacking on energy medicine in general and on craniosacral therapy.

In our experience, energy healing techniques are helpful in dealing with acute and chronic pain. Numerous conditions frequently associated with pain, such as connective tissue disorders and autoimmune conditions, and

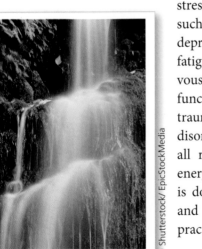

stress-related issues such as anxiety and depression, chronic fatigue, central nervous system dysfunction, and post-traumatic stress disorder (PTSD) can all respond well to energy healing—if it is done by a skilled and experienced practitioner.

An ACE Healing Treatment^{SM}

When we first started working with various complementary therapies at the Alliance Institute, we found that we got excellent results when we combined Acupuncture, Chiropractic, and Energy Healing. The treatments seem to be highly synergistic—they are more effective together than they are alone. In our experience, when a healing partnership is established and integrative therapies are used together, the cumulative effect can far exceed the benefit of any one of these therapies on its own.

We have fine-tuned that collaborative model into what we call an ACE Healing Treatment. In this treatment, patients are first seen by a chiropractor for a structural assessment and manipulative therapy. Chiropractic treatment is followed by acupuncture and then energy healing to further enhance the treatment.

These sessions can also include a tailored combination of deep stretches and trigger point massages, individualized to each patient's needs. The neurochemical benefits that occur during the chiropractic treatment are then augmented in the acupuncture treatment that follows.

During the acupuncture treatment, the patient is evaluated again. By listening to the patient's symptoms, hearing how he or she responded to the previous treatment, understanding the biopsychotype, and examining the patient carefully, our acupuncturists are able to quickly identify the correct treatment.

Finally, an energy healer treats the patient,

Barbara's Story

Barbara was 65 years old when she tripped and fell on a toy her grandchild had left lying around. As she fell backward, she grabbed for the stairway banister, only to hear a popping noise, followed by a searing pain in her shoulder. A trip to the emergency room followed. X-rays were negative, but the ER physician thought she had torn one of her rotator cuff tendons. An MRI the following day confirmed this. After meeting with an orthopedic surgeon, Barbara decided the best thing to do was to have her shoulder repaired surgically as soon as possible.

The surgery went well. As expected, she had significant pain afterward. For two weeks afterward, she could sleep only sitting upright on the couch, with her arm in a sling. She started physical therapy and rehabilitation exercises. Although the surgery was successful and Barbara followed a good rehab program, her shoulder was much stiffer than the therapist would have liked. In fact, it began to suddenly get worse. Her pain began to increase, and then

her shoulder range of motion got progressively worse. A trip back to the orthopedic surgeon established the diagnosis. She had a frozen shoulder, or what is medically known as an adhesive capsulitis. Physical therapy became unbearably painful, and cortisone injections didn't help. That's when she came to us.

Barbara responded well to the therapies we offered. Initial acupuncture and FSM treatment quickly calmed her pain. She had developed significant muscle spasm and myofascial pain in her neck and shoulders, which quieted with acupuncture and massage. Finally, ACE Healing Treatment[SM] helped mobilize her shoulder and treat her capsulitis and her pain. As she said when she finished her first treatment, "Why couldn't my orthopedic surgeon have included these therapies in my treatment regimen? They made the healing process go so much faster!" Our hope is that one day such a combination will be both commonplace and reimbursed by insurance.

---

placing his or her hands lightly on the body. Patients often feel a sense of warmth or energy from this treatment. Our energy healers are able to use the final part of the ACE Healing Treatment to deepen the patient's relaxation and the effect of the treatment. Patients often experience a profound sense of relief and rest during this phase.

As we explain to patients: Imagine your body as a water pipe. Chiropractic fixes the kinks. Acupuncture directs and pressurizes the water. Energy is the water!

Many patients come to our center as a last resort for pain relief, after having tried multiple medications and surgery. In a survey of four hundred patients, 79 percent reported that their medical condition improved, and 87 percent re-

ported that they would recommend this treatment to others.

Your Role in Your Treatment

We encourage our patients to come in for their appointments rested and hydrated. It is important to note that patients do not have to believe in these treatments for them to work. Ideally though, if you are having a treatment, you are in a state of physical and mental receptivity. This is different than lying there passively while treatment is done to you. Rather, it is a matter of relaxing, while being attuned to how your body is feeling at that moment. We like to call this "a state of willing openness." In this state of receptivity,

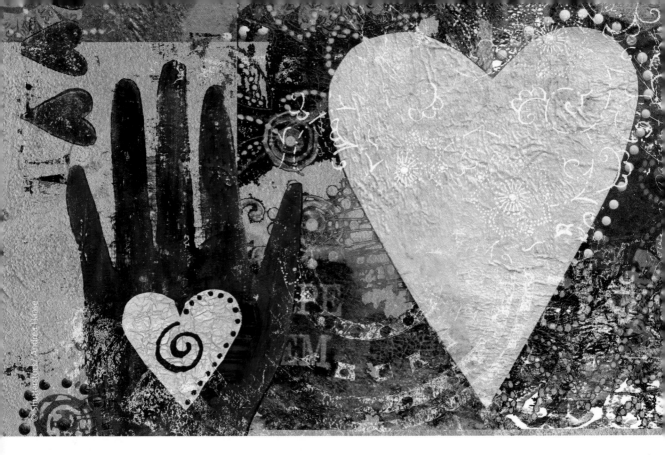

you have a heightened awareness of what is happening within and without your body and in your environment. Often, patients experience a sense of balance and equanimity. In this restfully alert state, you begin to appreciate the healing process and are better able to assist it. This heightened awareness will also give you greater control over your healing and vitality—helping you become yourself, once again.

After a treatment, we advise patients to drink plenty of water and get plenty of rest. The body seems to want to balance itself after a treatment. If, for instance, you have been in a sleep-deprived state, you may want to sleep. If you have been feeling sluggish and depleted, you may find yourself filled with energy as the body repletes itself. In any case, you should experience a sense of improvement after the treatment. Pain usually will diminish after a treatment, but sometimes symptoms may worsen slightly right after the treatment and then diminish within about twelve hours.

When the body undergoes a natural healing process, it will shunt its own chemicals to areas where it needs them. In order not to interfere with this process, we suggest only light physical activity after a treatment. In addition, we generally give patients the same advice acupuncturists have passed on to their patients for hundreds of years: Eat lightly. Avoid heavy meals, especially food that is very hot, very spicy or very cold. Drink lots of room-temperature water. Avoid alcohol, heavy exercise, or sexual activity for about six to twelve hours.

At our center, patients often tell us that healing starts the moment they walk through the door. We have made an effort to create a total therapeutic environment, with soft colors, soft music, and aromatic scents, rather than a sterile, hospital-type environment. As integrative physicians, we go out of our way to find staff who are warm and friendly.

Layla is a 47-year-old secretary who came to us with chronic daily headaches, fibromyalgia, and depression. Layla remembers being a vibrant, vivacious personality in her 20s, healthy except for intermittent migraines. She worked for a demanding CEO and considered herself exceptional at dealing with high-stress situations. In her early 30s, though, Layla found herself struggling with two young children and a husband who often had to travel out of town. Then she had the car accident. Rear-ended by a drunk driver as she sat stationary at a traffic light, Layla got out of her car, thankful that she was alive. She refused the paramedics suggestion to go to the emergency room, saying that all she had was a stiff neck. That night though, she developed severe pain in her neck, head, and shoulders, and the following morning took herself to the emergency room. X-rays revealed only some neck spasm. She was placed on anti-inflammatories and muscle relaxants. Not only did these medications do little to help her pain, but Layla also found her life "becoming a nightmare." The pain started spreading throughout her body. She began waking frequently during the night, then feeling exhausted in the morning. She found herself irritated by her young children and rejecting intimacy with her husband. Within six months, the pain was so severe that Layla had to stop working. She spent the next few years seeing neurologists, neurosurgeons, rheumatologists, physical medicine and rehabilitation specialists, physical therapists, and ultimately a psychiatrist. Her eventual diagnosis—fibromyalgia and chronic daily headache—seemed to make all health care professionals want to avoid her. Her psychiatrist assured her depression was secondary to all of this, but still felt she should be on antidepressants and have counseling.

Pain medications did little to help. Layla was grateful that she didn't like the feeling of being on narcotic drugs, as she was sure she would otherwise have become addicted to them. Ultimately, she was able to control her pain by taking two drugs simultaneously: duloxetine (Cymbalta®), an antidepressant, and pregabalin (Lyrica®), an anti-seizure medicine also used for pain. But on these medications, she gained sixty pounds, had severe sexual dysfunction, and "felt numb all the time." Despite this, Layla still suffered from a continual, low-grade daily headache that nothing seemed to relieve, along with persistent fatigue and achiness.

During her first consultation with us, we asked Layla if she would allow us to inject the back of her head and shoulders with some local anesthetic. This nerve block took less than two minutes. Layla's eyes widened, and then she began to cry as she realized her pain had gone away for the first time in years. We followed this with an acupuncture treatment lasting about thirty minutes. Layla stood up afterward, transformed. Giggling and jovial, she said this was the first time since her accident she had felt pain-free.

The first treatment gave her hope, but as we explained to her, the road to health had many twists and turns, three steps forward and then one step back. She had a mixture of acupuncture, ACE Healing Treatment, and massage. Some treatments flared her symptoms, while others left her in a state of pain-free euphoria.

We continually looked at Layla's other rings of diagnosis, correcting what we found as we moved ahead. Layla was in the "overwhelm" area on the stress chart, so we used the appropriate herbal formulas. We used nutritional supplements to support her neurotransmitters as we gradually weaned her from her medication. Her vitamin D was very low from never going outdoors. This was easily corrected with a supplement. Finally, a nutritional program aimed at supporting her detoxification processes helped her reduce her pain as well as shedding twenty pounds.

Today, Layla is essentially pain-free. She occasionally develops mild symptoms of what she calls a "preheadache" when she is stressed, but she now knows to deal with it by using a relaxation technique rather than reaching for pain medication.

What You Can Do for Yourself

Sometimes in the midst of a busy life, we forget to make time for ourselves. If we want to get well and stop getting sick or being in pain, however, we need to take the time for self-care. Forgetting to do so becomes self-defeating. If we don't look after ourselves, we ultimately cannot help those around us. Self-care should not be done in a self-centered or selfish way, but with a mindset that nurtures and nourishes us.

When we first visited Hong Kong and Taiwan, we were amazed to see hundreds of people practicing the slow, circular, rhythmic movements of tai chi each morning in the public parks. When we asked tai chi masters about why they did this practice, they typically explained to us that when they reached their 40s and 50s, they found themselves lacking in vitality and stamina. Their bellies and libido had begun to sag, and they tended to develop problems with their blood pressure and general health. After practicing tai chi for a few months, their health problems disappeared, and their vitality returned. As they continued the practice over decades, they found themselves doing better and better. Their bodies felt better, and their minds were clearer and sharper.

Adherents to yoga practice often report a similar return to health. These practices help reduce pain and improve stamina, mood, and vitality. Tai chi or yoga are not the only answers. Any type of regular, gentle exercise has broad and lasting benefits (see Star 1 and 2 for more suggestions on this).

The question is: What are you going to do to help yourself regain a positive sense of vitality? How can you restore an abundant sense of well-being? Are there ways you can restore your health without medication? We believe that a practical, balanced lifestyle, individualized to your condition, provides the foundation for almost any form of treatment.

Using Pain as a Guide

Our culture wants us to switch off pain as fast as we can, but pain isn't always a bad thing. If you have chronic pain, we encourage you to change your viewpoint and see your pain as something to work with, not against. We would like you to listen to your body as you learn to heal. If a certain exercise hurts—don't do it! There is a difference between what we call an "oooh" pain and an "owww!" pain. An "oooh" pain is one that says, "Go deeper." This is a typical sensation you may feel when a massage therapist works out a knot in your muscle or when you are enjoying a stretch. An "owww" pain is an important message from your body that says "Stop now." Patients often tell us about little "owww" pains that precede a much bigger one. These occur in golf games, yoga classes, and even bending down to put on socks. Learning to pay attention to the little pains—and then finding a way to get rid of them—can prevent much bigger problems later on.

Healing Your Feelings

In some cases, the body can help us understand suppressed emotions. Sometimes chronic pain can mask underlying issues caused by physical or emotional trauma that has been overlooked. When there is no physical cause of your pain that makes sense, you need to consider this as a possibility. In Star 2, we suggested ways to learn to be become mindful of underlying emotions.

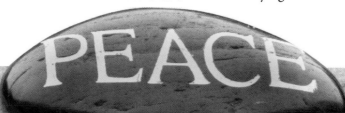

© Shutterstock/
Andrea Haase

Often the first stage in learning to heal emotions is by becoming aware of intense emotions that surface as you have bodywork done. In addition, by paying attention to what you are thinking and feeling every time your stomach hurts or your shoulders ache, you will begin to realize how your job, relationships, or other stresses are affecting you. You can become attuned to the way your body's responses serve as a barometer of your emotions. It is often the early warning radar system that is telling you about stress, long before your mind consciously realizes it.

Finding Help

When it comes to self-help, there are so many different practitioners and philosophies that it can be difficult to know where to start. If you are in pain or in poor physical shape, you may want to look for a physical therapist or personal trainer with expertise in this area. If you just want to improve your health, we suggest exploring the more popular gyms, personal trainers, exercise studios, yoga centers, and self-care practitioners in your area. No matter what the modality, you want to leave the class or session feeling alive, invigorated, inspired, and empowered. A good teacher should encourage you and stimulate your personal growth.

How Much Exercise?

How much exercise is right for you depends on where you are on the stress curve. (Check back to page 63 to see this diagram.) If you are on the left side of the curve (wired and tired), heavy exercise can be beneficial. It helps to burn off excess adrenaline and calm you down. As you head toward the right side of the curve (exhausted, inflamed, and depleted), heavy exercise can make you feel worse. How do you know? Go exercise and see how you feel. If you feel worse after you exercise, then your body is more run down than you think, and you need to use a more gentle form of exercise.

Pain and Discomfort as a Door to Transformation

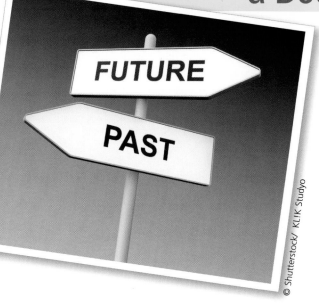

In the beginning of this book, we asked you how you *really feel* about your health. Some of you may have reported all kinds of problems, while others may have blissfully denied anything wrong, content to live in denial that something could be a problem. The truth is that we all have health issues to deal with. Wellness is a state we need to work at and live for. Pain and discomfort nudge us to change. As you go forward into your life, embrace this philosophy. Allow your body to give you feedback that you willingly act upon, making yourself healthier every day.

Our Stepwise Approach to Chronic Pain

We begin by thoroughly assessing the patient from a medical standpoint. We like to know everything about their pain. We look at MRIs, EMGs, and standard lab blood work including vitamin D, hs-CRP, and thyroid levels. We use standard medications and refer for physical therapy, epidurals, and surgery where appropriate. After that, we follow these steps:

1. Assess and treat what are called comorbid medical conditions. In other words, what else may be contributing to the pain?

2. Assess and treat depression. As we have seen already, neurotransmitters can play havoc with pain.

3. We like to know what the patient's stress level is and how they are dealing with it. Certain people have a tendency to somatize their pain. In other words, they take emotional pain and put it into their body. Other patients may have something called hypervigilance, which makes them anxious and unusually responsive to pain. We try to teach patients to observe rather than react to their symptoms. If necessary, we use psychological counseling in various forms for this.

4. We examine all of our patients carefully, looking for "invisible" or myofascial pain. Very often we can press on a trigger point and reproduce the very pain they are having. We treat this using massage, acupuncture, Rolfing, and occasionally muscle relaxant herbs or medications.

5. We look for and treat dysautonomia. This is especially important in patients who have reflex sympathetic dystrophies (RSD) and chronic regional pain syndromes (CRPS). RSD and CRPS are sometimes aggravated initially by direct therapy, so if they are severe, we will use energy healing modalities or acupuncture at different sites in the body. (Refer back to Ring 5 for a discussion of RSD and CRPS.)

6. We assess patients from a structural standpoint. We look both at the area of pain as well as the reciprocal area. For instance if a patient has neck pain, we look at the front of their neck, as well as their shoulders, lower back, pelvis, legs, and feet. We look for a "march of symptoms." Did the pain start in the right ankle, then move to the right knee, low back, shoulder, and finally to the neck? Treatment includes manipulative therapies, acupuncture, Rolfing, and massage.

7. We assess what is known as the biological terrain. In other words, we try and assess what kind of physiology a patient has. We use functional labs to further evaluate nutrient deficiencies, oxidative stress levels, mitochondrial dysfunction, dysbiosis in the gut, and hormonal and neurotransmitter levels. We treat this appropriately with supplements and/or medication.

8. We assess bioenergetic imbalance. We treat this using acupuncture, energy healing, and FSM (frequency specific microcurrent).

9. Finally, we like to understand the patient from a social and spiritual perspective. We want to know about their family and community life, and whether or not they are increasing or decreasing their stress and coping levels. Treatment for this aspect is obviously delicate, and it is of utmost importance that the therapist acts only as a guide and a reflector for the patient. It is important not to impose opinions or spiritual beliefs on a patient. We do know that when people are engaged in their own communities and feel a part of something larger than themselves, they do better. Our job is simply to facilitate this.

There Is Hope!

Transformational Medicine is about turning your life around. We see people get better every day. We see people improve their health every day. You can do the same.

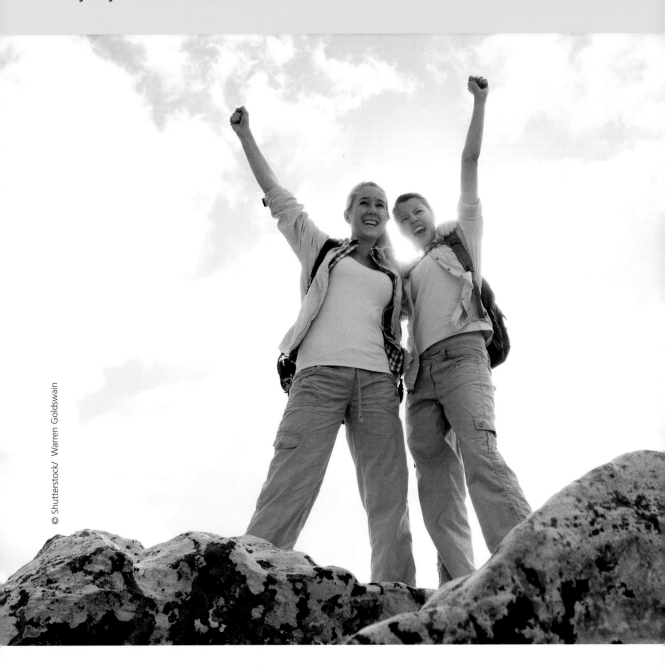

© Shutterstock/ Warren Goldswain

Alex Learns to Handle His Back Pain

Alex continues to pursue Health and Wellness

Alex was very proud of how he had transformed his life in just six months. Daily exercising had helped his back pain somewhat, but his back remained stiff in the morning. Sometimes, when he bent and twisted, such as when he picked up something from the floor, he would develop sharp back spasms. The pain could drop him to his knees.

Alex decided to come in for regular ACE Healing Treatment. The combination of acupuncture, chiropractic, and energy healing left him pain-free and relaxed, almost in a state of euphoria. He initially came in once a week. As his back pain appeared less and less, he dropped his treatment frequency down to every two weeks, then once a month. After coming in monthly for a few months, he noticed that he could not remember when he last had pain.

We encouraged him to keep coming once a month. He laughed. "Not only does this keep my pain away, but I hardly notice my allergies. I consider this the best type of prevention—it's enjoyable, restful, and invigorating all at the same time!"

Alex had learned to use his body as a barometer of his stress. He knew that when his knees ached, he was under too much stress and needed to modulate whatever he was doing. His back pain was related to mechanical issues, and he knew to come see us more frequently at times, especially when he played more golf.

Alex came to us seeking wellness. When he found he had significant health problems that needed to be addressed, he discovered true health. Alex is a success story of Transformational Medicine. You can be one, too!

To administer medicine to diseases which have already developed and thereby suppress bodily chaos which has already occurred is comparable to the behavior of those who would begin to dig a well after they had grown thirsty, or those who would begin to cast weapons after they have engaged in a battle.

Would these actions not be too late?

— Huang Di, The Yellow Emperor, 400 BC

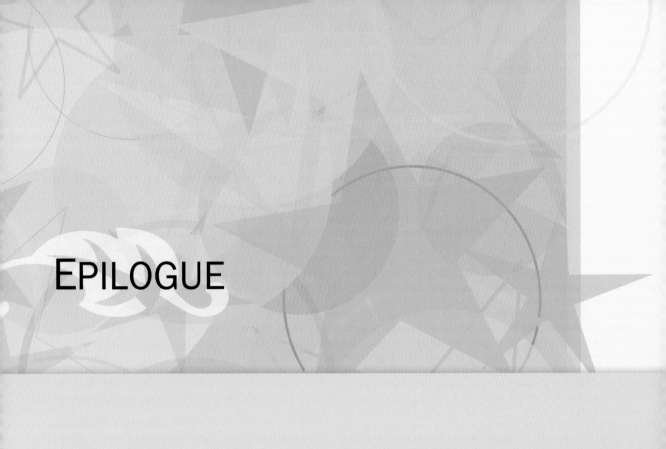

EPILOGUE

A Transformational
Medicine Story

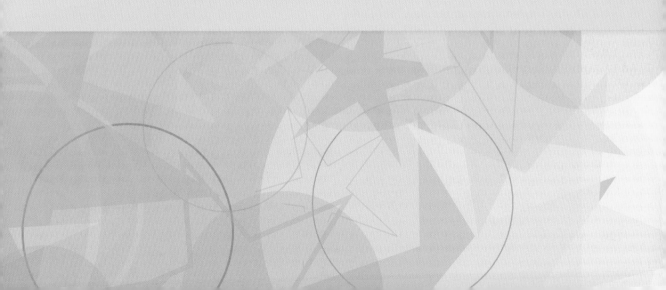

Our children loved watching the movie *The Wizard of Oz* when they were young. They never seemed to tire of it, so the characters became an indelible part of our household. Little did we realize how much we learned from them and this story.

To refresh your memory in case you were never subjected to this film, we will give you a short synopsis as we saw it.

Dorothy, the heroine of the story, lives in a black-and-white world. Like many of us stuck in our own lives, she dreams one day of going "over the rainbow" to a place that is much better. Little did she know how important this visualization of her dream would be! The next thing she knows, she and her dog Toto are swept from her world by a tornado into the magical Technicolor Land of Oz. Dorothy, like all of us who dream of bigger things, had no idea what she was getting into.

While she achieved what she wished for, she also suddenly realized that she was facing a dangerous, quirky, and unexplored new world. While not at all her fault, her house had landed on the Wicked Witch, killing her. The Wicked Witch of the West, sister of the dead witch, threatens to get rid of her. Dorothy is petrified. Strange little Munchkins dance around her, believing her to be a witch. You can only imagine how overwhelmed Dorothy must feel. Suddenly, Glinda, the Good Witch of the North, gives Dorothy the dead witch's enchanted ruby red slippers, and advises her that if she wants to get back to her home in Kansas, she should seek the help and advice of the Wizard of Oz, who lives in the Emerald City.

Dorothy sets off down the yellow brick road, accompanied by her dog Toto, and three flawed individuals who themselves are seeking something that they believe is missing in their lives. The Scarecrow is looking for a brain, the Tin Man is looking for a heart, and the Cowardly Lion is looking for courage. Together, they believe they can find the magical missing answers to their life quests.

Dangers abound. On the way to the Emerald City, the Wicked Witch of the West casts a spell on them by conjuring up a field of poppies that cause Dorothy, Toto, and the Lion to fall asleep. Glinda, the Good Witch, counteracts the effects of the poppies by making it snow, waking them up.

When they ultimately make it to their destination, they believe that the "great and powerful" Wizard of Oz will tell them what to do and how to fix themselves. This is not to be. The Wizard won't even see them before they perform a task for him—to bring the broomstick of the dreaded Wicked Witch of the West, the very person who had threatened Dorothy's existence. They set off again on a second quest, determined to bring back the broomstick. Little do they know that the evil witch is about to harm them. She sends winged monkeys to attack them before they reach her castle. The monkeys grasp Dorothy and Toto and bring them to the wicked witch. Unfortunately for the witch, she finds out that she cannot take the ruby slippers from Dorothy while she is alive. She simply turns her hourglass, threatening Dorothy that she will die when the sand runs out. Meanwhile, Toto has escaped. He runs out and finds Dorothy's three friends, bringing them back to the castle. Dressed as guardsmen they enter the castle, free Dorothy,

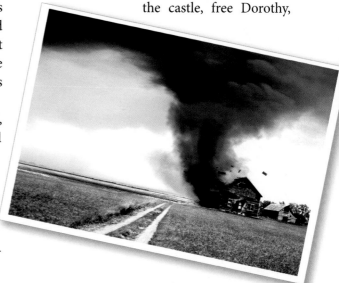

and hatch their escape. Before they can get very far, the Wicked Witch catches them and sets the Scarecrow on fire. Dorothy, in a fit of panic, picks up a pail of water and douses the Scarecrow. Serendipitously, she splashes the Witch, causing her to melt away. Happily, she takes the Witch's broomstick and returns to the Emerald City, eager to learn from the Wizard how to go home.

The Wizard appears furious to see them. Dorothy and her friends are frozen by the booming voice and the theatrical appearance of the Wizard. Not so Toto. He scurries around the side, then tugs away at a curtain to reveal a bumbling man pulling at levers and speaking into a microphone. Dorothy quickly realizes the Wizard is a con man, a fake. However, he too comes through, helping Dorothy to realize, and then convince her friends, that they in fact have always had the qualities which they sought. The Scarecrow did indeed use his brain, the Lion showed his courage, and the Tin Man showed he had a heart. The Wizard quickly realizes that he can add some benefit to the occasion, awarding a diploma to the Scarecrow, a medal of valor to the Lion and a heart-shaped watch to the Tin Man. Finally, he reveals that he too is from Kansas, and is about to return in his hot-air balloon, taking Dorothy and Toto with him. In his absence, he appoints the Scarecrow, Lion, and Tin Man as rulers of all of Oz.

Unfortunately, Dorothy is once again beset by disaster. Toto runs off just as they are about to leave. Then the Wizard flies off in his hot air balloon without Dorothy or Toto. Dorothy is distraught. Now she has no way to get home! Suddenly, Glinda appears, telling her she always had the power to get home. The only reason she hadn't told her was that she didn't think she would believe it. Tearfully, Dorothy performs the magical ritual of tapping her heels together three times, then repeating her mantra, "There's no place like home . . . There's no place like home . . . There's no place like home . . . ."

All of a sudden, Dorothy reawakens, back in her own bed. Everything back in Kansas is now in color instead of black-and-white. She is surrounded by her Auntie Em, who reminds her of Glinda, as well as her Uncle Henry. Right there is Professor Marvel, an itinerant magician who looks like the Wizard, and three farmhands who remind her of the Scarecrow, Lion, and Tin Man. She tries to tell them what happened. Although no one believes her, she is ecstatically happy.

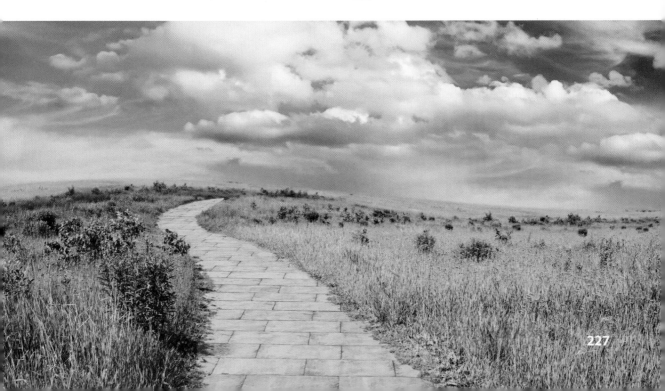

The Metaphor of Illness

Illness for most us is a tornado. It throws us from our mundane existence into a turbulence-filled, dangerous, uncertain future. Like Dorothy, we initially don't quite understand what just happened.

An illness essentially hands us our own pair of ruby red slippers, instilling in us the power to do things that we never would have wanted to do.

When we get sick, our emotions take over. Just like little Munchkins, they give us conflicting advice. Ultimately we need to follow the yellow brick road, representing the path of the intellect. We need facts as we journey toward the Emerald Castle, our place of intended healing. So we gather our data and off we go. We learn about our illnesses and glean facts from multiple sources. We meet fellow travelers along the way, all of whom are trying to heal themselves.

So off we go to the mystical Emerald Castle. Before we get there we too may be struck by the poppy-derived morphine-like power of addictive medication. We may have our own trials and tribulations, but we are sure that the "Wizard" of Medicine will know what to do. The Wizard may represent the ultimate surgeon, the hospital oncology ward, or even a mystical healer to whom we attribute superpowers. While the Wizard may fix some of us, that is not always the case. Too often we need to go on another quest, searching for something else. The procedure we thought could fix us perhaps doesn't.

In energy healing, green is associated with the heart, and the heart is associated with a quest. In mythology, the purpose for the quest is not usually what one comes back with. So too with Dorothy. She goes to get a broomstick. In the process she learns to deal with flying monkeys and eventually kills the Wicked Witch. She doesn't intend to do so. It just so happens that the water she uses to quench the fire and help her friend is exactly what she needs to kill the Witch. How often does that happen for us when we allow it? We think we're doing something for one reason, and then find out later that what we got out of it was so much richer and more profound—yet totally unexpected.

When Dorothy finds out the Wizard is a fake, she is forced to take further control, to speak out about her own truth. In doing so, she helps her fellow travelers understand that they already have what they are looking for. How true is that for most of our emotional needs? When we learn that what we are looking for is "in here," not "out there," it makes our lives so much better.

Finally, Dorothy is still at an impasse. Glinda, her spiritual companion, has been watching over her all along. It is only at the point of greatest stress that Dorothy starts to trust her own spirituality. By opening to this, she is finally able to return home. When she gets there, everything is as it always was, but now it is in color, filled with bliss and greater understanding!

Your Path to Healing

We have tried in this book to show you our understanding of healing and a new pathway to health. We hope it will offer you a new way to see the multidimensional, multifaceted miracle we call a human being. We hope too it will expand your paradigm of health, offering you new insights into how people get sick and how they can get well.

Ultimately, we wish you a safe and pleasant journey on your transformational trip *home!*

Transformational Medicine is about **rethinking your approach** to disease and discomfort, as well as your approach to health and well-being.

You can start transforming your health today!
Put the 5 Ring and 5 Star approach into action:

1. **Discover and deal with your medical problems. Change your exercise level and lifestyle to reawaken your sense of vitality.**

2. **Learn to transform stress into success.**

3. **Learn to use nutrition and supplements to optimize your metabolism, immune function, and body chemistry. You can begin to change your body chemistry in just 24 hours.**

4. **Learn to optimize your hormone balance with lifestyle, exercise, stress reduction, nutrition, and medications if and when needed.**

5. **Learn to heal your body. Learn what others can do for you, and what you can do for yourself.**

Transformational Medicine is about transforming your health every day.
The same approach that takes away your current problems can also help you heal old problems and prevent new ones.
So…
Get Well and Stay Well—*starting now!*

Transformational Medicine in a Village: A Story of H.O.P.E.

Changing lives and transforming health is more than working on ourselves—it is also about community. We learned this in a wonderful way through our daughters, friends, and family.

In 2003, we visited a rural village in the mountains of South Africa, near where Sandi's sister and her husband, Carol Anne and Chris Mumby, own and manage a hotel. Our children looked on aghast as we discussed the high unemployment and AIDS rate. Impoverished orphans ran around with few clothes on, playing in burned out cars. An area once rich in vegetation now lay arid. With no running water or electricity, diseases of all kind were rampant.

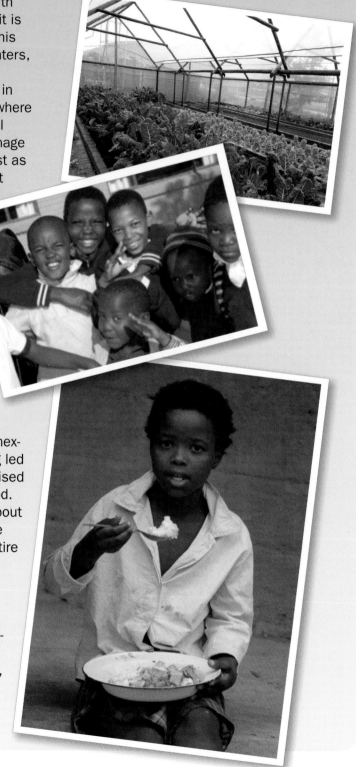

The experience prompted our younger daughter Maya and her friends at school in Cincinnati to form a charitable group called H.O.P. E.—Help Other People Endure. Their contagious enthusiasm for this project grew in unexpected ways. One serendipitous thing led to another. The outcome: H.O.P. E. raised over $1.4 million over a six-year period. Former President Bill Clinton wrote about the girls in his book, *Giving*. And more importantly than anything else, an entire village was transformed! The story is chronicled on their website: www.SouthAfricanHope.org.

Four years after H.O.P. E. began, under Carol Anne and Chris's stewardship, an impoverished preschool was totally refurbished, with running water, electricity, flushing toilets, vegetable tunnels, and boisterous schoolyards full of beaming children. The high school now has a library and a computer lab. Children began to know what it was like to grow and harvest produce and to eat seasonal, fresh, locally grown vegetables. Up to seven hundred kids would arrive at the preschool twice daily for meals. No one who was hungry was ever turned away.

While the success of H.O.P. E. was heartwarming and surprising for us all, this story teaches us more than just about one small village in a distant place. It teaches us how to transform health with simple lifestyle changes. During our first H.O.P. E. trip to South Africa, we depleted loads of antibiotics and medicines within a few days. Many of the children displayed clear symptoms of malnourishment. But after a few years of travelling to Langkloof, we noticed that we didn't use medicine anymore. Besides the usual playground scrapes, there was very little need for it. The signs of malnourishment were gone. The

good food, community support, hygiene, fresh air, and clean water were enough to keep the majority of the young population healthy! Our older daughter Misha, later to become a doctor, was profoundly influenced by this transformation as she worked with the children. It was she who noted how it was often the small changes that made the greatest differences.

And that is the point of transformational change. Making multiple, synergistic, small changes allows for a quantum leap in health!

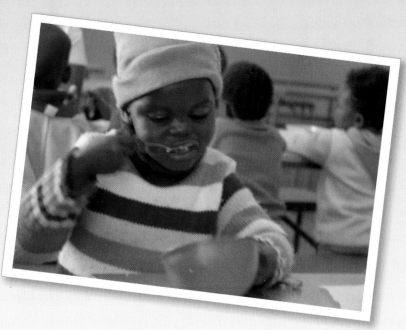

Acknowledgments

In Japanese, the word *sensei* means doctor, master, or teacher. A doctor should be a healer, displaying a mastery of the healing arts, as well as a teacher to his or her patients. We have been lucky to be mentored by wonderful senseis in the form of friends, healers, doctors, masters, and teachers during our careers. This book could never have been written without the support we have received. We attempt to thank just a few of these here.

Firstly, we would never have been able to do this without the encouragement of our friends and family. Their support was invaluable, especially when we left on a mission to pursue our dreams and explore the world of alternative therapies when it was not fashionable to do so. To our parents Arthur and Margot, Cecil and Yvonne, brothers Dennis and Phillip, and sisters Carol Anne and Denise—we are eternally grateful. Perhaps they thought we were crazy, but at least they didn't tell us. Our daughters Misha and Maya have been honest critics and fervent supporters, embracing and enhancing our philosophies. We are eternally appreciative for their presence and love in our lives.

We owe a great debt of gratitude to the friends and teachers who encouraged us to look further. Reg and Jon-Jon Park, Johnny Goldberg, Megan Draudsing, Jill Brodie, Dr. Tom Gormley, Roy Jensen, Andrew Watson, and of course Mii Sensei. Rosalyn Bruyere truly taught us to look at the world with new eyes. It was Rosalyn's interpretation of the story of *The Wizard of Oz* that allowed us to see what Transformational Medicine could become.

We will always be thankful to the founding fathers of functional medicine and medical acupuncture: Jeff Bland, Ph.D. and Joe Helms, M.D. The vision of these two men is helping to change medicine for the better. Their influence and support has allowed us to proceed with courage where we may otherwise have faltered. We would like to thank our colleagues at The American Academy for Medical Acupuncture for helping bring traditional wisdom to conventional medicine. We would like to acknowledge Dr. Clyde Wilson for introducing us to his concept of food groups. We also could not have survived without the patient and gentle prodding, teaching, and mentoring support of Dr. Patrick Hanaway, who allowed us to see the wisdom of functional lab testing.

We would also like to acknowledge Dr. David Jones and Dr. Mark Hyman for the pioneering work they are doing at the Institute for Functional Medicine. Also, to Dr. Andrew Weil and Dr. Dean Ornish, for the pioneering work they have done in the field of Integrative Medicine. It was Dr. Ornish's research data that provided us the "aha moment" of seeing that Transformational Medicine can and does work. His groundbreaking research showed that the same approach that works to reverse cardiovascular disease can also reverse prostate cancer while simultaneously lengthening telomeres. In other words, the same diet and lifestyle approach that reverses disease also prevents disease and lengthens life.

We could also never have achieved the outcomes we have without the incredible team of healers and therapists we have at the Alliance Institute for Integrative Medicine. They are truly amazing people. We would also like to express our special gratitude to our contributing authors: Steve Bleser, D.C., Claudia Harsh, M.D., Jim Leonard, M.D., John Sacco, M.D., Keith Wilson, M.D., and Liz Woolford, M.D. We would also like to thank Lisa Gallagher, N.D., Tiffany Gillam Lester, M.D., and Michelle Zimmer, M.D. for their thoughtful manuscript revisions.

The Bravewell Collaborative under the guiding light of Christy Mack and Penny George has helped everyone to see the value of Integrative Medicine. We would like to thank them and all our fellow members of the Bravewell Clinical Network for their courage, their leadership, and their support. We especially thank Brian Berman, M.D., who pioneered much of the research into Integrative Medicine, Dan Monti, M.D., for his support and guidance, and Mimi Guarneri, M.D. for her selfless and tireless stewardship of this field.

We would like to recognize the help of Nancy Faass and her team at The Writers Group (www.ProWritersGroup.com), whose editorial wisdom and support helped shape this book, and Kathy Coogan (www.writers-resources-cafe.com) for all her help and insights. To our editor, Sheila Buff (www.sheilabuff.com), we owe eternal gratitude for helping to bring this book to fruition. Sheila helped us hone down an enormous body of knowledge into something that is readable and inspiring. Our book designer Brenda Grannan (www.Grannandesign.com) understood our wish to make our readers use both brain hemispheres while reading this handsome book. She has remained gracious and resourceful during delays and deadlines, always calm and creative under the final pressure to get the book done. Kristin Luther (www.Luthermultimedia.com) did an exceptional job of taking our ideas and making illustrations of them, and Abbey Urbas (www.abbeyurbas.com) has continually inspired us with her creative graphic design. Dan Segal (www.skidogimages.com)—thank you for the photos.

We would also like to thank all our friends who read the book and shared their views, especially Tom Hattersley, who endured many questions while disguised as a cycling partner.

We would like to thank Chef Suzy DeYoung and La Petite Pierre not only for preparing the food you see on these pages, but also keeping us sustained during the many long hours of writing. Special thanks to Nancy Merrell, who helped with so many aspects of the administration and organization of this book.

Finally, we would like to thank the board of The Integrative Medicine Foundation for their support in getting this book published. Dan Bailey, Nate Bachman, Neil Bortz, John Burns, Fredric Holzberger, Scott Kadish, Craig and Frances Lindner, and Heather Theders—we don't know what we would have done without you!

We would especially like to thank Fredric and Julie Holzberger and the Holzberger Family Humanitarian Foundation for their absolute support for this book. Fredric first came to us years before we opened our center to tell us that we needed to do it. We told him then that it was impossible, but his persistence opened our eyes to new possibilities . . . and when he suggested to us we needed to write a book on what we do—we told him that was impossible too!

We would also like to add a special thank you to our friends, Craig and Frances Lindner, who have supported, encouraged, and inspired us to help make a difference in the world.

If there is one thing we have learned from all we have received, it is that it is often impossible to give back directly to the person that gave to us. We can ultimately only pay it forward. We hope that all that has been given to us will be paid forward manifold!

References

PROLOGUE

Angell M, Kassirer JP. Alternative medicine: the risks of untested and unregulated remedies. *N Engl J Med.* 1998;339(12):839-841.

Hoffman C, Rice D, Sung HY. Persons with chronic conditions: their prevalence and costs. *JAMA.* 1996;276(18):1473-1479.

Kroenke, K et al. Common symptoms in ambulatory care: incidence, evaluation, therapy, and outcome. *Am J Med.* 1989;86: 262-266.

RING 1

National Institute of Diabetes and Digestion and Kidney Diseases. *The Pima Indians: Pathfinders for Health.* NIDDKD, 1996. Available online at http://diabetes.niddk.nih.gov/DM/pubs/pima/obesity/obesity.htm.

Waterland RA, Jirtle RL. Transposable elements: targets for early nutritional effects on epigenetic gene regulation. *Mol. Cell. Biol.* 2003;23:5293-5300.

STAR 1

Ames, B. High dose vitamin therapy stimulates variant enzymes with decreased coenzyme binding affinity (increased Km): relevance to genetic disease and polymorphisms. *Am J Clin Nutr.* 2002;75: 616-658.

Ames, B. The metabolic tune-up: metabolic harmony and disease prevention. *J Nutr.* 2003;133: 1544S-1548S.

Benson, Herb. *The Relaxation Response* (William Morrow, 2000).

Fields, Wayne. *What the River Knows: An Angler in Midstream* (University of Chicago Press, 1996).

Kabat-Zinn, Jon. *Wherever You Go, There You Are* (Hyperion, 2005).

Norris JC, van der Laan MJ, Lane S, Anderson JN, Block G. Nonlinearity in demographic and behavioral determinants of morbidity. *Health Serv Res.* 2003;38:1791-1818.

Svetkey, LP et al. Comparison of strategies for sustaining weight loss: the weight loss maintenance randomized controlled trial. *JAMA.* 2008;299:1149-1148.

RING 2

Sapolsky, Robert. *Why Zebras Don't Get Ulcers* (Holt, 2004).

STAR 2

Cox T, Griffiths A, Rial-González E. Research on work-related stress. European Agency for Safety and Health at Work. 2000. Available at http://osha.eu.int, accessed 01/15/11.

Hölzelab BK et al. Bottom of Form Mindfulness practice leads to increases in regional brain gray matter density. *Psychiatry Res.* 2011;191(1):36-43.

Kabat-Zinn J, Wheeler E et al. Influence of a mindfulness meditation-based stress reduction intervention on rates of skin clearing in patients with moderate to severe psoriasis undergoing phototherapy (UVB) and photochemotherapy (PUVA). *Psychosom. Med.* 1998;60:625-632.

Kabat-Zinn, Jon. *Full Catastrophe Living: Using the Wisdom of Your Body and Mind to Face Stress, Pain, and Illness* (Delta,1990)

Venket Rao A, Bested AC et al. A randomized, double-blind, placebo-controlled pilot study of a probiotic in emotional symptoms of chronic fatigue syndrome. *Gut Pathog.* 2009;1:6.

STAR 3

Wilson, Clyde. *What, When & Water: Nutrition for Weight Loss Wellness* (Lulu.com, 2007).

RING 3

Buettner, Dan. *The Blue Zones: Lessons for Living Longer From the People Who've Lived the Longest* (National Geographic, 2009).

Diamanti-Kandarakis E et al. Endocrine-disrupting chemicals: an Endocrine Society scientific statement. *Endocr Rev.* 2009;30:293-342.

Goodarz D et al. National, regional, and global trends in fasting plasma glucose and diabetes prevalence since 1980: systematic analysis of health examination surveys and epidemiological studies with 370 country-years and 2.7 million participants. *Lancet.* 2011;378:3- 40.

Jiang Q et al. ApoE promotes the proteolytic degradation of Abeta. *Neuron.* 2008; 58:681–693.

Nguyen T, Nioi P, Pickett CB. The Nrf2-antioxidant response element signaling pathway and its activation by oxidative stress. *J Biol Chem.* 2009; 284:13291–13295.

Schubert J, Riley EJ, Tyler SA. Combined effects in toxicology—a rapid systematic testing procedure: cadmium, mercury, and lead. *J Toxicol Environ Health.*1978;4:763-776.

Sinha R, Anderson DE et al. Cancer risk and diet in India. *J Postgrad Med.* 2003;49: 228-238.

STAR 3

Ames B. The metabolic tune-up: metabolic harmony and disease prevention. *J Nutr.* 2003;133:1544S-1548S

Ames B. High dose vitamin therapy stimulates variant enzymes with decreased coenzyme binding affinity (increased Km): relevance to genetic disease and polymorphisms. *Am J Clin Nutr.* 2002;75:616-658.

Arkadianos I et al. Improved weight management using genetic information to personalize a calorie controlled diet. *Nutr. J.* 2007; 6:29.

Buettner, Dan. *Thrive: Finding Happiness the Blue Zones Way* (National Geographic, 2011).

Campbell, Colin T. *The China Study: The Most Comprehensive Study of Nutrition Ever Conducted and the Startling Implications for Diet, Weight Loss, and Long-term Health* (BenBella Books, 2006).

Ghanim H, Sia CL, Abuaysheh S, Korzeniewski K, Patnaik P, Marumganti A, Chaudhuri A, Dandona P. An antiinflammatory and reactive oxygen species suppressive effects of an extract of Polygonum cuspidatum containing resveratrol. *J Clin Endocrinol Metab.* 2010;95(9):E1-8.

Interleukin Genetics. The Science Behind the Weight Management Genetic Test. www.inherenthealth.com/media/4759/wm_scientific%20summary.pdf .

Knoops KT et al. Mediterranean diet, lifestyle factors, and 10-year mortality in elderly European men and women: the HALE project. *JAMA.* 2004;292(12):1433-1439.

Kris-Etherton P, Eckel RH, Howard BV, St Jeor S, Bazzarre TL. AHA Science Advisory: Lyon Diet Heart Study. Benefits of a Mediterranean-style, National Cholesterol Education Program/American Heart Association Step I dietary pattern on cardiovascular disease. *Circ.* 2001;103(13):1823-1825.

Smith, Jeffrey. *Genetic Roulette: The Documented Health Risks of Genetically Engineered Foods* (Chelsea Green, 2007).

Nestle, Marion. *What to Eat* (North Point Press, 2007).

Wansink, Brian. *Mindless Eating: Why We Eat More Than We Think* (Bantam, 2010).

U.S. Department of Health and Human Services. *Cancer and the Environment: What You Need to Know, What You Can Do.* NIH Publication No. 03–2039, 2003.

Zahid M et al. Prevention of estrogen-DNA adduct formation in MCF-10F cells by resveratrol. *Free Radic Biol Med.* 2008:45(2):136–145.

Zahid M, Saeed M, Beseler C, Rogan EG, Cavalieri EL. Resveratrol and N-acetylcysteine block the cancer-initiating step in MCF-10F cells. *Free Radic Biol Med.* 2011:50(1):78-85.

Zinczenko, David. *Eat This, Not That! The No-Diet Weight Loss Solution* (Rodale Books, 2011).

RING 4

Cavalieri E, Chakravarti D, Guttenplan J, Hart E, Ingle J, Jankowiak R et al. Catechol estrogen quinones as initiators of breast and other human cancers: implications for biomarkers of susceptibility and cancer prevention. *Biochim Biophys Acta.* 2006;1766(1):63-78.

Cavalieri E, Rogan E. Catechol quinones of estrogens in the initiation of breast, prostate, and other human cancers: keynote lecture. *Ann N Y Acad Sci.* 2006;1089:286-301.

Cavalieri EL, Rogan EG. Depurinating estrogen-DNA adducts in the etiology & prevention of breast and other human cancers. *Future Oncol.* 2010;6(1):75-91.

Cavalieri EL, Rogan EG. Is bisphenol A a weak carcinogen like the natural estrogens and diethylstilbestrol? *IUBMB Life.* 2010:62(10):746-751.

Cavalieri EL, Rogan EG. A unifying mechanism in the initiation of cancer and other diseases by catechol quinones. *Ann N Y Acad Sci.* 2004;1028:247-257.

Chakravarti D, Zahid M, Backora M, Myers EM, Gaikwad N, Weisenburger DD et al. Ortho-quinones of benzene and estrogens induce hyperproliferation of human peripheral blood mononuclear cells. *Leuk Lymphoma.* 2006;47(12):2635-2644.

Gaikwad NW, Yang L, Muti P, Meza JL, Pruthi S, Ingle JN, Rogan EG, Cavalieri EL. The molecular etiology of breast cancer: evidence from biomarkers of risk. *Int J Cancer.* 2008;122(9):1949-1957.

Gaikwad NW, Yang L, Rogan EG, Cavalieri EL. Evidence for NQO2-

mediated reduction of the carcinogenic estrogen ortho-quinones. *Free Radic Biol Med.* 2009;46(2):253-262.

Gaynor M. *Environmental Epigenetics: Integrative Medicine and the health of the public. A summary of the 2009 Institute of Medicine Summit conference* (National Academies Press, 2009).

Grundy SM et al. Diagnosis and management of the metabolic syndrome: An American Heart Association/National Heart, Lung, and Blood Institute scientific statement. *Circ.* 2005;112:2735–2752.

Kim T, Park H, Yue W, Wang JP, Atkins KA, Zhang Z et al. Tetramethoxystilbene modulates ductal growth of the developing murine mammary gland. *Breast Cancer Res Treat.* 2011;126(3):779-789.

King H, Keuky L, Seng S, Khun T, Roglic G, Pinget M. Diabetes and associated disorders in Cambodia: two epidemiological surveys. *Lancet.* 2005; 366:1633–1639.

Lu F, Zahid M, Saeed M, Cavalieri EL, Rogan EG. Estrogen metabolism and formation of estrogen-DNA adducts in estradiol-treated MCF-10F cells. The effects of 2,3,7,8-tetrachlorodibenzo-p-dioxin induction and catechol-O-methyltransferase inhibition. *J Steroid Biochem Mol Biol.* 2007;105(1-5):150-158.

Markushin Y, Gaikwad N, Zhang H, Kapke P, Rogan EG, Cavalieri EL et al. Potential biomarker for early risk assessment of prostate cancer. *Prostate.* 2006;66(14):1565-1571.

Muti P, Rogan E, Cavalieri E. Androgens and estrogens in the etiology and prevention of breast cancer. *Nutr Cancer.* 2006;56(2):247-252.

Ravdin PM et al. The decrease in breast-cancer incidence in 2003 in the United States. *N Engl J Med.* 2007;356:1670-1674.

Robson M, Offit K. Clinical practice:

management of an inherited predisposition to breast cancer. *N Engl J Med.* 2007;357:154-162.

Rogan E. Xenoestrogens, biotransformation, and differential risks for breast cancer. *Altern Ther Health Med.* 2007;13(2):S112-121.

Saeed M, Higginbotham S, Gaikwad N, Chakravarti D, Rogan E, Cavalieri E. Depurinating naphthalene-DNA adducts in mouse skin related to cancer initiation. *Free Radic Biol Med.* 2009;47(7):1075-1081.

Saeed M, Higginbotham S, Rogan E, Cavalieri E. Formation of depurinating N3adenine and N7guanine adducts after reaction of 1,2-naphthoquinone or enzyme-activated 1,2-dihydroxynaphthalene with DNA. Implications for the mechanism of tumor initiation by naphthalene. *Chem Biol Interact.* 2007;165(3):175-188.

Saeed M, Rogan E, Cavalieri E. Mechanism of metabolic activation and DNA adduct formation by the human carcinogen diethylstilbestrol: the defining link to natural estrogens. *Int J Cancer.* 2009;124(6):1276-1284.

Saeed M, Rogan E, Fernandez SV, Sheriff F, Russo J, Cavalieri E. Formation of depurinating N3Adenine and N7Guanine adducts by MCF-10F cells cultured in the presence of 4-hydroxyestradiol. *Int J Cancer.* 2007;120(8):1821-1824.

Santen R, Cavalieri E, Rogan E, Russo J, Guttenplan J, Ingle J, Yue W. Estrogen mediation of breast tumor formation involves estrogen receptor-dependent, as well as independent, genotoxic effects. *Ann N Y Acad Sci.* 2009;1155:132-140.

Sephton SE, Sapolsky RM, Kraemer HC, Spiegel D. Diurnal cortisol rhythm as a predictor of breast cancer survival. *J Natl Cancer Inst.* 2000; 92:994–1000.

Singh S, Zahid M, Saeed M, Gaikwad NW, Meza JL, Cavalieri EL,

Rogan EG,Chakravarti D. NAD(P)H:quinone oxidoreductase 1 Arg-139Trp and Pro187Ser polymorphisms imbalance estrogen metabolism towards DNA adduct formation in human mammary epithelial cells. *J Steroid Biochem Mol Biol.* 2009;117(1-3):56-66.

Sripathy SP, Chaplin LJ, Gaikwad NW, Rogan EG, Montano MM. hPMC2 is required for recruiting an ER-beta coactivator complex to mediate transcriptional upregulation of NQO1 and protection against oxidative DNA damage by tamoxifen. *Oncogene.* 2008;27(49):6376-6384.

Welsh JA, Sharma A, Abramson JL, Vaccarino V, Gillespie C, Vos MB. Caloric sweetener consumption and dyslipidemia among US adults. *JAMA.* 2010;303(15):1490-14977.

Yang L, Gaikwad NW, Meza J, Cavalieri EL, Muti P, Trock B, Rogan EG. Novel biomarkers for risk of prostate cancer: results from a case-control study. *Prostate.* 2009;69(1):41-48.

Zahid M, Saeed M, Ali MF, Rogan EG, Cavalieri EL. N-acetylcysteine blocks formation of cancer-initiating estrogen-DNA adducts in cells. *Free Radic Biol Med.* 2010;49(3):392-400.

Zahid M, Saeed M, Rogan EG, Cavalieri EL. Benzene and dopamine catechol quinones could initiate cancer or neurogenic disease. *Free Radic Biol Med.* 2010;48(2):318-324.

Zhang Y, Gaikwad NW, Olson K, Zahid M, Cavalieri EL, Rogan EG. Cytochrome P450 isoforms catalyze formation of catechol estrogen quinones that react with DNA. *Metabolism.* 2007;56(7):887-894.

STAR 4

Gaikwad NW, Rogan EG, Cavalieri EL. Evidence from ESI-MS for NQO1-catalyzed reduction of estrogen ortho-quinones. *Free Radic Biol Med.* 2007;43(9):1289-1298.

Kaszkin-Bettag M, Beck S, Richardson A, Heger PW, Beer AM. Efficacy of the special extract ERr 731 from rhapontic rhubarb for menopausal complaints: a 6-month open observational study. *Altern Ther Health Med.* 2008;14:32-38.

Kawano H et al. Dehydroepiandrosterone supplementation improves endothelial function and insulin sensitivity in men. *J Clin Endocrinol Metab.* 2003;88:3190-3195.

Kawano H et al. Vitamin D receptor genetic polymorphisms and prostate cancer risk: a meta-analysis of 36 published studies. *Int J Clin Exp Med.* 2009;2(2):159-175.

Kyrou I, Chrousos GP, Tsigos C. Stress, visceral obesity, and metabolic complications. *Ann NY Acad Sci.* 2006;1083:77-110.

Lu F, Zahid M, Wang C, Saeed M, Cavalieri EL, Rogan EG. Resveratrol prevents estrogen-DNA adduct formation and neoplastic transformation in MCF-10F cells. *Cancer Prev Res (Phila).* 2008;1(2):135-145.

Montano MM, Chaplin LJ, Deng H, Mesia-Vela S, Gaikwad N, Zahid M, Rogan E. Protective roles of quinone reductase and tamoxifen against estrogen-induced mammary tumorigenesis. *Oncogene.* 2007; 26(24):3587-3590.

Rogan EG. The natural chemopreventive compound indole-3-carbinol: state of the science. *In Vivo.* 2006;20(2):221-228.

Shames RL. Nutritional management of stress-induced dysfunction. *Applied Nutritional Science Reports.* 2003; no. 576.

Yang CZ, Yaniger SI, Jordan VC, Klein DJ, Bittner GD. Most plastic products release estrogenic chemicals: a potential health problem that can be solved. *Environ Health Perspect.* 2011;119:989-996.

Zahid M, Gaikwad NW, Ali MF, Lu F, Saeed M, Yang L, Rogan EG, Cavalieri EL. Prevention of estrogen-DNA adduct formation in MCF-10F cells by resveratrol. *Free Radic Biol Med.* 2008;45(2):136-145.

Zahid M, Gaikwad NW, Rogan EG, Cavalieri EL. Inhibition of depurinating estrogen-DNA adduct formation by natural compounds. *Chem Res Toxicol.* 2007;20(12):1947-1953.

Zahid M, Saeed M, Lu F, Gaikwad N, Rogan E, Cavalieri E. Inhibition of catechol-O-methyltransferase increases estrogen-DNA adduct formation. *Free Radic Biol Med.* 2007;43(11):1534-1540.

RING 5

Amoils S, Kues J, Amoils S et al. The diagnostic validity of human electromagnetic field (aura) perception. *Journal of Medical Acupuncture.* 2002;13:25-28.

Committee on Advancing Pain Research, Care, and Education, Institute of Medicine. *Relieving Pain in America: A Blueprint for Transforming Prevention, Care, Education, and Research* (National Academies Press, 2011).

Helms, Joseph. *Getting to Know You: A Physician Explains How Acupuncture Helps You Be the Best You* (North Atlantic Books, 2007).

STAR 5

Audette J. Acupuncture energetics: clues to an expanded view of somatovisceral homeostasis. *Pain Practitioner.* 2011;3:21.

Audette JF, Ryan AH. The role of acupuncture in pain management. *Phys Med Rehabil Clin N Am.* 2004; 15:749-772.

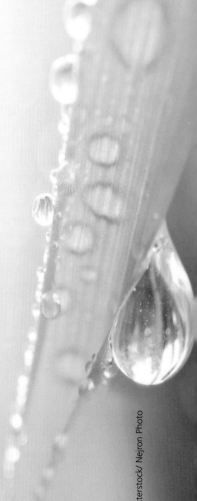

Glossary

A

ACE Healing Treatment^{SM}. A combination of acupuncture, chiropractic, and energy healing developed at the Alliance Institute for Integrative Medicine. An ACE Healing Treatment is particularly helpful for chronic pain; it also helps restore overall health and balance.

Acupuncture. The ancient Asian art of painlessly inserting very thin needles into specific points on the body to relieve pain and improve health. In traditional Asian medicine theory, energy (qi) flows through channels in the body called meridians. A blockage or imbalance in the natural flow of the meridians causes illness; acupuncture unblocks the qi and restores balance to the body. The scientific theory is that acupuncture stimulates the body to heal in various ways, affecting the fascia, muscles, spinal cord, and brain. The needles also reduce muscle spasm and cause a healing response at the site of insertion.

Adaptogenic herbs. Herbs such as ginseng and ashwaganda that help strengthen the body, improve immunity, and increase the ability to withstand stress and fatigue.

Adduct. See Quinones.

Aerobic exercise. Lower intensity physical activity such as swimming, brisk walking, jogging, and biking whereby the body uses oxygen efficiently, improving endurance and fitness.

Anabolic. Anything that builds up the tissues of the body. Hormones such as testosterone are anabolic because they build muscles.

Anabolic steroids. Drugs that resemble the chemical structure of testosterone. These drugs stimulate the growth of muscle tissue.

Anaerobic exercise. Intense exercise such as sprinting or weight-lifting that forces the body to create energy without using oxygen, leading to lactic acid buildup in the muscles. In general, anaerobic exercise builds muscle strength and size.

Androgens. A group of chemically related steroid hormones, including testosterone, cortisol, and dehydro-epiandrosterone (DHEA), that create male sex characteristics.

Andropause. The time in a man's life when his body produces fewer androgen hormones.

Antioxidant. An agent, such as vitamin C or the flavonoids in foods, that counteracts damaging oxidation from free radicals and other substances created by normal metabolism.

Autoimmune disorders. Diseases such as rheumatoid arthritis caused when the body's immune system mistakenly attacks healthy cells.

B

Bioidentical hormones. Hormones that are identical in molecular structure to the hormones made by the body.

Biopsychotype. The physical and personality characteristics of an individual. Based on the work of Joseph Helms, M.D., the three biopsychotypes are Will/Spirit, Vision/Action, and Nurture/Duty.

Bodywork. Therapies that work with the body, including manipulative therapies such as chiropractic, massage, and Rolfing, and non-touch energy therapies such as reiki, tai chi, and yoga.

C

Catabolic. Relating to catabolism, the metabolic breakdown of large molecules in the body into smaller ones. The Wear and Tear Phase of the body.

Chi. See Qi.

Chiropractic. The science and art of restoring and maintaining health through the gentle, careful manipulation of the body joints and spine, to restore normal nerve function. Chiropractic adjustments to the spine and other parts of the body correct alignment problems, alleviate pain, and improve function.

Complex regional pain syndrome (CRPS). Also called Reflex Sympathetic Dystrophy (RSD), this chronic pain condition usually affects an arm or leg, although it can affect any part of the body. It is probably caused by nerve damage that affects blood flow, sensation, and temperature in the affected area.

Cortisol. A steroid hormone produced in the adrenal glands and needed for glucose metabolism, regulating blood pressure, and inflammation. Cortisol is also released in response to stress. Constant high levels of cortisol can cause insulin resistance, high blood pressure, and weight gain.

Costochondral pain. Chest pain caused by irritation or inflammation of the cartilage where one or more ribs attach to the spine or the sternum.

C-reactive protein. *See* High-sensitivity C-reactive protein.

CRPS. *See* Complex regional pain syndrome.

D

Dermatome. A localized area of skin that gets its sensation from a single nerve radiating from a single nerve root in the spinal cord.

Detoxification. The process of converting damaging byproducts of metabolism into less toxic molecules. Detoxification takes place in the liver, kidneys, skin, lungs, and gut.

Dehydroepiandrosterone (DHEA). The body's well-being hormone, DHEA is produced in the adrenal glands and, in men, in the testes. It is the precursor to testosterone and estrogen.

DHEA. *See* Dehydroepiandrosterone.

Diabetes mellitus. A disease that causes blood sugar (glucose) levels to rise too high. Type 1 diabetes is an autoimmune disease that stops the body's production of the hormone insulin. Type 2 diabetes occurs when the cells of the body become resistant to insulin.

Dysbiosis. An imbalance between the beneficial and harmful bacteria of the digestive tract.

E

Energy healing. Channeling healing energy in order to correct imbalances in the body's energy field. Energy healing techniques include Reiki, Healing Touch, and Therapeutic Touch.

Endocrine-disrupting chemicals. Environmental chemicals that affect hormone receptors in the cells and disrupt their normal action.

Epigenetics. Environmental factors that change how a gene is expressed without changing its structure.

ERT. *See* Estrogen replacement therapy.

Estrogen. The main female hormone. In women, estrogen is made primarily in the ovaries; in men, small amounts of estrogen are made in the testes.

Estrogen-disrupting chemicals. Environmental chemicals that disrupt the action of estrogen receptors in the cells. Also called endocrine-disrupting chemicals.

Estrogen replacement therapy (ERT). *See* Hormone replacement therapy.

Estrone (E1). A metabolite produced when estradiol, the body's primary form of the hormone estrogen, is broken down.

Estradiol (E2). The body's primary form of the hormone estrogen.

Estriol (E3). A weak form of estrogen, produced in higher amounts during pregnancy. A metabolite of 16-OH estrone.

F

Fascia. The fibrous connective tissue that surrounds muscles, blood vessels, and nerves.

Fibromyalgia. A chronic disorder characterized by widespread pain, diffuse tenderness, and fatigue. Associated with cognitive and memory problems, sleep disturbances, and other functional disorders such as migraine and irritable bowel syndrome.

Free radical. A highly reactive molecule that is a normal byproduct of metabolism. Free radicals can cause cell damage and DNA damage; antioxidants in the body limit the damage.

Frequency specific microcurrent (FSM). A subsensory microcurrent applied via graphite gloves or directly through acupuncture needles to reduce inflammation and heal injuries faster.

FSM. *See* Frequency specific microcurrent.

Functional medicine. Science-based personalized medicine that focuses on primary prevention and treating underlying causes rather than symptoms of chronic disease.

G

Genomics. The study of all of a person's genes (the genome), including interactions of those genes with each other and with the person's environment.

Glycemic index (GI). A measure of the quality of a carbohydrate food based on its immediate effect on blood sugar levels. The higher the GI number, the faster the food raises blood sugar.

Glycemic load (GL). A way to predict the effect of a carbohydrate food on blood sugar by looking at the GI of the food and the serving size.

H

High-sensitivity C-reactive protein (hs-CRP). A protein, detected by a blood test, that is a marker for inflammation. High levels of hs-CRP reveal an increased risk for heart disease, as well as many other illnesses.

Hormone. A natural chemical produced in one part of the body, such as the thyroid gland, that acts on other parts of the body. The pancreas, for example, produces the hormone insulin, which affects all cells in the body.

Hormone replacement therapy (HRT). *See* Hormone Therapy (HT).

Hormone therapy (HT). Using hormones such as estrogen, progesterone, and testosterone to alleviate the symptoms associated with menopause, andropause, and aging.

hs-CRP. *See* High-sensitivity C-reactive protein.

I

Iliotibial band (ITB). A thick band of fascia that starts on the outside of the hip, passes down the outside of the thigh and inserts into the side of the patella (knee-cap) and the tibia (shin bone).

Iliotibial band syndrome. Pain on the outside of the knee that occurs with running, walking, or going up and down stairs. The pain is caused by repeatedly bending and straightening the knee, which can cause irritation of the area where the ITB slides over the side of the knee.

Insulin. A hormone, produced by the pancreas, which stimulates the passage of sugar (glucose) from the blood into the cells, where it can burned for energy.

Insulin resistance. A condition that occurs when the body's cells become resistant to the action of insulin. Insulin resistance causes blood sugar to rise and can lead to type 2 diabetes.

Integrative medicine. Healing-oriented medicine that looks at the whole person (body, mind, and spirit), including all aspects of lifestyle. It emphasizes the therapeutic relationship and makes use of all appropriate therapies, both conventional and alternative.

ITB. *See* Iliotibial band.

L

Leaky gut syndrome. Damage to the intestinal lining that allows gut bacteria and incompletely digested food particles to leak from the intestines and enter the bloodstream, resulting in an altered immune response. May be associated with multiple diseases. Also called gut or intestinal hyperpermeability.

M

Manipulative therapy. Physical treatments utilized by chiropractors, osteopaths, and physical therapists to treat soft tissue, muscle, and joint pain. Also called manual therapy.

Maximum heart rate (MAX HR). The highest heartbeat rate an individual can safely achieve during exercise. The MAX HR is used to determine aerobic and anaerobic exercise levels

MBSR. *See* Mindfulness-based stress reduction.

Mindfulness-based stress reduction (MBSR). A form of meditation based on mindfulness, or paying attention to the inner self as a form of stress reduction and healing.

Mediators of illness. Factors that produce disease symptoms, damage body tissues, or behaviors associated with illness. These include biochemicals such as cytokines and free radicals, subatomic particles such as ionizing radiation, and emotional problems such

as fear and helplessness, as well as cultural issues related to the sick role or lack of health-care resources.

Menopause. The period in a woman's life, usually beginning in her late 40s, when egg production, estrogen production, and menstruation slow and finally stop. Menopause is complete when a woman has not had a period for a year.

Metabolic syndrome. A group of risk factors that occur together and increase the risk for heart disease, stroke, and type 2 diabetes. The risk factors include central obesity, insulin resistance, and elevated blood pressure.

Myofascial pain. Pain and inflammation in the soft tissues of the body, including the muscles and fascia.

N

Neurotransmitters. Chemicals in the nervous systems that transmit signals from one nerve to another. The major neurotransmitters in the body include serotonin, epinephrine (adrenaline), norepinephrine, melatonin, and acetylcholine.

Norepinephrine. A neurotransmitter that affects the rate at which the heart beats. It is one of the stress hormones released in the fight-or-flight response.

Nutrigenomics. The study of how genes interact with nutrients on an individual level.

O

Obesogens. Endocrine-disrupting chemicals that lead to weight gain by interfering with the normal regulatory pathways that control body weight.

Osteopathy. An approach to medicine that emphasizes the connection between structure and function in the body and the body's ability to heal itself. Osteopathic physicians are fully trained in standard medicine and practice just as medical doctors (M.D.s) do. Also called osteopathic medicine.

Oxidation. In the body, the loss of an oxygen electron from a molecule through normal metabolism or by exposure to toxins such as cigarette smoke. Oxidation creates free radicals, which can cause cell damage.

P

Perimenopause. The time in a woman's life when estrogen levels begin to drop before menopause.

Prebiotics. Nondigestible food ingredients, such as soluble fiber, that promote the growth of beneficial bacteria in the gut. *See also* Probiotics.

Probiotics. Live microbes, such as *Lactobacillus* and bifidobacteria, used as supplements to restore healthy levels of good bacteria in the intestines.

Progesterone. A female steroid hormone. Works in concert with estrogen.

Prolotherapy. A nonsurgical treatment for damaged ligaments and tendons that injects a dextrose solution into the tissue where it attaches to the bone. Localized inflammation from the injections increases blood flow to the area and stimulates the tissue to repair itself. Also called regenerative therapy.

PSA (prostate-specific antigen). A natural chemical produced by the prostate gland in men and detected by a blood test. An elevated PSA level may indicate an infected or enlarged prostate or prostate cancer.

PTSD (post-traumatic stress disorder). Long-term symptoms that may result from a psychologically traumatic event. Symptoms can include depression and pain syndromes.

Q

Qi. Pronounced *chee;* also written as chi. In traditional Eastern medicine and philosophy refers to life force or energy.

Quinones. Toxic organic compounds produced when estrone, a metabolite of estradiol, is oxidized. Quinones are found in high amounts in cancerous breast and prostate tissue. Also called adducts.

R

Reflex sympathetic dystrophy syndrome (RSD). *See* Complex regional pain syndrome.

Reiki. A traditional Japanese form of energy healing that promotes stress reduction and relaxation. See also Energy healing.

Regenerative therapy. *See* Prolotherapy.

Relaxation response. A physical state of deep rest that helps moderate the body's response to stress and promotes physical and emotional relaxation. The relaxation response can be created through regular practice of a short, simple meditation technique.

Rolfing. Named after its founder, Dr. Ida P. Rolf, Rolfing is a form of bodywork that uses deep massage and other techniques on the fascia to realign and balance the body.

RSD. *See* Complex regional pain syndrome.

S

Serotonin. A neurotransmitter that helps relay messages in the brain. An imbalance in serotonin levels may cause depression and anxiety.

SNP (single nucleotide polymorphism). An individual variation or switch in a single nucleotide, the basic building block of DNA in a gene. The SNP (pronounced snip) in the gene causes a change in the morph, or shape, of the gene, which then affects its action. Polymorphism refers to normal genetic variation.

Steroids. A large group of natural chemicals the body manufactures from cholesterol, including hormones such as cortisol, estrogen, and testosterone.

Stress. The body's response to physical, emotional, or mental demands, such as threatening or upsetting events, overwork, illness, financial worries, relationship problems, and other pressures.

Stress curve. The predictable physical and emotional problems that develop as the body faces increasing stress over a long period.

Stress hormones. Hormones such as cortisol and nor-epinephrine released as the body's response to stress. Long-term stress and high levels of stress hormones raise blood pressure, suppress immunity, cause weight gain, increase the risk of heart attack and stroke, and contribute to anxiety and depression.

Stressor. Anything that places high demands on the body, including illness, major life changes, threatening situations, worry, exhaustion, and relationship problems.

Synergy. Two or more systems, processes, or agents working together to produce a result greater than the sum of these individual things together.

Systems biology. A way of looking at the complex interactions of the human body to see the major factors that influence health and disease, including genetics and social, disease, metabolic, and bioenergetic networks.

T

Tai chi. A traditional Chinese movement system based on gentle, repeated movements that increase energy (qi) flow and improve health.

Tensegrity. A combination of the words tension and integrity; refers to the push and pull of muscles, connective tissues, and bones that balance the body.

Testosterone. The primary male hormone, produced mostly in the testes. Women also produce very small amounts of testosterone.

Thyroid gland. A butterfly-shaped gland found in the neck that produces the thyroid hormones that control the body's metabolism.

Thyroid-stimulating hormone (TSH). A hormone produced by the thyroid gland that in turn causes the gland to make the hormones triiodothyronine (T3) and thyroxine (T4). These hormones help control your body's metabolism. A blood test for TSH can show if the thyroid gland is underactive or overactive.

Transcendental meditation (TM). A simple, easily learned meditation technique that provides deep relaxation and can help relieve stress.

Transformational medicine. A combination of conventional medicine with exercise, mind-body techniques, and integrative therapies to treat current health problems, heal old ones, and prevent future ones.

Trigger point. A specific point or area on the body where stimulation by touch or pressure produces a painful response.

TSH. *See* Thyroid-stimulating hormone.

Index

Patient Stories Index